HEALTHY
FOR LIFE

Dr. Richard F. Heller, M.S., Ph.D.

Professor, Mount Sinai School of Medicine, New York;
Professor, Graduate Center of the City University of New York,
Department of Biomedical Sciences;
Professor Emeritus, Bronx Community College of the City University of New York,
Department of Biology and Medical Laboratory Technology

and

Dr. Rachael F. Heller, M.A., M.Ph., Ph.D.

Assistant Clinical Professor, Mount Sinai School of Medicine, New York;
Assistant Professor, Graduate Center of the City University of New York,
Department of Biomedical Sciences

HEALTHY FOR LIFE

The Scientific Breakthrough Program for Looking, Feeling, and Staying Healthy Without Deprivation

A DUTTON BOOK

DUTTON
Published by the Penguin Group
Penguin Books USA Inc., 375 Hudson Street,
New York, New York 10014, U.S.A.
Penguin Books Ltd, 27 Wrights Lane, London W8 5TZ, England
Penguin Books Australia Ltd, Ringwood, Victoria, Australia
Penguin Books Canada Ltd, 10 Alcorn Avenue, Toronto, Ontario, Canada M4V 3B2
Penguin Books (N.Z.) Ltd, 182–190 Wairau Road, Auckland 10, New Zealand

Penguin Books Ltd, Registered Offices:
Harmondsworth, Middlesex, England

First published by Dutton, an imprint of Dutton Signet,
a division of Penguin Books USA Inc.
Distributed in Canada by McClelland & Stewart Inc.

First Printing, March, 1995
10 9 8 7 6 5 4 3 2 1

 REGISTERED TRADEMARK—MARCA REGISTRADA

LIBRARY OF CONGRESS CATALOGING-IN-PUBLICATION DATA:
Heller, Richard F. (Richard Ferdinand)
Healthy for life : reversing the single most important health
risk factor of your life / Richard F. Heller and Rachael F. Heller.
p.   cm.
Includes bibliographical references and index.
ISBN 0-525-93733-1
1. Health.   2. Low-carbohydrate diet.   3. Insulin.
I. Heller, Rachael F.   II. Title.
RA776.5.H42   1995
613—dc20   94-32988
                                               CIP

Printed in the United States of America
Set in Garamond Light
Designed by Eve L. Kirch

This book is dedicated to Dr. Ignaz P. Semmelweis
and to all others who dare to ask why

CONTENTS

ACKNOWLEDGMENTS

We wish to express our deep appreciation to the following people:

Deb Brody—our editor, whose insightful suggestions and sage advice have proven invaluable—and her fine and capable assistant, Jennifer Moore.

Lisa Johnson—our publicist for hardcover, who worked so hard on the first of our projects, and whose energy, fine professional judgment, and assistance will be important in making this book another best-seller.

Neil Stuart—Penguin's Vice President and Art Director of Hardcover and Trade Books, for his fine eye, his commitment and talent.

Elaine Koster and Arnold Dolin—our publishers, for their continued integrity and commitment to bringing their readers the very best in publishing.

Mel Berger of the William Morris Agency—the best agent and counselor known to woman or man. His years of experience, thoughtful and incisive advice, common sense, creativity, patience, and very, very hard work have helped make "stone soup" every step of the way.

Claudia Cross—Mel Berger's exceptional assistant.

Professor Paul Gilbert, M.D., Associate Professor and Acting Chairman of Medicine, Mount Sinai Medical Center—one of the finest minds and best hearts in medicine, for his insightful advice and recommendations, and for providing us with the best health care possible.

Norman Katz (whose office we share), Supervising Technologist of Electron Microscopy, Department of Pathology, Mount Sinai Medical Center, and his wife, Madeline—whose suggestions, comments, and encouragement were most important to this project.

Professor Alan L. Schiller, M.D., Chairman, Department of Pathology, Mount Sinai School of Medicine—for his insights, enthusiasm, and total support.

Irwin Neus, D.D.S.—whose interest, support, comments, and contributions to our research were welcomed and valued.

Ana Luisa Vazquez, Sharon Althea Smith, and Audrey Stedford—the finest of research assistants, whose industriousness, intelligence, commitment, and unending hours in the library made our research possible and our lives most enjoyable.

Betty Lincoln—a cherished friend, whose unswerving efforts in the reading of every single word of the original manuscript—and whose intelligent, incisive responses, comments, and suggestions—were invaluable to our writing.

Deborah Heller DeLisa—the love of our life, for her encouragement, friendship, caring, insights, wonderful talks, and unfailing support.

The Apple Computer Company—for development of the powerful, user-friendly Powerbook 170 and 180 computers, which can be taken on planes, trains, buses, and out under the apple tree in our backyard, and for their repair team, who make sure our Powerbooks stay in good working order. Our Powerbooks have been invaluable tools in the preparation of all our written and graphic materials as well as in the compilation and organization of research data. Without Apple's hard work, our work would never have been the same.

FIVE BLIND MEN

Five blind men set about their task of describing an elephant.

"An elephant," declared the first as he felt the animal's trunk, "is quite long and thick. It is flexible and wrinkled and, to some extent, capable of manipulating the world around it."

"I disagree," declared the second blind man, his hands sliding over the elephant's ears. "It is obvious to anyone that an elephant is smooth, not wrinkled, and very thin and flat rather than thick. Furthermore, it flaps in the wind."

"How can you say that?" questioned the third as he touched the elephant's foot. "Anyone can see that an elephant is a thick, round animal. It's heavy and wrinkled. No wind could ever budge it."

"Don't be silly," declared the fourth as he ran his hand over the animal's ample side. "An elephant is as broad as a house and as wide as a wall."

"You are all wrong," declared the fifth as his fingers surrounded the animal's tail. "It is plain as the nose on your face that an elephant is flexible and tapered. It is not large in size and though it moves easily, it does not seem to have much purpose."

The five men argued much of the day and, as night approached, each retired to his own home, amazed at the stupidity of his fellowman and convinced of the rightness of his own perceptions.

So it may be in the study of medicine. Each, schooled in his own specialty, may describe the physical traces that he observes, blind to or isolated from the knowledge of others and denying their observations.

And so it has come to pass that heart disease, atherosclerosis, hypertension, obesity, diabetes, and the like are seen as distinct diseases, different beasts, though they may, in fact, be varying features of the same creature. That one animal, that single united disease that is perceived so differently by so many, we have come to identify as Profactor-H.

part one

PROFACTOR-H: YOUR PERSONAL PROFILE

Introduction: The Chance of a Lifetime in a Lifetime of Chance

You are about to greatly improve your chances for living a long and healthy life, a life with far fewer demands on your time, fewer restrictions on your eating, and, at the same time, a life with fewer health concerns than you ever thought possible.

The ground-breaking scientific discovery that follows has already begun to change the way we think about disease, about risk factors, about illness, and about health. It will provide you with an easy, enjoyable way to increase your likelihood of living long and well, and enjoying your life without deprivation or struggle. Most important, it is available to you now, right here, in the pages that follow.

This book will help you understand what Profactor-H is and why it may be the most important risk factor in your life. We will help you determine your probable risk for Profactor-H and what you can do to best prevent it or reverse it. The information that you will find in the chapters that follow is based on the current work of thousands of the world's most well-respected scientists as well as research that we have personally directed for over ten years.

The discovery of Profactor-H* answers questions that have stumped scientists and physicians for decades:

Why do some people do all of the "right things" and still become ill?

Why do some people do all of the "wrong things" and still live to be a hundred?

Why are some people able to eat eggs and red meat and other high-fat foods and still maintain normal blood levels of cholesterol and triglycerides?

Why does it become harder to control your weight as you get older, and why do some of us gain weight more easily than others?

What can be done to break the link between stress and illness?

Why are so few of us able to consistently follow our physician's health recommendations (even though we know they are for our own good)?

Why has medicine failed to help us prevent or really control:
atherosclerosis and heart disease
adult-onset diabetes
high blood pressure and stroke
hypoglycemia
overweight
polycystic ovary disease
vascular disease
and many forms of cancer?

Until the discovery of Profactor-H, answers to these questions have remained as isolated reports in scientific journals, buried in the stacks of medical school libraries.

The demands of our research and teaching require us to keep up with these reports—the findings of scientists from around the world. It is not an easy task, even for the two of us working together. We know

---

*Physicians and research scientists often refer to the hormonal imbalance we call Profactor-H in a variety of ways, including insulin resistance, insulin (implying hyperinsulinemia), hyperinsulinemia, etc. Since all of these conditions describe different aspects of the same process, which results in a chronic excess level of insulin in the bloodstream, throughout this book Profactor-H will be used as a specific term in place of any or all of these conditions. In addition, within direct quotes, this term as well as common lay terms will be used in place of medical or Latin terminology.

now that the coordination of these many research studies, coming from several different areas of specialty, was essential in providing the key pieces to the discovery and understanding of Profactor-H.

A Single Purpose

When we began our research program, our sole intent was to discover and correct physical problems that caused people to lose control of their eating and to gain weight. We quickly found that the most common of these problems was a hormonal imbalance called *hyperinsulinemia* (meaning too much insulin). At first, we found that this excess of insulin appeared to affect up to 75 percent of the overweight and many normal-weight individuals as well. As our research continued, however, we became aware that hyperinsulinemia was much more widespread than we had previously thought.

Our research, as well as that of other scientists, revealed that hyperinsulinemia appeared to affect the majority of Americans—in fact, a far greater number of people seemed to have this "excess of insulin" than did not. And what was most important to us was that many people were not even aware that they were hyperinsulinemic and so they were unaware of the impact it had on their health and their lives.

As our work continued, it became increasingly clear that while some people with hyperinsulinemia showed signs of carbohydrate addiction (a recurring or intense craving for starches, snack foods, or sweets), others showed no outward signs that they had this hormonal imbalance. At the same time, other scientists were beginning to report the power of this silent killer. Research results documented the millions of people who were experiencing poor health and, in some cases, might be needlessly dying from an excess of the hormone insulin—a hormonal imbalance they did not even know they had.

Millions of people may be experiencing poor health
and might, in some cases, be needlessly dying
from a disorder that they do not even know they have.

The Twin Discovery:
The Common Denominator

For most of our lives, both of us had unknowingly suffered from hyperinsulinemia, so we had a personal as well as a professional stake in conquering this medical mystery.

At first our work focused on correcting our research subjects' insulin imbalances in order to eliminate their addiction to carbohydrates and to help them to lose weight and permanently maintain their new weight levels. By reducing their insulin levels, up to 80 percent of our subjects were able to reach their goal weight and to maintain it, struggle-free. This was, in itself, a scientist's dream come true. But then something unexpected happened. As the number of our readers and research subjects passed half a million, report after report documenting remarkable improvements in health and well-being, in addition to weight loss, began to emerge.

Letters poured in. Over and over, research subjects, readers, researchers, nutritionists, and physicians reported great and unexpected improvements in health:

Physicians reported that their patients' cholesterol and triglyceride levels had decreased by as much as 25 to 60 percent.

Blood pressure levels that had been dangerously high for years were approaching normal.

HDL-cholesterol levels (which are best kept high) were rising and the LDL-cholesterol levels (which are best kept low) were, in fact, going down.

Adult-onset diabetics were showing the same improvements as others, along with weight loss, improved blood sugar levels, and, in some cases, the ability to greatly reduce or stop insulin therapy.

Men and women suffering with hypoglycemia (low blood sugar) were reporting far better control of their sugar levels, and in many cases, their experiences of weakness, headache, irritability, and fatigue were greatly reduced or, in some cases, had disappeared.

Excess insulin levels such as those associated with breast cancer, cancer of the ovary and uterus, and polycystic ovarian disease were greatly decreased.

Case after case bore witness to the fact that by both their own and others' standards, our readers and research subjects were not only looking better and feeling better, but they were *getting* better. Laboratory and physicians' reports confirmed they were, indeed, showing important signs of becoming healthier.

> **By both their own and others' standards, our readers and research subjects were not only looking better and feeling better, but they were *getting* better.**

At first we attributed the unexpected bonus of health to their loss of weight; some of our readers and subjects had lost thirty, fifty, even a hundred or more pounds. But weight loss alone did not explain the 40 percent of the people we saw who were *within* normal weight limits. Though these people had come to see us because of their strong carbohydrate cravings and battles with food, they had little or no weight to lose. Still, as they continued on the Program, they reported the same health benefits as others who had lost far more weight. Since even normal-weight subjects were showing significantly lower levels in health risk, we could not attribute our subjects' new and welcome health benefits to a simple decrease in weight.

We looked for a different factor, a common denominator that all of our people shared. It wasn't age or sex or ethnic group or socioeconomic level. Our people came from every background and from every walk of life. It was not their contact with us or something we were unconsciously doing or saying; many of the health improvements that were being reported came from nutritionists, physicians, and readers who had never met us!

The only feature that all of our people shared was that they had been following a program that was designed to reduce excess levels of insulin. The evidence had become undeniable. Reduction of excess insulin levels leads to improved health. Other scientists were predicting the same results and we were witnessing it ourselves—firsthand.

As its widespread importance became even more evident, hyperinsulinemia could no longer be viewed as a freestanding disorder. It was much more than a simple hormonal imbalance. Its far-reaching effects on so many diseases and risk factors qualified it as what we call a *profactor*—the first, or underlying, disorder that can lead to many other diseases and health problems. With an understanding that it may well be the parent disorder to a whole host of health- and life-threatening diseases, we now refer to chronic hyperinsulinemia as Profactor-H.

We had come upon a remarkable twin discovery. First, our research confirmed what other scientists were reporting: that Profactor-H was a major link to many risk factors for the major illnesses in the world today (qualifying it as a profactor). Second, and most important, we had uncovered a simple way to greatly reduce or reverse this profactor. The Program that we had originally designed to reduce cravings and weight appeared to correct the hyperinsulinemia itself.

It now became clear why, virtually effortlessly, the Profactor-H Program led to surprising improvements in health. The lifesaving gains that were taking place were free and added benefits to our people, no matter how little or how much weight was lost, simply because they were reducing their excess levels of insulin.

It was a chance of a lifetime—for us as scientists as well as for us as people, and now, after a bit of good luck and a lot of hard work, we had the results to prove it.

In the years that have followed we, along with much of the scientific community, have come to recognize that Profactor-H (or hyperinsulinemia, as it is sometimes still referred to by many physicians and researchers) appears to be one of today's most important and deadly risk factors.

Many Faces

Quickly and quietly, Profactor-H has been spreading through this country. It has many faces. We see it in the mechanic losing his sight because his diabetes is out of control; we see it in the semiparalyzed body of a young mother struggling to recover from a stroke;

we see it in the worried face of a working father when he is told that he needs coronary bypass surgery.

Profactor-H may appear as a "simple" case of high blood pressure or high cholesterol or triglyceride levels. It may reveal itself as a few extra pounds that need to be lost or the weakness or headache or irritability that often accompanies low blood sugar levels. Many of these may be early symptoms of a much more lethal problem that must be addressed. If uncorrected, these problems will most likely progress toward greater illness and an increased chance of early death.

Along with the discovery of Profactor-H came the good news: This major health risk factor, this common denominator to many of this country's illnesses, this silent killer, as well as its many effects, can be prevented and, indeed, in many cases reversed! The Profactor-H Program is simple and easy to follow, it requires no sacrifice, and, best of all, it is available not only to the scientist or to the physician but to all who need it—today.

▽

CHAPTER 1

New Bodies, New Hopes, New Lives

They must change who wish to be constant in happiness,
health, and wisdom. —Confucius

This book is about a medical discovery that would normally have taken another twenty years to make its way into your doctor's office. It is about a potentially lifesaving breakthrough that links nine of this country's top killer diseases and risk factors to a *single* basic physical imbalance. It is about how to know if you have this imbalance, and most of all, what to do about it.

This book is about how we, ourselves, used the Profactor-H Program to break free of our family's risk for illness and early death and become healthier than we ever imagined we could be. This book is about the many others who have come before you and how they used this Program to help reverse their risk for heart disease, heart attack, and atherosclerosis; for diabetes and vascular disease; for high blood pressure and stroke; and for several forms of cancer. Most of all, this book is about how you can do the same.

This book is about how the Profactor-H Program
can help you break free of the
health risks and illnesses that rule your family.

Escape from the Brink:
Dr. Rachael Heller's Story

The physician's thick dark hair stood in stark contrast to his perfectly white lab coat and he looked more like some movie star playing the part of a doctor than he did a real physician. He stared at the wall-mounted light box. As I entered the room, he looked up, nodded, and flashed a brilliant, reassuring smile that seemed a bit too wide. He went back to studying the X rays of my brain lit up against the wall light box. I slipped into the chair across from his desk and waited. Finally, he half turned and pointed to the X ray.

> He half turned and pointed to the X ray.
> "There it is," he announced triumphantly.
> "They missed it."

"There it is," he announced triumphantly. "They missed it." I sat motionless. I didn't know what to say. He beckoned me closer. "Look," he said excitedly, "there it is, right there. Can't you see it?"

He pulled a ballpoint pen out of his pocket and pointed to a gray ball about the size of a small grape. I wasn't sure where the gray ball ended and the rest of my brain began. "I'm not sure," I mumbled. He paid no attention to my reply, and continued.

"It's most certainly larger by now and it's probably benign." My heart began to pound. I could barely hear his voice. During the long wait in his office, I had prepared myself for the verdict, but now my body responded as if I were witnessing a car accident. The world was moving in slow motion and my every thought was crystal clear.

"It's okay," I told myself. "He said that it's benign. There's nothing to worry about. Just stop it and listen to what he's trying to tell you. Don't jump to conclusions." I took a breath and tried to concentrate on his words.

> "... the tumor is very close to the carotid artery
> and that means that there is an increased chance
> of hemorrhage when we remove it.
> Still, we don't have any choice. ..."

He was several sentences ahead of me. "... the tumor is very close to the carotid artery in the brain and that means that there is an increased chance of hemorrhage when we remove it. Still, we don't have any choice. ..."

"Tumor?" I screamed to myself. "Who said anything about a tumor? I thought he said that it was benign!"

"*Probably* benign," a voice inside reminded me. My heart trip-hammered again.

"Hemorrhage? Did he say something about hemorrhage?" My mind quickly changed the subject and focused on more practical matters. "Oh, my God," I thought. "What am I going to do? I have no one to help me. I have twenty bucks in the bank. I won't be able to work. I won't have any money to pay the rent. I'm going to be out on the street." And then the fear took over. "Oh, my God. Oh, my God, I have a brain tumor."

> "Oh, my God. Oh, my God, I have a brain tumor."

Suddenly, a calm washed over my body.

I listened coolly as he went on regarding details of the length of hospital stay and recuperation. With an objective manner he detailed my probabilities of becoming paralyzed or blind or of death, and then explained that although I was only thirty-seven years old, my high blood pressure and obesity "complicated an already less-than-optimal surgery." I quietly asked for a sheet of paper and pen and then, dispassionately, began to take notes.

As I wrote, a deep and penetrating sadness overtook me. I could barely move. I had been running from illness and death almost all of my life and now it had overtaken me. I wasn't ready. I wasn't ready to die. I didn't want to die. Oh, God, how I didn't want to die. I had fought so hard, so many times, but each time I had always regained control before any "real" damage had been done. I guess I figured it would always be like that. Somehow, I thought, it would always turn out okay. Now it had finally caught up with me. I wasn't going to be able to talk my way out of this one.

I assured the doctor that I would make all the arrangements necessary for admission to the hospital. I then headed for the privacy of the nearest bathroom. Sitting in the stall, I waited for the tears to flow. None came. I pulled out the piece of paper and pen that I had absentmindedly stuck in my pocketbook and started to list the necessary calls and details that would fill my days to come.

I waited for the tears to flow. None came.
I methodically started to list the necessary calls and details that would fill my days to come.

My mind refused to move forward; I could not deal with all that had to be done. I could not figure out how I would handle it all. As I sat, mentally paralyzed in the bathroom stall, the struggles of my past crowded into my tiny space—pulling me twenty-five years back in time.

I saw myself sitting cross-legged on the hospital bed, trying in vain to pull the short hospital gown over my two-hundred-pound body. Two young doctors stood beside my bed.

"How old are you?" one doctor asked.

"Twelve and a half," I mumbled, trying desperately to cover my short fat legs with a gown that barely reached to my knees.

One after the other, the two doctors took turns asking for details that a twelve-year-old could not possibly supply. I felt stupid and ashamed, but I soon found that their difficult questions were nothing compared to the humiliating physical examination that was to follow.

Drawing my clothes aside, their hands exposed my body to full view, commented on it in words that I barely understood, and then committed these words, irrevocably, to my chart.

Every part of me was probed and pinched and, even worse, was commented on. I did not need to know Latin to understand that they were shocked at my obesity; the looks in their eyes and their tone of disapproval and disdain crossed all language barriers. Though it was the curse of my childhood, I would have welcomed the outright teasing of my classmates to the humiliation that I experienced as their hands exposed my body, commented on it in words that I barely understood, and then committed these words, irrevocably and in writing, to my chart.

On admission to the hospital, they found my blood pressure to be 220/120, dangerously high even for a person five times my age. I was carrying the equivalent of more than another person's weight on my developing body, and though I had been told how important activity was to my health, the burden of the weight made it virtually impossible for me to exercise.

My blood pressure was 220/120 and I was twice my normal weight. At the tender age of twelve, I was already a "high-risk patient."

It was not as if I had not been "trying." I had been battling with my weight and hunger as long as I could remember, though it seemed as if I were always hungry. I had started to "watch my weight" by the time I was eight years old and had begun the useless rounds of diet doctors and diet pills by age eleven.

Diet after diet, nothing worked. I would lose a few pounds and put back twice as many. I tried new doctors, new diets, new pills. Though I had been noticeably chubby at eight, I was clearly obese by twelve, and the pills, dieting, and weight were already taking their toll on my young body.

I had become knowledgeable about death and illness before I knew anything about life and love.

Long before I ever kissed a boy, I had become familiar with terms such as *hypertension, stroke,* and *coronary artery disease*—warnings, said the doctors, of things to come. I had become knowledgeable about death and illness before I knew anything about life and love. At a time when I should have been concerned with friends and dresses and parties, I was trying to cope with staying alive.

Upon my discharge from the hospital, I was given no medication and virtually no help. "Lose weight and bring down that blood pressure," cautioned one doctor, "or you'll never . . ." Embarrassed, he looked up into my young face, ruffled my hair, and walking down the hall, called back, "Take care now, hear?"

Not knowing of any other alternatives, I did what most adults do. I continued the same practices that had proved unsuccessful in the first place, with the promise to myself that this time I would try harder.

I failed at diet after diet and, by the time I was seventeen, I weighed well over three hundred pounds. I ached for a life that was no longer limited by obesity and illness. Over the years, my high blood pressure resulted in a heart murmur and an irregular heartbeat. Each night, I prayed for only one thing: "to be normal." To me, a typical adolescence would not have been a time of turmoil and distress. It was the wish of my life.

My family could offer me no help. My parents were themselves in poor health. My father was overweight and suffered from high blood pressure, emphysema, and borderline diabetes. He died of a stroke at the age of fifty-two, when I was only nineteen years old.

My mother was overweight and had three heart attacks by the time she hit her mid-forties. A borderline diabetic, she was to die at age fifty-four. My brother had inherited my family's genetic predisposition to obesity and he tried desperately to control it with diet pills. He managed to keep his weight down, but in the end, the pills took their toll. He was dead before his fortieth birthday. It seemed as if there was no way of winning; either the weight made you ill or the cure killed you.

There was no way of winning;
either the weight made you ill or the cure killed you.

With all the illness in my immediate family, still I did not come from "bad stock." My great-grandmother and great-grandfather, having lived most of their lives in "the old country," survived to 107 and 109 years, respectively. Except for one grandfather who died of complications related to diabetes, my grandparents lived into their late seventies and eighties. With each successive generation, the life expectancy in my family was being cut by twenty or thirty years, with my parents dying in their fifties and my brother in his late thirties.

A genetics professor once commented that it appeared my family was doing something terribly wrong, something that was getting worse with each generation, something that my great-grandparents had not done, and that this "something" was literally killing us. His simple observation was to foretell the discovery of Profactor-H.

In the meantime, my health continued to worsen. I registered and reregistered for commercial diet programs but found they led to the yo-yo dieting and weight gain cycle. I would follow their advice, at times I would feel like I was literally starving myself—but I was determined. Eventually, no matter how I tried, I would fail. I went to a hypnotist, twice; and for behavioral modification, twice. I tried liquid fasts and water fasts. I went to holistic doctors and to nutritionists. Each time I took off twenty, fifty, even a hundred pounds at a throw, only to gain it back . . . and more. I had three or four sets of clothes in varying sizes. My self-confidence and happiness, even my good health, were dependent on whether I was climbing up or down the ladder of success.

In the beginning, each weight gain would lead to a worsening of health, a shortness of breath, chest tightness, and heart palpitations. All of these symptoms would then fade with each new bout of weight loss. As I approached my thirties, my body's resiliency seemed to fade and new weight-loss schemes seemed to have no impact on bettering my health and well-being.

When I would take off weight, my triglycerides remained in the range of 350 (twice the optimal level), and as my physician became knowledgeable about such things, we found that my cholesterol level was close to 300 as well. After a while, my blood pressure did not seem to respond to weight loss. My irregular heartbeat had become worse. I could feel the murmur whenever I exerted myself. I began having gallbladder attacks and my knees and feet hurt all of the time.

> The whole thing blew apart when, at the age of thirty-four,
> I suffered a heart "episode" while at work.

The whole thing blew apart when, at age thirty-four, I suffered a heart "episode" while at work. It came on suddenly. I was late for the class I was teaching and I took a halfhearted jog in the hall to get to the classroom on time. Suddenly, I couldn't catch my breath and my heart went wild. It felt like a frightened animal struggling to get out of my chest.

Repeatedly I lost consciousness, regained it and lost it again, but each time I "came to" I refused to let them call an ambulance. A co-worker sat by my side begging me to let her call the rescue squad.

I was terrified. I was going to die, never having really lived. I bargained with God. "Please," I said. "Let me live. I have important things to do," although at the time I had no idea what they were. Still, I didn't want to have them carry me out on a stretcher. I didn't want to see the knowing looks as they struggled to carry my bulk.

Finally, my terror got me to my feet. I made my way to the street and together my friend and I hailed a passing police car to take me to the hospital. EKGs and heart monitors told the story. The emergency room physician explained that my heartbeat had become un-coordinated; for a time it was no longer able to effectively pump blood. He said that it foretold of a coming heart attack in clear and certain terms. This was my last chance, he told me sternly, "to turn my life around and get it together." He turned and left the emergency room without a clue as to how I was to make this miracle happen.

> My body was falling apart.
> No, I knew I was tearing it apart,
> but I didn't know how to stop.

In the years that followed, I had to be readmitted to the hospital about once a year for some sort of health-related problem: irregular heartbeat, high blood pressure, heart murmur, loss of consciousness related to possible stroke, pericarditis, possible meningitis, pleurisy, hepatitis, even gout. My body was falling apart. No, I knew I was tearing it apart, but I didn't know how to stop.

By my mid-thirties, I had been well on my way to following my parents' history of very early death. With each doctor's visit or hospital discharge, I was cautioned to watch my weight and restrict my diet, but diets left me hungry and I invariably found myself cheating. Exercise regimes were boring and exhausting and, try as I might, I was simply unable to radically change my lifestyle to the one they said would save my life. I truly wanted to do it, but I simply could not.

My body seemed to be some kind of "fat machine," pushing me to crave breads, starches, snack foods, and sweets, and even when I restrained myself, leading me to gain weight on the amount of food that caused others to shed pounds.

My body seemed to be some kind of "fat machine."

I was determined to find the cause and cure to my problems, and, at over three hundred pounds, I made it into an excellent doctoral program.

I used my new research skills to search the book stacks for clues to my problem, but my first trip to the library proved quite enlightening in a surprising way. Most of the articles and books carried recommendations based on what *should* be rather than what *was*. They continued to give the same advice that I had been given for the past twenty years. Eat sensible meals, they advised. Exercise, eat small meals, eat slowly, keep fat levels low, etc., etc., etc. All this advice had one thing in common—it offered no insight into what was *causing* my cravings, my weight and health problems, in the first place.

Though the authors of all of these books were well aware that millions of people had, in good conscience, attempted to follow their same old advice and had failed over and over again, they offered the same advice once again as if no one had ever thought of it before. I remember reading yet another article: "To lose weight eat low-fat, sensible meals and exercise."

But I knew that the same old tried-and-untrue advice simply did not work—not in the real world. The most commonly accepted advice was, at best, unlivable, and when I was unable to follow it, I blamed myself for not being able to stick to what seemed like "sensible" recommendations.

But what my physicians had recommended for simple good health was beginning to look more and more like an act requiring impossible strength and discipline and doomed to eventual failure. Surely there had to be a better answer.

> What my physicians had recommended for simple good health
> was beginning to look more and more
> like an act requiring impossible strength and discipline and
> doomed to eventual failure.
> Surely there had to be a better answer.

The answer I so desperately sought, the solution that brought me a life of health, happiness, and freedom, came from a sequence of discoveries. Each new discovery gave me a piece of the puzzle that, when fully uncovered, became the Profactor-H Program.

I discovered the first piece of the Program when I realized that once I began to eat carbohydrate-rich foods such as breads and other starches, snack foods, and sweets, I had a very difficult time controlling myself. When I discovered that, by saving these foods for one of my three daily meals, I could enjoy all of the carbohydrates I loved and needed without suffering the hunger and weight gain, I was well on the way to freedom. The pounds fell away, my blood pressure dropped, my heart murmur disappeared, my blood fat levels plunged to normal, and, by the time I had achieved a 150-pound weight loss, friends and strangers alike were flocking to me for help.

To top it off, Richard dropped into my life. He, too, had discovered the same carbohydrate link to weight loss, and in addition to dropping thirty-five pounds and four inches off his waist, his blood pressure had become normal.

Our joint appointments as professors at New York's Mount Sinai

School of Medicine opened up research possibilities on a wide scale. As word of success spread, the research program was swamped. Not only were our overweight subjects losing weight but, by objective criteria, our overweight and normal-weight subjects alike were becoming healthier. Because of the Profactor-H Program, they looked better, they felt better, and their health risk levels dropped—and stayed down.

Today, I stand before you, a healthy woman full of life, energy, and joy. At a time when most people feel as if their bodies are beginning to wear and to age, I feel reborn.

Today, I stand before you, a healthy woman
full of life, energy, and joy.
I eat the foods I love every day—
with never a thought of measuring or counting.
Without sacrificing my health,
I live a life without deprivation or sacrifice.

Today, my blood pressure rarely varies from its 122/70 level. My cholesterol is in the low 150s range and I have an ideally low LDL level. My HDL-cholesterol level is ideal and my cholesterol profile puts me in the lowest 5 percent risk range for coronary heart disease in the country. Not bad for a woman over forty-nine years of age! I have the strength and vitality of someone half my age (our students actually complain that they can't keep up with Richard and me), and what is most important, I truly enjoy my life, my health, and my body.

At a time when most people feel as if their bodies
are beginning to wear and to age,
I feel reborn.

I eat the foods I love every day, in portions that are neither measured nor counted. I maintain an active lifestyle but do not have to engage in formal exercise regimes. My physical well-being is *not* the hard-earned result of trading away my pleasure, my joy, or my time. It is a natural result of correcting an underlying physical disorder that usually goes unrecognized and uncorrected.

I enjoy the food I love; I live the life I always wanted. I follow a few simple guidelines that make it possible to get what I always wanted out of life.

**Our bodies are amazingly resilient.
When we stop hurting them, they stop hurting us.**

Our bodies are amazingly resilient. When we stop hurting them, they stop hurting us. The long battles of my past are over. I have no trace of a heart murmur. My heart irregularity has long been reversed. There remains no damage to my body at all.

I have been healthy, happy, and a size six for over ten years—struggle-free! The Profactor-H Program is not a miracle; it is simply good science.

**The Profactor-H Program is not a miracle;
it is simply good science.**

The Spiral of Denial:
Dr. Richard Heller's Story

My story is quite different from Rachael's. I was a healthy, happy child, a stocky teenager, and a strapping young man. I worked hard and enjoyed the fact that I was strong and active. I struggled to keep my weight in line and was irritated by my slowly expanding waist and my "love handles." Still, I was young and healthy; and, I assumed, I would always be.

My parents had been healthy all of their lives, too; or at least their rare visits to doctors never revealed any obvious problems.

> I was young and healthy; and, I assumed, I would always be. As I reached my mid-forties, however, my illusion of immunity began to crumble.

As I reached my mid-forties, however, my illusion of immunity began to crumble. My father, a strong and powerful man, who had started to put on a bit of middle-aged spread in his later years, suffered a heart attack followed almost immediately by a stroke. He died in a matter of days. I was away at the time and my mother chose to allow me to continue my "well-earned vacation" without interruption. I never got a chance to say good-bye to my father, and in many ways not being there for his funeral allowed me to deny a very important lesson: that there was no longer a generational buffer between me and my own mortality.

By the time I returned home, my mother had buried her grief. When I visited her, it felt as if my dad was out visiting a friend or at work. His bed and clothes remained untouched and it was easier for both of us to act as if nothing had changed. She missed him, she would say, and she would cry. I would hold her but, at the same time, neither of us ever forced the other to face the finality of his leaving.

Not fully experiencing my father's death was only a sign of a much greater denial on my part, the denial that I, too, was mortal and that as time passed I was showing signs of a lessening of strength, health, and well-being.

As a full professor, my full-time position held me responsible for only five classes a week. In order to earn additional monies for the growing needs of my family, I took on four additional part-time teaching jobs at three other colleges. My now ex-wife had returned to school and I took on most of the child-care responsibilities as well. I worked like a maniac. I was on the go from 6:30 in the morning (preparing for lectures, marking papers) and continued without a break until midnight (when I finished the laundry and packed the kids' sandwiches for the next day).

In between, I made hot dinners, taught cool lectures, and lived a lukewarm existence. To myself and others, I was a superman. My power was undeniable; my ability was legend . . . and I rarely stopped to listen to the exhaustion and the pain that I was feeling.

**By the time I literally dropped into bed at night,
I was so tired that I had neither the desire nor the
ability to think or to care about anything.**

By the time I literally dropped into bed at night, I was so tired that I had neither the desire nor the ability to think or to care about anything. And so the cycle repeated day after day, month after month, year after year. During the day, I grabbed whatever was quickest to eat in order to keep up my energy, and as the meals-on-the-run took their toll, my expanding waist became a full-fledged belly.

**I rarely stopped to listen to the exhaustion
and the pain that I was feeling.**

The surprise anniversary party that I been planning for my wife turned out to be a double surprise. The party was truly wonderful and she was very happy. Friends and family gathered; it was a time of joy, straight out of a Hallmark advertisement. The only problem was that I had been having pains in my chest for at least a week, and though I had tried hard to pretend that they were just "muscle cramps," I knew they were the typical signs of a heart problem that could have come straight out of a medical school textbook.

The night of the party, I dragged myself home, my body screaming for rest. I had been eating even more poorly than usual; there simply was not enough time to do everything. The kids had sore throats that week and two unplanned trips to the doctor pushed my already impossible schedule past endurance.

It was around 5:00 in the evening; I had completed food shopping for the week and for the party, the laundry was finished, and I had just picked up the kids from their friend's house. "Now," I thought, "a quick dinner, a bath, and they're done." The kids were quieter than usual and I was concerned that they might be getting sick again. I had to admit, I didn't feel so good myself, and with the long evening and party ahead, every inch of me ached for sleep.

I had fought off a bout of pain while driving to work a few days before and now, as I felt the same ache deep in my chest, I pushed aside the warning and hustled the kids into the house.

The guests arrived and the evening looked like it was going to be a solid success, but as I reached down to pick up my daughter to carry her off to bed, a giant fist closed around my chest. I couldn't breathe, I couldn't move, I could barely stay focused. I was struck by the thought of being carried out of my own anniversary party on a stretcher.

For weeks I had been thinking of increasing my life insurance coverage, and all I could think of now was how I had screwed things up by putting it off. I was going to die and I should have better taken care of my family.

I reached down to pick up my daughter and a giant fist closed around my chest.

I still don't know how I did it but I continued to smile and say all the right things. In a few moments, the grip on my chest loosened but a feeling of deep soreness remained.

When the guests had departed, I dropped into bed—barely able to think or talk. The next day was filled with cleaning up from the party and a promised zoo trip for my children, so any visit to the doctor was put on hold. Besides, the pain had subsided . . . for the moment.

In the weeks that followed, the tightness in my chest became a familiar companion. I filled out the necessary forms for more life insurance, but when I realized that I would have to get a physical exam, I panicked; not for fear of facing the state of my health but for fear of being turned down for a larger policy.

I told myself I was too young to have a heart attack but decided to hold off applying for the extra insurance until I was in better shape.

"After all," I concluded,
"I'm too young to be having a heart attack."

The pain did not go away. It continued, and in time grew worse. I knew that I had to get some help. I wanted to find out what was wrong before I told my wife, so I picked a new doctor out of the phone book and went to see him.

He confirmed my fears. "You're exhausted and you're treating your body like #!!*#!." My blood pressure was dangerously high and he was willing to bet my cholesterol was through the ceiling (lab tests confirmed that he was right). I was eating poorly, putting on weight, and slowly, though not too gently, committing suicide. I was helping to raise a family that I would probably never enjoy in my old age.

I was doing everything right for everyone else
and everything wrong for me.
I was helping raise a family that
I would probably never enjoy in my old age.

I was doing everything right for everyone else and everything wrong for me. "If your children or your wife needed good food or rest or exercise, you would stop everything else and do it; you'd probably even do it for your dog, but for yourself . . ." The doctor didn't need to finish.

Though the electrocardiogram did not reveal any damage, he felt sure that the pain was serious. "The recurring pain is a sign. How much more do you need before you believe that your body is trying to tell you something?" he asked.

It should have "told me something" but, as usual, I wasn't listening. I heard what I wanted to hear and did what I thought best. I added exercise to my already insane schedule.

Every morning between 6:00 and 7:10, I ran about six miles. I started taking the time to eat the hot meals that I prepared for the family and went for regular checkups. And except for adding medical bills to my expenses, little changed.

My cholesterol and triglycerides were high (we didn't know much about HDL- and LDL-cholesterol then) and my blood pressure was out of control. It would peak to dangerous levels, then return to almost normal within a few minutes. "Not a good sign," my doctor remarked in his usual understated manner.

> ## As long as I went back to the doctor for regular checkups, I felt protected.

I kept my medical visits a secret, wanting to deny that there was any real problem. The pains in my chest came and went, but as long as I returned for regular checkups, I felt protected.

As I approached my late forties, my weight went up by leaps and bounds. I was more than thirty-five pounds over my desired weight and was clearly headed skyward. My pants were feeling the strain and so were my knees. With the added weight and years, running was becoming a risky business, and after my second knee injury, my doctor recommended that I stop running. My shell of denial was beginning to crumble.

> ## My shell of denial was beginning to crumble.

I was up against a stone wall and it was getting harder. Denial and halfway measures would no longer do. My choices were decreasing and a life of increasing medications and decreasing health seemed inevitable.

The answer to all my prayers came, ironically, when I finally tackled the problem that was hardest for me to deny—my weight. In the weeks that followed, I ate only when I was hungry and noticed which foods increased my hunger and tiredness levels.

To the trained scientist in me, it was obvious that large meals that contained carbohydrates—starches, snack foods, fruits, and sweets—were often followed by hunger, cravings, and a sort of drugged feeling. At times these feelings were subtle, at other times they were not.

I had been told to "carbo load" when running, but if I carbo loaded more than once a day, I felt bloated and lethargic. I coined the termed "carbohydrate sensitive" for myself and found that when I carbo loaded only *once* a day and then ate high-fiber, low-fat, low-carbo meals during the rest of the day, I felt terrific. Better than I had in years.

My weight dropped. The chest pains disappeared and I looked younger and healthier than I had when I was running. I was encouraged by the way I looked and felt and, for the first time in my life, began to believe that I could really make a difference. I read up on the importance of stress reduction and added it to my routine. I forced myself to take time for myself. It was no longer a matter of indulgence. At first, taking the time I needed had become a matter of life and death; now it was a source of pride.

My blood tests confirmed my hopes. I was getting healthier. Suddenly, my health and my life were precious to me in a way that I had never let myself admit.

The program I had designed for myself was improving not just my weight but my overall health as well. The crucial test came when I returned to my doctor's office. I had lost nearly twenty pounds in a little over two months and my blood pressure was better than he had ever seen it. The blood tests confirmed what I already knew. I was getting healthier.

Though my diet was not particularly low in fat, the fats in my blood were dropping steadily. Though my diet was not very low in salt, my blood pressure was normalizing. Though my diet provided me with the food I loved, in the more-than-generous portions that I required, I was easily shedding pounds. I could not deny it. Neither could my doctor, though he resisted at first. The numbers were going down, and with every pound lost I was looking and feeling better.

In the past, when I had tried so hard to follow his recommendations, I had failed. Now, virtually effortlessly, I was succeeding in becoming healthier. My health and my life had become precious to me in a way that I had never let myself admit. I wanted to live and be healthy and enjoy my life and now it looked as if I finally knew how.

Shortly after my marriage ended, I found Rachael. Together we learned that we were not alone in our discoveries. Thousand of scientists had already uncovered the hormonal imbalance that had led to my overweight and ill health: the overrelease of insulin that would have, in most probability, led to my early and unnecessary death.

We had, each in our own way, discovered the Profactor-H Program that corrected this imbalance. Our Program has stood the test of time. At over fifty-eight years of age I am far, far healthier than I was at forty. I take no medication and have the strength and health that men half my age would envy.

I do not take it for granted. I know that I owe my health and happiness to the Profactor-H Program. It has changed my life and the lives of more people than Rachael and I will ever know.

A personal success is a wonderful victory, but a success that can help others gives meaning to life. Rachael and I are proud and happy to share our successes, our victories, and our lives and our Program with you.

CHAPTER 2

$\triangledown$

A Matter of Life and Health

Balance is the basis of all good health. Everything in moderation. —Benjamin Franklin

Your body is in a never-ending battle for survival. As you work or eat or sleep, the struggle continues. The warriors in this internal battle are insulin and insulin's arch opponent, glucagon. These two hormones, glucagon and insulin, literally rule your life, and in the battle, if you are lucky, both sides will win.

When most people hear the word *insulin* they think of diabetes. But each second of every day, insulin affects your every movement and every breath. Insulin is your body's saving hormone. It is a miser in the truest sense of the word.

As you take in energy in the form of food, insulin loves nothing more than to save that energy and put it away "for a rainy day." Although a small portion of incoming food is sent to cells that require energy to stay alive, insulin channels most of the energy, in the form of fat, deep within your fat cells. If insulin had its way, it would save and save, our fat cells would grow larger and larger, and insulin would never spend the energy it so carefully put into storage.

> Without your ever knowing it,
> insulin and glucagon literally rule your life.

Glucagon, on the other hand, is the body's spending hormone. Glucagon's job is to bring energy out of storage—out of the fat cells—so that it may be used to repair and to fuel the body. Insulin puts energy into the fat cells; glucagon takes it out.

In the best of all possible worlds, insulin and glucagon complement each other and maintain a perfect balance. All too often, however, this ideal balance becomes a hormonal tug-of-war with insulin having the upper hand. The outcome of this battle will often mean the difference between a long and healthy existence and a life plagued by disability or cut short by disease.

The outcome of this battle will often mean
the difference between
a long and healthy existence and
a life plagued by disability or cut short by disease.

The Essential Insulin Link

Many decades ago, long before the current talk of risk factors and profactors, scientists were beginning to suspect that insulin might be the invisible connection among several diseases that had, in the past, been viewed as separate and unrelated.

As far back as 1936, in the British medical journal *The Lancet,* Dr. H. P. Himsworth first wrote about the central imbalance that we have now identified as Profactor-H and identified it as an important cause of disease. At the time, Dr. Himsworth called on his fellow researchers and the physicians of the time to more intently study this vital imbalance.

It was obvious to Dr. Himsworth, almost sixty years ago, that an insulin imbalance lay at the base of several different and devastating diseases. Unfortunately, the lack of available technology at the time kept this discovery from being confirmed in Himsworth's lifetime. The experiments that were needed to confirm his ideas and bring them into medical practice were, in his day, simply not possible.

It took another five decades for researchers to acquire the tools and knowledge to begin to discover the profactor that Dr. Himsworth described and that has since been linked to so much needless illness and death.

It was not until 1988, in an article published in the medical journal *Diabetes,* that Dr. G. M. Reaven could finally report that, after fifty years, Dr. Himsworth's understanding of insulin's great impact on human disease has been proved and that "it now seems quite clear that Himsworth was correct, and the point of view he introduced has become well established."

For lack of the technology needed to confirm his discovery, five decades of help were lost to the untold numbers who could have benefited from Dr. Himsworth's breakthrough. But today the tide of scientific understanding has turned. In the last few years alone, Profactor-H has been identified, examined, investigated, and researched by thousands of scientists.

In the past, when researchers studied Profactor-H, they often used the term *hyperinsulinemia*—meaning too much insulin. In the beginning physicians and scientists alike thought of it as a simple excess of insulin, a not-too-common disorder that had some effect on the body but was not yet fully understood. In the last ten years, however, a virtual explosion of research articles has emerged reporting the connection of hyperinsulinemia to an extraordinarily wide variety of diseases. Day by day, the reports of vital discoveries and connections to hyperinsulinemia (or Profactor-H, as we call it now) continue to grow.

In 1983, the number of scientific articles relating Profactor-H as an essential link to other diseases numbered around three hundred. Ten years later, more than three thousand articles have explored and reported this important and potentially lifesaving discovery.

In articles in the top medical research journals from around the world, Profactor-H is being reported as the underlying link, the unifying factor, that connects many of the most prevalent and devastating of this country's top killer diseases. *Profactor-H has been implicated in over half of this country's deaths each year.*

Today, the finest scholarly journals and most respected reports include, on a regular basis, groundbreaking research on the effects of the sweeping impact of Profactor-H. Such reports and journals include *The Surgeon General's Report on Nutrition and Health, The*

New England Journal of Medicine, The Lancet, Clinical Nutrition, Annals of the New York Academy of Science, Journal of Clinical Endocrinological Metabolism, Journal of Human Hypertension, American Heart Journal, Journal of the American Medical Association (JAMA), and innumerable others.

The Profactor-H Facts, Clear and Simple

Scientist after scientist has linked Profactor-H to atherosclerosis, heart disease, stroke, and diabetes mellitus, as well as to many of this country's major health risk factors such as high blood pressure, excess weight, and undesirable blood fat levels. Several new studies link Profactor-H to a number of forms of cancer. Behind each of these diseases and risk factors lies the same crucial connection: Profactor-H.

In the chart that follows, the negative impact that untreated Profactor-H can have on health and long life speaks for itself. The good news is that the facts of the past are no longer the sentence of the future. Today, we are able to correct the very cause of Profactor-H, reduce our exposure to the many diseases and risk factors it can help promote, and live Profactor-H free at last.

Leading Causes of Death in the United States in Which Profactor-H Has Been Identified as a Major Cause[1, 2]

Heart disease (coronary and other)
Cancer (several forms)
Stroke
Adult-onset diabetes mellitus
Chronic liver disease and cirrhosis
Atherosclerosis

Health Risk Factors in Which Profactor-H Has Been Identified as a Major Cause[2]

Undesirable levels of lipids (fats) in the blood
High blood pressure
Excess weight

[1] Adapted from *The Surgeon General's Report on Nutrition and Health,* 1988.
[2] As reported in medical and/or scientific journals.

Health Risk Factors That Have Been Shown to Lead to Profactor-H²

Smoking
High-fat, high-salt, or high-sugar diets
Low activity/exercise levels
Physical or psychological stress
Increased age

Where Credit Is Due

In the past, uncovering Profactor-H's many connections was a monumental task; it took untold years of work and the concentrated effort of countless numbers of biologists, biochemists, endocrinologists, cell biologists, and nutrition researchers in the world's most prestigious medical schools and universities. No one person or group of scientists was responsible. But credit for the discovery is unimportant. What matters now is getting this knowledge to you, so that you and your physician can use it—now, when you need it most.

In the pages that follow, you will learn how Profactor-H can impact on your life and health and how to save yourself and those you love from the ravages of this biological tyrant. You will meet some of the people who have been through the program themselves and who are far healthier and happier than they ever dreamed they could be.

The old "no pain, no gain" philosophy is a bunch of muck!
You do *not* have to suffer to be healthy.

The old "no pain, no gain" philosophy is a bunch of muck! You do *not* have to suffer to be healthy. That antiquated belief is simply not true. The people we help are not deprived of the food they love, the leisure they enjoy, or the health they have a right to. They are living proof that good health does not have to come from deprivation or frustration. Your health and well-being are gifts that are yours for the taking. You have a right to claim them.

> Your health and well-being are gifts that are yours for the taking.
> You have a right to claim them.

CHAPTER 3

What Is Profactor-H?

Nothing is more powerful than an idea whose time has come. —Anonymous

What Is a Profactor?

For centuries, physicians and scientists have dreamed of finding a *unifying factor,* a single, central cause that would explain all of the diseases that plague the human race and that, when corrected, would relieve mankind of the pain and suffering that have come to be accepted as a part of life and aging.

Amazingly, today, without fanfare or flourish, science has uncovered not one single factor but, rather, *several* important imbalances in the body, each of which seems to be responsible for a whole host of diseases and risk factors.

We call these imbalances *profactors,* because each one appears to be the first factor, the underlying cause, of several diseases and risk factors.

Profactor: the "first factor" or underlying cause.
A central imbalance of the human body
that will often lead or contribute
to a wide variety of diseases and risk factors.

At this very minute, three different profactors are being studied intensely by scientists and physicians alike. The first imbalance is Profactor-A.*

Profactor-A is responsible for many of the autoimmune diseases, such as rheumatoid arthritis, rheumatic fever, pernicious anemia, and lupus erythematosus. In the diseases caused by Profactor-A, the body literally attacks itself. Unfortunately, the process responsible for Profactor-A has not yet been positively identified, though current research in the area of *cytokines,* substances secreted by immune cells as they fight disease, may soon provide some answers. The prevention and alleviation of autoimmune diseases still awaits positive identification of this important profactor.

The second imbalance, Profactor-C,* is responsible for the abnormal growth of cells, the set of diseases we call cancer. Cancer cells grow out of control, stealing nourishment and vital space needed by normal cells. Again, the prevention and eradication of cancer awaits the discovery and correction of its underlying malfunction, Profactor-C.

Both Profactor-A and Profactor-C are being actively studied and, while some strides have been made in understanding these two profactors, no final breakthrough and no correction, as yet, have been uncovered.

But the third profactor, Profactor-H, has a far happier story to tell.

What Is Profactor-H?

Profactor-H is the term we use for the silent but deadly imbalance that comes from having too much insulin in your bloodstream. An excess of insulin can occur when your body releases too much insulin (after eating or during stress, for instance), or it can come from your body's inability to use the insulin that you have, or it can come from a combination of both.

*Profactor-A and Profactor-C have not, as yet, been positively identified; these profactor designations are temporary and are terms we are using for the time being, until specific causal processes are uncovered. These terms are being used as labels for the communication of concepts.

Most people never suspect they have too much insulin, but over time, without your knowing it, high insulin levels can cause great damage to your body and lead to the development of many serious health risk factors and diseases. If your insulin level remains high for extended periods of time, it can become a profactor for disease— Profactor-H.

Though scientists again and again describe Profactor-H's power to cause illness and early death, at this time Profactor-H may still go unrecognized and uncorrected. In many cases, physicians and other health professionals attempt to treat or eliminate disease, disorders, or risk factors without correcting the underlying cause—the profactor itself. What is worse is that Profactor-H's impact is mounting by the day and if it were a contagious disease it would be classified as "epidemic."

Profactor-H: A continuous excess of insulin that is often undiagnosed and can lead or contribute to heart disease and atherosclerosis, stroke, adult-onset diabetes mellitus, polycystic ovary disease, some types of cancer, and vascular disease, as well as many health risk factors such as undesirable levels of fats in the blood, excess weight, and high blood pressure.
Physicians and researchers alike may still refer to Profactor-H as *chronic hyperinsulinemia.*
Our research shows that once Profactor-H risk is recognized it may be preventable as well as reversible.

THE PROFACTOR-H WARNING LIST

Signs and Symptoms of Profactor-H:

Are you overweight? Do you find that maintaining a normal weight is
a struggle?
Do you often experience carbohydrate cravings (cravings for starches,
snack foods, fruits, or sweets)?
Are you tired and/or hungry in the mid-afternoon?
Do you feel very sluggish after eating dinner?
Have you experienced the signs of low blood sugar (headache,
weakness, irritability, shakiness, sweats)?
Do you have a tendency to retain fluid?
Do you have high blood pressure?
Do you have undesirable levels of fat in your blood?
Do you have adult-onset diabetes or peripheral vascular disease?
Do you have atherosclerosis or coronary heart disease?

Any one of these signs taken alone may indicate that you have Profactor-H,
but the greater number of signs you show, the more probable it is that
you are, indeed, Profactor-H Positive. It is important for you to take the
Profactor-H Evaluation in chapter 4 and determine your personal level
of risk for Profactor-H and, most important, find what your score means
to *you*.

The greater number of signs you show, the more probable
it is that you are Profactor-H Positive. It is important for you
to take the Profactor-H Evaluation in chapter 4.

Risk Factors—Probable Cause

Scientists and physicians have long known that the greater the
number of risk factors you have, the greater your chances of getting
an illness, and with each additional risk factor, the probability of im-
pending illness greatly increases. Unfortunately, the relatively new

concept of risk factors is often misunderstood and people may come to think that risk factors actually cause the diseases and disorders in question.

It is important to understand exactly what the term *risk factor* means. By common use of the term, a risk factor is a condition, disorder, or disease that has been found to predict the future occurrence of another condition, disorder, or disease.

A risk factor is a condition, disorder, or disease that has been found to predict the future occurrence of another condition, disorder, or disease.

High blood pressure, for example, is a risk factor for heart disease. Those who have high blood pressure will have a higher *probability* of developing heart disease in the years to come than those who do not have high blood pressure. This is not to say that everyone who has high blood pressure will get heart disease or that *not* having high blood pressure assures you of never getting heart disease. It simply means that high blood pressure makes the possibility of heart disease more likely (in statistical terms).

Most important, this risk factor connection does *not* necessarily mean that high blood pressure *causes* heart disease. And here is where a great deal of confusion and misunderstanding occurs.

In some cases, a risk factor may be the cause of a disease; in other cases it is not. Knowing the difference can be critical to your health.

While, in some cases, a risk factor may be the *cause* of a disorder or disease, in other cases the risk factor is simply a co-existing condition. Sometimes the connection is obvious. Being Jewish, for instance, is a risk factor for the genetic disease Tay-Sachs, which means that if you are Jewish you have a greater probability of having a child with Tay-Sachs than someone who is not Jewish.

It is obvious that being Jewish does not cause Tay-Sachs, but it may be reflective of having an Eastern European heritage, from which this disease springs. Since being Jewish is a risk factor for Tay-Sachs disease, *and not a cause,* trying to change the risk factor—in this case, converting to a different religion—makes absolutely no sense and would not, of course, change your child's probability of having the disease.

When a risk factor is *not* the cause of the disease, trying to avoid it or change it *cannot* reduce your chances of getting the disease. All of your efforts will be wasted, and worse, you may be ignoring the very things that may make you more vulnerable to other problems. While the futility of changing noncausal risk factors seems obvious when we look at the example above, the clarity often fades when it comes to risk factors that are, in themselves, diseases or disorders.

Consider the risk factor of obesity for diabetes. If obesity causes changes in the body that can lead to adult-onset diabetes, then obesity is a *causal* risk factor for the disease and it makes sense to do whatever is necessary to reduce your weight in order to avoid this disease.

If, on the other hand, obesity and diabetes both come from a single—and perhaps undiscovered—cause, it is essential to uncover the mutual cause of both the excess weight *and* diabetes. If, indeed, there is a common cause to both conditions, then trying to lose weight will do little or no good since being overweight is not a *causal* risk factor but simply a risk factor that happens to appear before the onset of diabetes.

Noncausal risk factors may predict the future occurrence of a disease but they have nothing to do with causing it. Obviously, putting your energy into reducing noncausal risk factors—reducing your weight, in this instance—may make no logical sense. Instead, your energy may be better focused on finding and correcting the *cause* of both the excess weight and the diabetes.

Many of today's health problems, called *diseases of civilization,* including heart disease, coronary artery disease, high blood pressure, undesirable blood fat levels, adult-onset diabetes, excess weight, some forms of cancer, and others, are often said to be risk factors, one for the other. In addition, lifestyle choices such as diet, activity level, smoking, alcohol intake, age, and stress are also cited as risk factors for these same diseases.

The greatest contribution that Profactor-H research provides is the discovery of a common link, a causal connection, between all of these diseases and their risk factors. This underlying imbalance is Profactor-H, which, when corrected, can reduce your probability of getting not just one but all of these diseases.

The Invisible Bridge

In addition to its direct link to this country's top killer diseases and risk factors, Profactor-H has been named by some of the most respected researchers from around the world as the invisible bridge that connects:

Smoking and heart disease
Smoking cessation and weight gain
Pregnancy and excess weight gain
Stress and heart disease
Stress and weight gain
Stress and some forms of cancer
Aging and weight gain

In the best of all possible worlds, the discovery of Profactor-H should have spelled the end to its powerful and deadly reign. Not so, for although scientists have repeatedly tied Profactor-H to un-necessary ill health and suffering, its discovery is so ground-breaking and new that, at this time, most physicians have not been trained to recognize its clear and obvious signs, nor do they properly test their patients for Profactor-H.

The truth is, at this time, most physicians and other health profes-sionals do not know how to help you prevent Profactor-H or how to reverse it.

Over the past ten years, Profactor-H has truly emerged as the uni-fying factor of which all scientists dream. Personally, however, we came face-to-face with the very real possibility that this breakthrough, like so many medical discoveries of the past, could be destined to lie silently on medical school library shelves for many, many years.

We realized that, if something was not done, the important health benefits that would come from preventing or reversing Profactor-H would be available only to the lucky patients of physicians who happened upon a relevant research article.

The thought that this vital information could go to waste was simply unacceptable to us, and we felt that we had no choice but to bring the research on Profactor-H to the people whose health and lives might be, literally, at stake.

This book was written for you, so that you can share what we have discovered; so that you can recognize the signs of Profactor-H in you and your family, well before it is too late; so that you might reverse the dangers and risk factors that need not be accepted as part and parcel of your family's heritage; and most of all, so that you and your physician can work together—to give you a long and healthy life. A life that is Profactor-H free.

CHAPTER 4

What Is Your Profactor-H Score?

A man's wellness or illness stem equally from his parents, himself, and the world around him.
—Ancient Chinese proverb

Profactor-H Positive: At greater risk for Profactor-H and the many diseases and risk factors linked to it.
A score of 12 or above on the Profactor-H Evaluation places you in the Profactor-H Positive category.

How do you know if you are at risk for Profactor-H and for the diseases that are linked to it? How can you tell if you, or someone you know, is Profactor-H Positive? Each day, in readers' letters, on hospital floors, in medical school classrooms and corridors, we are asked these questions.

As physicians and their patients become aware of the importance of Profactor-H, the question as to which is the best way to test for Profactor-H, to see if a patient is Profactor-H Positive, is inevitable.

In the pages that follow,
you can take a simple quiz that will help you determine if you are Profactor-H Positive and,
if you are, how great your risk may be.

In the pages that follow, you can take a simple quiz that will help you determine if you are Profactor-H Positive and how great your risk may be. Still, many people find the idea of a simple blood test for Profactor-H very appealing. In our letters and lectures and consultations, we explain that blood tests that evaluate patients' fasting insulin levels *do not* test for Profactor-H. These tests can, in fact, be tragically misleading.

Blood tests that evaluate patients' fasting insulin levels *do not* test for Profactor-H.
These tests can, in fact, be tragically misleading.

Remember that if you have Profactor-H, you have unusually high insulin levels that, usually without your ever knowing it, may remain high for a prolonged period of time. Insulin levels rise after eating or drinking or during periods of intense stress.

Now imagine this: The most commonly ordered blood test for determining your insulin level takes only a single reading after you have had no food or drink for a period of eight to twelve hours. In addition, you are usually told to come for testing early in the morning, the time at which your stress levels are often the lowest. The blood taken at this time determines your *fasting insulin level.*

Since Profactor-H insulin levels usually rise in response to eating or drinking or stress, if they are tested after you have had *no* food or drink or stress for a good period of time they may *appear* normal. In addition, a single sample says nothing about how high your levels remain over a period of hours. The fasting insulin test is absolutely the worst test for determining your Profactor-H level. Unfortunately, it is usually the only insulin test given, if it is given at all. To make matters even worse, if you show normal levels on your fasting insulin test, you are likely to be told that there is nothing wrong. Many of our Profactor-H Positive research subjects showed absolutely normal fasting insulin levels—yet after more appropriate testing they were shown to clearly have Profactor-H.

Relying on a fasting insulin test to determine if you are Profactor-H Positive is like being tested for a strawberry allergy when you have been instructed to avoid strawberries for several days before the test. Chances are, after staying away from strawberries, your skin will show no rash and you will report no congestion or headache. It is likely you will have no signs or symptoms of strawberry allergy at all and you will, in all likelihood, be found allergy-free.

You might protest that the test was invalid because the instructions that you had been given eliminated any way for your body to show this allergy. It is the same for using a fasting insulin test when testing for Profactor-H; it is totally illogical to look for high levels of insulin that occur in reaction to food or drink or stress in a person who has had no food or drink and minimal stress. It simply makes no sense. This is, however, the way in which most people are currently tested. To add possible injury to error, patients are often told that, since their insulin levels are normal, they do not need to be tested again. For the Profactor-H Positive patient, these can be very wrong and potentially dangerous conclusions.

Most of us do not think twice about fasting before a blood test; it is done all the time. In the case of Profactor-H, however, the information you get from a fasting insulin test is the absolute *opposite* of what physicians *should* be looking for when they test for Profactor-H.

Ideally, testing for Profactor-H involves testing for the results that come from *your* body's response to food, drink, changes in the environment, stress, and general hormonal and menstrual cycle changes.

Profactor-H insulin levels can vary greatly, especially in response to:

The kinds of foods you eat
How frequently you eat
Stress
Medications
The time of day
The time of month
Your current health status
Your age
Many other factors

A single insulin sample cannot give a meaningful measure of how *your* particular body responds to all of these factors, and testing your insulin level after fasting tells you nothing about how your body releases insulin in response to food or drink.

Due to the many factors that affect Profactor-H, there is currently no reliable, standardized laboratory test for evaluating Profactor-H levels. Scientists and physicians are still debating the positives and negatives of a whole battery of laboratory tests used for research purposes alone.

The good news is that, in our research, we have developed a simple quiz that will allow you to discover your risk for Profactor-H.

The good news is that, in our research, we have developed a simple quiz that will allow you to discover your risk for Profactor-H. The quiz has been revised several times in the last eight years; each revision has improved its accuracy and validity. We have added risk factor indicators from *The Surgeon General's Report on Nutrition and Health,* along with the finest medical research available. When compared with the most intricate blood tests, our quiz has been shown to reliably indicate risk for Profactor-H.

We call our quiz "The Profactor-H Evaluation," and it will help you to evaluate your own particular level of risk for Profactor-H.

The Profactor-H Evaluation

Before You Begin

The Profactor-H Evaluation will take only a few minutes to complete. It takes into account the contributions of your family genetics, your personal medical history, your environment, and your lifestyle. It will guide you through an individualized assessment that will help you to determine if you are Profactor-H Positive.

At the end of the Evaluation, you will be given a subscore in each of the four areas of risk factors:

Your Family and Medical History
Your Nutritional Profile
Your Activity Level
Your Stress Level

You will also be given an overall score that will indicate your personal overall Profactor-H Risk level.

You are about to begin an exciting and enlightening journey. You will discover, right now, how your health, well-being, and happiness may be influenced by Profactor-H.

As you complete the Profactor-H Evaluation, you will begin to understand why each of your four subscores, along with your overall score, is essential in helping you lower your risk for Profactor-H, and best of all, as you begin the Profactor-H Program, they will help you keep track of your own progress and success.

THE PROFACTOR-H EVALUATION

Part 1: Your Family and Medical History

Place a check next to all that apply. If more than one family member has had the same disorder, still place a single check next to that item.

One or more of my grandparent(s) have or had:

_____ high blood pressure	(1 pt.)
_____ adult-onset diabetes	(1 pt.)
_____ a stroke	(1 pt.)
_____ heart disease or atherosclerosis	(1 pt.)
_____ cancer of the ovary, breast, or uterus	(1 pt.)
_____ difficulty controlling their weight	(1 pt.)

One or more of my parent(s) have or had:

_____ high blood pressure	(2 pts.)
_____ adult onset diabetes	(2 pts.)
_____ a stroke	(2 pts.)
_____ heart disease or atherosclerosis	(2 pts.)
_____ cancer of the ovary, breast, or uterus	(2 pts.)

____ difficulty controlling their weight   (2 pts.)
____ undesirable fat levels in the blood   (2 pts.)

I have or had:

____ high blood pressure   (4 pts.)
____ adult-onset diabetes   (4 pts.)
____ a stroke   (4 pts.)
____ heart disease or atherosclerosis   (4 pts.)
____ cancer of the ovary, breast, or uterus   (4 pts.)
____ difficulty controlling your weight   (4 pts.)
____ undesirable fat levels in the blood   (4 pts.)

Check if the following applies to you:

____ I regularly take birth control pills or female
hormone replacement medication.   (2 pts.)

Check the *one* sentence that applies to you:

____ I am under 35 years of age.   (0 pts.)
____ I am between 35 and 49 years of age.   (1 pt.)
____ I am between 50 and 64 years of age.   (2 pts.)
____ I am over 65 years of age.   (3 pts.)

Family and Medical History Subscore: ▢

Part 2: Your Nutritional Profile

Check any of the following that apply:

____ During the day, I snack between meals.   (1 pt.)
____ I often snack at night.   (1 pt.)
____ I often chew gum or eat mints or hard candies
(regular or artificially sweetened).   (1 pt.)
____ Between meals, I drink coffee or tea that
contains milk, creamer, sugar, or artificial
sweeteners.   (2 pts.)
____ Between meals, I drink soda or other beverages
sweetened with sugar or artificial sweeteners.   (2 pts.)
____ At least one meal a day usually lasts for more
than an hour.   (1 pt.)

_____ When I feel like snacking, I will often eat either
a piece of fruit or some snack food (chips,
cookies, crackers, or candy).   (4 pts.)

_____ I eat high-fat foods almost every day.   (2 pts.)

_____ I usually include at least one of the following in
every meal: bread, pasta or some other starch,
fruits, or sweets.   (4 pts.)

_____ I often eat when I am not really hungry.   (2 pts.)

Nutritional Subscore:

Part 3: Your Activity Level

Check the *one* sentence that describes you, in general:

_____ I am a very active person.   (0 pts.)

_____ I am a moderately active person.   (2 pts.)

_____ I am not active.   (4 pts.)

Activity Subscore:

Part 4: Your Stress Level

In each of the following groups, check *one* sentence in any group *if* it
applies to you.

I experience a great deal of stress:

_____ rarely or not at all   (0 pts.)

_____ at my job but not at home   (2 pts.)

_____ at home but not at work   (3 pts.)

_____ at home *and* at work   (5 pts.)

I smoke:

_____ not at all   (0 pts.)

_____ less than one pack of cigarettes a day   (2 pts.)

_____ between one and two packs of cigarettes a day   (4 pts.)

_____ more than two packs of cigarettes a day   (8 pts.)

_____ cigars or a pipe   (2 pts.)

I drink beer, wine, or mixed drinks:

_____ very rarely   (0 pts.)

_____ on occasion, but then in pretty large amounts (1 pt.)
_____ once or twice a week (1 pt.)
_____ once a day (2 pts.)
_____ twice a day or more (4 pts.)

I am:

_____ not overweight (0 pts.)
_____ less than 20 pounds overweight (2 pts.)
_____ 20–50 pounds overweight (3 pts.)
_____ 51–100 pounds overweight (4 pts.)
_____ over 100 pounds overweight (6 pts.)

Stress Subscore: [   ]

Scoring

To the right of each of the questions you will find the point value for that item.

For each section separately—Parts 1, 2, 3, and 4—total the points for all of the items that you checked. Each of these totals is that area's subscore. Fill in the subscore at the end of each section.

In addition, place each of the four totals (subscores) in the appropriate areas marked below.

Add all four subscores together to get your overall Profactor-H Score.

	Your Subscores	Total Possible Points
Part 1: Family and Medical History	_____	(0–53)
Part 2: Nutritional Profile	_____	(0–20)
Part 3: Activity Level	_____	(0–4)
Part 4: Stress Level	_____	(0–23)
Overall Profactor-H Score	_____	total (0–100)

What Your Profactor-H Scores Mean

Your overall Profactor-H score indicates your general risk level for Profactor-H as it stands today. The higher your overall score, the greater your risk for Profactor-H *if you were to take no risk-reducing action.*

Your overall Profactor-H score will place you in one of four ranges: Doubtful Risk (probably Profactor-H free), or one of three Profactor-H Positive levels: Mild Risk, Moderate Risk, or High Risk. A High Risk score suggests that you are at greater immediate risk than someone with a Moderate Risk score, though depending on changes in lifestyle or stress, unexpected illness or trauma, anyone can quickly move to a higher level of risk. As you grow older, most overall scores will naturally rise, so if your score places you in the Mild or Moderate range, use this program and this time wisely.

YOUR PROFACTOR-H RISK LEVEL

Profactor-H Free:

Doubtful Risk   Overall Score: 0–11

Profactor-H Positive Scores:

Mild Risk   Overall Score: 12–18
Moderate Risk   Overall Score: 19–36
High Risk   Overall Score: 37 and over

Doubtful Risk

A score of 11 or less suggests that you are probably not at risk for many of the Profactor-H–related diseases or risk factors. Please remember: Being at Doubtful Risk for Profactor-H does *not* mean that you are somehow immune from these and other diseases that might stem from factors other than Profactor-H.

Although some people who score in the Doubtful Risk level have improved their general health condition and risk factor indicators while on this Program, the Profactor-H Program was not specifically designed for those who fall into the Doubtful Risk range. In any case, it would certainly be advisable to maintain a sensible and balanced lifestyle.

Mild Risk

An overall Profactor-H Score in the 12–18 range indicates that you have a small but significant family or lifestyle risk for Profactor-H. Your mild risk for Profactor-H may be the result of a mild genetic tendency for the imbalance—a scattered family history, for instance—where one parent or grandparent shows signs of Profactor-H but other family members do not. In this case, your Risk-Reducing Choices may well make the difference between a healthy life or one plagued and shortened by Profactor-H–related problems.

A Mild Risk for Profactor-H may also be the result of a moderate or strong family risk for Profactor-H in combination with your own healthy lifestyle choices. In this way, you may be counteracting your family's tendency toward Profactor-H by your own strength of commitment to your health and well-being. You literally may be holding Profactor-H–related problems at bay, at least for the time being.

In order to keep your risk in the Mild range, however, you will most likely need a program that does *not* require the sacrifice and deprivation you may have been enduring. You need a program that will allow you to make health-promoting choices while you enjoy your well-earned peace of mind.

If you are at Mild Risk for Profactor-H, this Program will offer you easy alternatives to help you to continue to keep your risk in the Mild range and your life filled with enjoyment and pleasure.

Moderate Risk

An overall Profactor-H Score in the 19 to 36 range indicates that you have a moderate but significant family and/or lifestyle risk for Profactor-H.

Depending on how young you are, a Moderate Risk level may reflect the fact that your relatively young age is compensating for stronger Profactor-H Positive genetic and lifestyle factors. In that case, you can almost surely expect your risk level to rise dramatically as the years go on. Starting your Profactor-H Program now may well help you avoid progressing to higher risk levels and many of the health problems that might have come with growing older.

A Moderate Risk for Profactor-H may also be the result of a strong family history of Profactor-H–related disorders, which you are keeping "in check" by your own healthy lifestyle choices. Compensating for a strong genetic predisposition toward Profactor-H can be difficult at best, especially when you do not know the key guidelines for correcting the imbalance. You will probably find the Program a delight, giving you the health benefits you have been working for without the deprivation you might have thought was inevitable.

A Moderate Risk level can also be the result of a mild genetic predisposition for Profactor-H in combination with nutritional, stress, and/or activity choices that increase your basic level. In some cases, risk-raising choices may have been made without your knowing it— by following the media's one-size-fits-all recommendations, for instance. In other instances, you may have found that the self-denial of most programs was simply not livable. You may have come to the conclusion that, though you wanted to follow a health-promoting program, most programs were not, in reality, an enjoyable or practical way to live.

If you are at Moderate Risk for Profactor-H, this Program can provide you with an easy way to lower your risk for Profactor-H while enjoying the simplicity and pleasures that make a healthy life worth living.

High Risk

An overall Profactor-H Score of 37 or over indicates that you have a strong and significant family and/or lifestyle risk for Profactor-H.

If you are in your twenties or thirties, a High Risk level indicates that, as you grow older, your genetic and/or lifestyle factors appear to make you a strong candidate for Profactor-H and its related disorders. Finding the Profactor-H Program may have been a very important discovery to you, and following the Program may well make the difference between a life plagued and shortened by Profactor-H–related problems and one filled with pleasure, enjoyment, health, and peace of mind.

If you are middle-aged or older, a High Risk level indicates that you have a strong genetic predisposition for Profactor-H or that you have begun to show some of the signs of Profactor-H, or both. The good news is that we know what causes it and, best of all, we know how to correct it. Your biology is not your destiny, and the damage you might have done by making unwise or misinformed choices can, in many cases, be reversed.

If you are at High Risk for Profactor-H, the guidelines in this book may well make the critical difference between a life shortened and dominated by limitations and illness and a life of freedom and vitality. We are glad you found this Program.

What Do My Subscores Tell Me?

Your subscores will show you how your genetics, nutrition, activity, and stress work in combination to affect your personal overall risk for Profactor-H. As you begin the Profactor-H Program, your subscores along with your overall score will help guide you in making the easiest and most beneficial choices that are right *for you.*

You can get a clear picture of the forces pushing you toward and away from Profactor-H by looking at your subscores. Go back to the "Scoring" section on page 50. To the right of each of the four scores you will find the number of points—the highest and the lowest scores—that are possible in each of the areas.

If any of your subscores fall in the lower end of a range, this class of risk factor may be counteracting the risks associated with higher subscores in other areas. A low subscore in the Family and Medical History range, for instance, may counteract a high Stress subscore. You can witness this "helping hand" risk phenomenon in the person with a low-scoring family history of Profactor-H who is able to handle high levels of stress without suffering physical repercussions.

On the other hand, if a particular subscore is very high, it may cancel out much of the positive effect of a lower subscore in a different area. If, for example, your Stress subscore is low, it may be virtually canceled out by a very high subscore in your Family and Medical History. In this case, you might find that you have no noticeable physical problems in low-stress situations but start to have difficulties when you find yourself under stress. For you, exposure to prolonged stress might take a great and deadly toll on your particular body, given your particular subscore profile.

The impact of two or more high subscores is "equal to more than the sum of their parts." Subscores do not stand alone but are compounded by the influence of other subscores. If you have several high subscores, the combined impact will probably increase your risk for Profactor-H more than if you had each one separately. Happily, though, as you reduce your subscore levels, the effect is also multiplied, so that reducing two or more subscores will have greater impact in reducing your overall risk level.

In the chapters that follow, the Profactor-H Program will take you, step by step, through a plan that will help you reduce your risk by making the changes *you* prefer to make. If you are a sports lover, Activity Options will help you lower your risk level by reducing your Profactor-H level through movement or exercise alternatives. If you hate to exercise but are willing to make nutritional changes, you will find you can make reductions in your Profactor-H risk level without involving yourself in long or complicated exercise regimens.

For a program to work, *for life,* it must come to live with you, listen to your needs, and be adaptable to your preferences and time limitations. Any program that says that all people must make the same choices simply does not work in the long run.

As you begin the Profactor-H Program, we will show you how you may dramatically lower your chances for Profactor-H and how to best reverse its impact if it has already begun. We will show how to use the Profactor-H Program to help correct what has been called the *pathologic link* to atherosclerosis, high blood pressure, excess weight, coronary artery disease, diabetes, heart disease, different forms of cancer, and many more. And we will help you reduce your Profactor-H risk while taking into account your individual preferences. Most important, you will greatly improve your peace of mind along with your chances for a long and healthy life—all without deprivation or sacrifice.

CHAPTER 5

The Thrifty Gene: Right Bodies, Wrong Time

Humans living today are Stone Age hunter-gatherers dis-
placed through time to a world that differs from that for
which our genetic constitution was selected.
                                        —S. B. Eaton, 1988

You may have inherited a "survivor's metabolism." If you are Profactor-H Positive, chances are your body has been very well designed
to keep you alive and healthy . . . in a caveman's world.

> Your survivor's metabolism has been designed
> to keep you alive and healthy . . .
> in a caveman's world.

In the times of feast or famine for which *your* body was constructed, the balance of insulin and glucagon worked in perfect harmony. Take a moment and imagine yourself back in a Stone Age
setting. As you hear that your clan has made a new kill or discovered a ripe field of berries, you feel increasingly hungry; that hunger
comes from insulin sending you strong and compelling messages to
"get out and get some food."

You follow your body's natural impulses and eat your fill, consuming large amounts so that you can survive until the next feast.
Feeling satisfied, you crawl back to your cave and fall asleep, con-

serving energy until it is needed. As you lie sleeping, the insulin in your body begins to move some of the food energy you have just eaten to your muscles and liver, where it fuels and repairs your body. The greater portion of the food, however, is moved to your fat cells, where it is stored for future use.

In the long hours or days that pass until more food is hunted or found, the insulin levels in your blood decrease dramatically. Now your body begins to release the opposing hormone, glucagon. Glucagon goes to work releasing the energy that you stored in your fat cells so that it can be used when no other food supply is available.

The harmony of your body matches the balance of your environment. In times of feast, insulin saves; in times of famine, glucagon spends—supplying you with needed energy. Each hormone does its part in perfect complement—their sole purpose is to keep you alive and well.

**In caveman times, the survivors
were those who inherited the *Thrifty Gene*.**

In caveman times, the survivors of this feast-and-famine existence were those who inherited what scientists now refer to as the *Thrifty Gene*. The Thrifty Gene gave its owners a bonus of extra insulin so that their drive to eat was greater than that experienced by others. In many cases, those possessing the Thrifty Gene had more intense hungers that lasted longer, were harder to satisfy, and were more easily triggered than those who did not possess this gene. When food was available, those having the Thrifty Gene were able to eat more and store more of what they ate. In times of famine, the food they stored, in the form of fat, was changed into life-giving food energy. When supplies were short, or nonexistent, the Thrifty Gene was a giver of life.

**When supplies were short, or nonexistent,
the Thrifty Gene was a giver of life.**

Today, the Thrifty Gene has outlived its usefulness, and instead of giving life, it may take it from us. In our world of constant plenty, the Thrifty Gene now leads to Profactor-H and the whole host of diseases and risk factors associated with it.

In their notable report in *The New England Journal of Medicine* in 1988, Dr. S. B. Eaton and his colleagues reported that the genetics that helped us to survive in a Stone Age environment act in today's environment as "a potent promoter of chronic illness," including atherosclerosis, high blood pressure, excess weight, adult-onset diabetes, and some cancers, among others. These "diseases of civilization," say Dr. Eaton and his colleagues, may cause 75 percent of all deaths in this country and other Western nations.

Within the few years that followed Dr. Eaton's report, many other noted scientists published articles confirming and supporting his work and connecting the Thrifty Gene to Profactor-H. In 1992, Dr. L. C. Groop and his colleague Dr. J. G. Eriksson reported in the *Annals of Medicine* that, in keeping with the Thrifty Gene theory, the Profactor-H gene had been useful in Stone Age times in protecting individuals during long periods of starvation by storing energy as fat rather than burning it up in muscles. They added an essential point similar to Dr. Eaton's— that today's lifestyle has now turned this once-protective gene into a harmful one. At particular risk, these scientists concluded, are those whose genetics make them unable to handle today's eating lifestyle.

In a powerful article in 1992, Dr. M. Wendorf added to the growing list of reports with his fine description of the impact of the Thrifty Gene in today's environment. It may have once allowed populations to survive feast and famine conditions of several generations, said Dr. Wendorf, but he added that with today's eating and activity lifestyle, the Thrifty Gene becomes a *dis*advantage, leading to Profactor-H and to overweight and adult-onset diabetes.

If you are Profactor-H Positive, your survivor's metabolism probably comes from inheriting the Thrifty Gene. For you, a typical day of eating, working, communicating, and sleeping may not bring about the same hormonal balance that other people experience and take for granted.

**If you are Profactor-H Positive,
you have probably inherited the Thrifty Gene.**

When people *without* Thrifty Genes, let's call them *spenders,* move through their daily activities, their insulin and glucagon levels rise and fall in an even flow. One hormone goes up as the other goes down. Spenders eat and store energy; when they refrain from eating for a while, their fat cells release the energy they had been storing. Spenders experience a rather steady state of blood sugar, alertness, strength, and mood.

After eating, spenders feel satisfied and are rarely concerned about food until the next appropriate time to eat. If they are offered food, they will often refuse it, or if they do snack, they eat small amounts—without exerting any willpower. They can indulge in a snack or "goodie" without feeling that they must finish what they have started to eat and go back for seconds—or thirds. Spenders may seem like paramounts of will and virtue to those of us who sometimes feel overpowered by our cravings, hunger, mood swings, or lack of energy, but it is really only a matter of genetics—and one that we, happily, know how to correct.

For the moment, however, let's compare the spender's day with a typical day in the life of those of us who have, indeed, inherited a Thrifty Gene. If you have a Thrifty Gene, chances are, when you eat a full breakfast, you begin your day by releasing an excess amount of insulin. Too much insulin leads to an imbalance in your blood sugar, which, in turn, can make you feel sluggish or hungry by mid-morning. After a full breakfast, you probably find that you are hungrier by 11:00 A.M. than you would be if you had skipped breakfast altogether or had only had a cup of coffee.

After eating a full breakfast,
you probably find that you are hungrier by 11:00 A.M.
than you would be if you had skipped breakfast altogether
or had only had a cup of coffee.

A moderate lunch may perk you up, but by mid-afternoon you may be craving a snack or a nap or both. Inside your body, insulin is wreaking havoc. Blood sugars are out of balance, leaving you moody, hungry, and/or tired. By the middle of the afternoon, you probably hit a low and feel unmotivated and sluggish.

A mid-afternoon nap might make you feel better—if you could get one—but most of us grab a snack instead, and while most snack foods help restore your blood sugar balance for a short time, they quickly put you back on a hormonal roller coaster. Chances are, you push yourself through the day, wishing you could concentrate better, feel better, or be in a better mood—all signs of Profactor-H and the changes in blood sugar it can bring.

If something happens to excite you and adrenaline is released, you may find you feel better, as adrenaline temporarily compensates for your insulin overload. But when the excitement of the moment passes, your newfound motivation and clarity will probably disappear with it.

As you eat dinner, you may feel a sense of relief and relaxation, but chances are it is short-lived. As you complete the meal, you may begin to feel tired, almost drugged. The well-intentioned plans you had for the evening fall away and you find that all you want to do is doze in front of the television or listen to the stereo. If you try to work, you have trouble keeping focused; you may fall asleep as you try to read. The thought of leaving the house, especially during the week, holds little reward if it means trying to overcome the sluggish feeling that overwhelms you, especially when you know you face the same routine the next day.

> As you complete your dinner, you begin to feel tired, almost drugged, and the well-intentioned plans you had for the evening fall away.

As your evening progresses, you may rouse yourself and wander to the kitchen for a snack, or force yourself to work a bit, but, chances are, you really would prefer to settle down and do nothing. Your evening slips away as Profactor-H, without your knowledge or consent, takes control of your body and your life.

Though, for some, these Profactor-H patterns may lift a bit during the summer months, they often grow worse again as winter approaches. This pattern is sometimes referred to as the "hibernation response" by scientists who recognize that during the fall and winter our experiences simply reflect nature's way of conserving energy. As it does in the hibernating animal, as the shorter months and cold winter approach, in anticipation of a smaller food supply, your body signals you to take in more food and then channels the food energy to fat cells. At the same time, it signals you to sleep more and more, so that you will use less energy.

You may have been told that much of your tiredness or hunger or lack of motivation is "psychological," but the overwhelming evidence bears witness to the fact that for most of us there is a *physical reason* for the rise and fall in energy, hunger, and mood. In today's world, your body, so beautifully built for a life of feast or famine, faces unexpected foods and stress—for which it was never built.

You may have been told that much of your tiredness or hunger or lack of motivation is "psychological," but for most of us there is a *physical reason*.

A look inside your body may easily explain the hunger, moods, and feelings that you often experience. Your typical breakfast—made up of carbohydrate-rich foods such as cereal, bread, bagels, fruit, juice, milk, and sugar (or their low-calorie or low-fat alternatives)—triggers your Profactor-H levels to rise.

You body was designed for meals made up of low-fat wild animal protein and, on occasion, roots and wild berries. You were never meant to consume dairy foods like milk or cheese past the first two years of life, and in prehistoric times, fruit was not available at all, or for only a few weeks out of each year. The rise in Profactor-H levels that your breakfast triggers in the morning can sweep the blood sugar from your bloodstream within a few hours, which is why, by mid-morning, you may be left feeling weak or hungry or both.

Your lunch can again trigger Profactor-H levels, leaving you tired and craving a snack or nap by mid-afternoon. The kinds of foods you eat at lunch play a key role in raising your Profactor-H levels, but more important, your body is simply not built to have *frequent* meals of these foods.

Remember, your body was constructed to consume and store great amounts of food when the food was available and to go for long periods of time, in between feasts, when there was nothing to eat. Your body was not built with twenty-four-hour groceries, refrigerators, and prepackaged snack foods in mind. In prehistoric times, you would have eaten only what you could kill or find. (By the way, this does not mean that when you are on our Program we are going to ask you to eat wild animals and unmilled grains or that you may not eat for prolonged periods. We only want you to understand that you have a wonderful body—that happens to be living in the wrong time.)

The stress and inactivity that are part and parcel of most of our lives raise your Profactor-H levels even more, and with each rise the foods you eat are turned into fat. The fat is meant to go into storage in your fat cells, though if Profactor-H levels get too high, doorways to the cells may close down and much of the fat may remain in your bloodstream—and that is where a great many health problems can begin.

Your body was designed to consume
low-fat wild animal protein and roots and wild berries.
It was not built with twenty-four-hour groceries, refrigerators,
and prepackaged snack foods in mind.

As your day continues, a stressful commute home, time demands, family pressures, and a typical modern-day dinner bring on another Profactor-H boost. This latest Profactor-H "insult" to your body triggers your after-dinner tiredness and late evening snacking. After a good night's sleep, you are ready to begin the hormone roller coaster ride all over again.

Each day, steady high Profactor-H levels mean that you are in a constant state of saving, turning much of your food energy into fat that is dumped into your bloodstream. The high levels of Profactor-H usher the fat from your bloodstream into waiting cells through doorways called *receptor sites.* If you are lucky, you will move most of the fat to cells that can burn it. In the Profactor-H Positive person, far more of the fat tends to go to the fat cells than to the muscles or organs.

Though you may not be happy with the added pounds that come when the fat is siphoned into your fat cells, the extra weight that this tends to make you gain is much preferred to the alternative—that is, becoming insulin resistant. If you become insulin resistant, many of the doorways to your cells close down in order to reduce Profactor-H overload to cells. When the cells' doors close, the fat is no longer able to move into the cells and high levels of both Profactor-H and fats are trapped in your bloodstream. This deadly combination can do great damage to your blood vessels, heart, liver, and kidneys, and lead to many complications, including stroke, heart attack, diabetes, and peripheral vascular disease.

If you are lucky, you will store energy in your fat cells.
Though you may not be happy with the added pounds,
the extra weight may be much preferred to the alternative.

Six hundred thousand years ago or so the Thrifty Gene and the Profactor-H level it helped to produce would have insured your survival when food supplies were scarce. Your body was well suited to a hunting-and-gathering lifestyle. In this world of continuous plenty, however, your Thrifty Gene can produce a Profactor-H Positive cycle that can lead to ill health and, in some cases, a far higher risk for early death. As you grow older or find yourself under increasing stress, *if no specifically designed Profactor-H risk-reducing actions are taken,* the chances for an unhappy outcome can grow even greater.

The cravings, mood swings, periods of low motivation,
tiredness, or weight gain that often come with
inheriting the Thrifty Gene *are not your fault*—
they are simply signs of Profactor-H.

SIGNS OF THE THRIFTY GENE

A Focus on Eating or on Your Weight

Do you find that the more food you eat, the more you want?

Do you gain weight easily, or regain it once it's lost?

As you grow older, do you find that you gain weight on the same amount of food that used to keep your weight steady?

Do you find that you get hungry about two hours after eating?

Does thinking about food or dieting take up more of your time than you would like?

Mood Swings

Do you find that you get angry easily or that your feelings are easily hurt?

Do you sometimes feel suddenly irritated or sad or weepy over little things?

Do you sometimes feel anxious or hopeless without knowing why?

Do your feelings sometimes change from moment to moment?

Do you often hide what you are really feeling?

Blood Sugar Blues

About two hours after you eat:
   Do you feel light-headed?
   Do you feel shaky?
   Do you get headaches?
   Do you feel weak?
   Do you feel unfocused or unmotivated?

And does a snack make most of the blood sugar symptoms go away—for the moment?

If you recognize several of these symptoms, you may be showing signs of Profactor-H caused by the Thrifty Gene. Each of these signs can have a *physical cause*, which we will help you learn to correct—for life.

The cravings, mood swings, periods of low motivation, tiredness, or weight gain that often come with inheriting the Thrifty Gene *are not your fault*. They, along with high blood pressure, high fat levels in your blood, and changes in blood sugar, are some of the signs of Profactor-H. And though Profactor-H may be "in your genes," it does not have to be your destiny. The Profactor-H Program can increase your chances of living well and living long in *today's world*.

CHAPTER 6

▽

Propelled Through Time

Doctors would do well to name less and treat more.
—Benjamin Franklin

Your body has been propelled through time to a world that it barely recognizes. Coping with the stress, food, and conflict of a modern lifestyle with a prehistoric body requires a period of adjustment. We might catch up if we had a few hundred thousand years of evolution at our command. But we don't.

As scientists, we have spent more than nine years studying Profactor-H from the perspective that Profactor-H is your body's ingenious and adaptive way of coping with a world in which it was never intended to exist. Our research has been successful beyond our imagination and has given us ways to help your body handle this challenging new environment.

Profactor-H: The Cause

Where does Profactor-H come from? How do you get it? How bad is it? How do you get rid of it? The answers are becoming clear and straightforward. First, in order to maintain high levels of insulin in the blood, Profactor-H depends on help from its two cofactors.

A cofactor is a contributing factor, a second imbalance, that makes the larger profactor possible. Without its cofactors, a profactor could not exist. Imagine a great river overrunning its banks, flooding the towns and cities for miles around. That great flood—like a profactor—is dependent on secondary or contributing events. In this case, the flood's cofactor could be either a great amount of rainfall in a short period of time or some blockage preventing the river from flowing freely into the ocean.

Without one or both of these contributing factors, the main event would never happen. The flooding, the damage, even the loss of lives, does not come from the rain or the prevention of the river's free flow to the ocean *directly*, but one or both of these contributing events is essential; without them, the damage would never occur and the flood—or profactor—would never exist.

Cofactor: a contributing factor.
An imbalance in the body that can contribute, through a profactor, to many other diseases and risk factors.

Cofactor-p: The Producer

Like the flood, Profactor-H is dependent on one or both of two cofactors. We call the first cofactor *Cofactor-p* because it is the *production* or release of too much insulin that can lead to Profactor-H.

Depending on their areas of specialty, scientists and physicians have many different names for Cofactor-p. It has been referred to as insulin hypersecretion, overrelease or overproduction of insulin, hyperinsulinemia, and other terms. In some cases, the same terms have been used to refer to Cofactor-p and Profactor-H itself. No wonder there is such confusion. No standard scientific term has existed until now.

In our research reports, we use the term *Cofactor-p* so that we can begin to establish a common term for the overproduction or overrelease of insulin that leads to Profactor-H.

Cofactor-p: the overproduction or overrelease of insulin, which can lead to Profactor-H (continuous excess levels of insulin).

Cofactor-r: The Resistor

In addition to its Cofactor-p, Profactor-H depends on a second cofactor, which we call *Cofactor-r*. Cofactor-r occurs when cells become *resistant* to insulin. When cells become insulin resistant, less insulin is able to move out of the bloodstream into the cells and insulin remains trapped in the bloodstream.

Cofactor-r: the body's ability to resist insulin and block insulin from leaving the bloodstream.

Profactor-H's first cofactor, Cofactor-p, occurs when too much insulin is produced or released—pouring excess amounts of insulin into the bloodstream. Its second cofactor, Cofactor-r, resists or blocks insulin from leaving the bloodstream.

Unfortunately, just as in the case of Cofactor-p, scientists and physicians may use a wide variety of terms to refer to Cofactor-r. In scientific and medical research reports alike, Cofactor-r and its impact have been referred to as insulin resistance, carbohydrate intolerance, glucose intolerance, impaired glucose tolerance, carbohydrate insensitivity, insulin insensitivity, down-regulation, and other terms. These many terms for Cofactor-r and its effects can be confusing, to say the least.

As knowledge of the importance of Profactor-H continues to grow, scientists and physicians no longer have the privilege of describing its cofactors in nonspecific and ill-defined ways. In order to best pool their knowledge, researchers must now use clear and distinct terms to refer to a continuous excess of insulin (Profactor-H), caused by:

The overrelease or overproduction of insulin (Cofactor-p), and/or
The body's ability to resist or block insulin from leaving the bloodstream (Cofactor-r)*

* In order to begin to establish singular and specific terms, throughout this book Cofactor-p and Cofactor-r will be used in place of any or all of those conditions that have previously been used to describe them. In addition, within direct quotes these terms as well as common lay terms will be used in place of medical or Latin terminology.

The Cofactor Epidemic

Either alone or in combination, Cofactor-p and Cofactor-r, and the levels of insulin in the blood that they lead to, have caused scientists to describe Profactor-H as fertile ground for the development of life-threatening diseases.

After reviewing the research of over three hundred scientists, in 1991 Dr. Ralph DeFronzo and Dr. Eleuterio Ferrannini concluded that Cofactor-r is a common disorder and that it occurs with high frequency in the general population. It can be viewed as "a large iceberg submerged just below the surface of the water." "The physician recognizes only the tips of the iceberg" and may see only the conditions we call diabetes, excess weight, high blood pressure, undesirable blood fat levels, and atherosclerosis, they added. Though these individual disorders are often diagnosed by the physician, say Drs. DeFronzo and Ferrannini, the underlying problem of Profactor-H may be completely missed.

Years of hard work have led other scientists to the same conclusion. In their research, published in *The New England Journal of Medicine,* Dr. A. Garg and his colleagues concluded that Profactor-H has been found "to be an independent risk factor for coronary heart disease." Dr. H. R. Black of Yale University of Medicine described Profactor-H, and in particular its Cofactor-r connection, as the link between high blood pressure, excess weight, and adult-onset diabetes, and went on to conclude that Profactor-H has been shown to be a "potent" risk factor for heart disease.

In a landmark conference in Denmark in 1990, Dr. Henning Beck-Nielsen and his research team concluded that Cofactor-r may induce not only high levels of blood sugar but also high blood pressure, excess weight, and undesirable levels of fat in the blood, "all variables that add to the risk of coronary heart disease." Articles too numerous to list here support and agree with Dr. Beck-Nielsen's research, including a 1991 article published in the *American Journal of Medicine* in which Dr. G. M. Reaven concluded that Profactor-H and its contributing cofactor, Cofactor-r, may play a central role in the cause and progress of adult-onset diabetes, high blood pressure, undesirable levels of fat in the blood, and coronary heart disease.

Profactor-H continues to be identified as the key connection in a greater number of diseases than ever thought possible. In a corner-stone article published in the journal *Clinical Nutrition,* Dr. Faiz Kakar and his research team connected a higher rate in breast cancer growth to Cofactor-p, which can be stimulated in response to dietary sugar. This new area of research relating Profactor-H and its cofactors to cancer growth is currently being explored, and many recent reports by other scientists in the field confirm these observations.

Even in the area of excess weight, though not necessarily life-threatening in itself, Cofactor-p has been named as a "common feature."

The Illusion of Safety

If you think that being healthy means you are not at risk for Profactor-H, think again. The healthy are not immune to the effects of Profactor-H. After studying normal-weight men and women with normal blood pressure, Dr. Ivana Zavaroni and her colleagues concluded that healthy persons with Profactor-H had an increase in risk factors for coronary artery disease compared to those without Profactor-H. So if you have Profactor-H but show no ill effects *yet,* don't be fooled. Having normal blood pressure and normal blood fat levels are by no means a guarantee that you are not at greater risk in the near, or not-so-near, future.

It is clear that Profactor-H and its cofactors hold the key to understanding, and to helping to put a stop to, the diseases that plague our bodies and trouble our minds. If you or your physician are interested in learning more about medical research on Profactor-H, the reference list at the back of the book shows where you can get copies of these research reports.

THE THREE CLASSES OF PROFACTOR-H

Depending on your family's genetics, your diet and medications, your lifestyle, your age, and the stress you experience, your Profactor-H levels can come from your overproduction of insulin (Class 1), from your body's natural resistance to removing insulin from your bloodstream (Class 2), or from overproduction and resistance *in combination* (Class 3). Whether you are an overproducer, a resistor, or an overproducer-resistor, the Profactor-H Program will help you reduce *your* personal risk for Profactor-H.

Class 1—The Overproducer

Your Body:

Cofactor-p rules your body, producing or releasing more insulin than your body can use. When food is available, Profactor-H sends strong messages telling you to eat.

About two hours after eating, your blood sugar levels may drop sharply, as the sugar is swept from your bloodstream into the fat cells. Additional snacks of fruit, breads and other starches, sweets, or other carbohydrates may cause your blood sugars to rise and fall in a roller coaster fashion throughout the day.

Class 1 Profactor-H is often accompanied by an increased tendency to gain weight. Your body is open to damage from repeated Profactor-H insults; blood sugar swings can prove to be a problem as well.

In time, Class 1 often leads to Class 3, as the muscles, liver and other organs, and fat cells begin to resist the flood of insulin.

Your Feelings:

Strong but passing cravings for carbohydrate-rich foods, especially breads and other starches, fruit or juice, snack foods, or sweets or artificially sweetened foods.

Intermittent periods of tiredness, shakiness, headaches, irritability, and/or weakness.* Periods of lowered motivation, lack of interest or feeling. Mood swings and feelings of heightened emotion.

*Headaches, tiredness, weakness, shakiness, mood swings, and depression may have multiple causes. Check with your physician to confirm that Profactor-H, chronic hyperinsulinemia, is the base cause of your symptoms.

Your Thoughts:

Self-blame for weight gain. Self-recrimination for what is wrongly perceived of as a lack of willpower or periodic laziness or loss of motivation. Concerns regarding a physical cause of hunger or blood sugar swings may be fleeting and are often not heeded.

Class 2—The Resistor

Your Body:

Cofactor-r rules your body, blocking insulin from leaving your bloodstream. Insulin levels continue to rise and may continue to signal your body to eat.

Your muscles, liver, and other organs may not get appropriate energy supplies. Your blood sugar levels may rise beyond normal limits.*

In time, Class 2 Profactor-H often leads to Class 3, as your body tries to compensate for lack of energy supplies to your muscles, organs, and fat cells by producing and releasing additional insulin.

Your Feelings:

Recurring and/or intense cravings to eat. After eating, the resistor may experience feelings of great tiredness, illness, panic, or depression.*

After finishing large meals, resistors often report feeling exhausted or that "something just doesn't feel right."

You may notice a low interest in exercise or activities.

Your Thoughts:

Because Class 2 Profactor-H may bring with it a vague feeling of some ill health, resistors may be uncomfortable with the state of their health although reluctant to talk about it. They may know that they are not feeling right but be unable to describe exactly what is wrong.

Resistors may notice that they are eating more than they intended, perhaps *without* great satisfaction, but may blame their eating on what they perceive as their "lack of willpower."

In some cases, Class 2 Profactor-H is misdiagnosed as depression or attributed to family, relationship, or work-related problems.

*High blood sugar levels, feelings of tiredness, illness, panic, or depression may have multiple causes. Check with your physician to confirm that Profactor-H (chronic hyperinsulinemia) is the base cause of your symptoms.

Class 3—The Overproducer-Resistor

Your Body:

Both Cofactor-r and Cofactor-p rule your body together, producing more insulin than your body can use and, at the same time, blocking it from leaving your bloodstream.

Your body receives strong and recurring messages to eat but cannot regulate the storage and use of your food energy. High levels of sugar may remain in your bloodstream, and muscles, liver, and fat cells do not get appropriate food supplies.

The stage is set for damage to your body from excess insulin in your blood in combination with excess levels of sugar.

Your Feelings:

At times, you may experience strong cravings for carbohydrate-rich foods, especially breads and other starches, fruit or juice, snack foods, or sweets. A "heightened sense of sweetness" may make food taste intensely satisfying although, after eating, the overproducer-resistor may be left feeling tired or hungry or both.

Many Class 3 Profactor-H Positives report that they feel vaguely out of sorts, though they may not be able to explain their feelings.

You may experience episodes of tiredness, hopelessness, or a lack of energy. You may experience a decrease in the desire for activities of all kinds, including sexual intimacy.* You may experience moments of panic on entering or leaving sleep.

Your Thoughts:

In your self-blame and self-anger, you may focus your worries about health on what you falsely perceive of as your lack of willpower or lack of motivation. If you are overweight, you may blame your overeating or overweight for your lack of energy and disinterest in activities and/or sex.

Though you think you should make plans for change, you find it very difficult to get started or your plans are very short-lived. You talk or think about your concern for your health from time to time, but the concerns remain vague and unfocused. At times, you may rouse your determination for change, but you find it difficult or impossible to make any real lifestyle changes.

*Episodes of tiredness, hopelessness, lack of energy, panic, decrease in desire for activity or sexual intimacy, and concerns about health may have multiple causes. Check with your physician to confirm that Profactor-H (chronic hyperinsulinemia) is the base cause of your symptoms.

CHAPTER 7

Fats and Fiber: Fears, Facts, and Fallacies

We fear the most that which we little understand.
—Confucius

In the realm of nutrition, there are few areas more filled with myths and superstition than that of dietary fats. Like some great, unfounded rumor, our fear of fats has become the overriding concern of most Americans, from the very young to the very old. We live in terror of some ill-meaning fat gram waiting to pounce on us and clog our arteries. And in our dread, we may be eating and doing the very things that may jeopardize our health even more.

> In trying to stay or get healthy,
> you may be eating and doing the very things that may
> jeopardize your health even more.

The Good, the Bad, and the Terrifying

To most Americans, the world of dietary do's and don'ts seems very simple and very clear, but it may, in fact, prove to be very wrong. High fats in the blood have been linked to heart attacks, strokes, atherosclerosis, and some forms of cancer—and it is therefore *assumed* that eating fat is bad, eating carbohydrates is good, and eating protein . . . well, eating protein is somewhere in the middle (as long as it does not contain fat, in which case protein becomes bad).

This kind of thinking, while it may be comforting and may give the illusion of control, may do little to help you live longer. At best, you may be sacrificing the food you love for nothing; on the other hand, you may inadvertently be eating the worst things possible for *your particular* health risk profile.

Compare Adriene C. and John W., for instance. Adriene has a strong family history for breast cancer. She is in her early forties and very few members of her family have had heart disease, though several grandparents, aunts, and uncles have acquired adult-onset diabetes in their forties and fifties. Adriene is about thirty pounds overweight and loves bread and sweets with a passion. She has a tendency to snack between meals and loves a treat during the evening or before she goes to bed. Her cholesterol levels are slightly elevated, but her blood pressure and triglyceride levels are far higher than they should be. Adriene is quite active but does not follow a regular exercise program. She tends to get upset at small things, though she can well manage the more serious problems in her life.

John W., on the other hand, is in his thirties. His father and grandfather died in their early fifties from their first heart attacks. John is slender and has no family history of diabetes, though several other male members of John's family, uncles and a brother, have had heart attacks. John does not smoke or drink. He exercises regularly. John dislikes sweets and has no passion for pasta, bread, or snack foods, but he has a "weakness" for buttery and greasy foods such as bacon, olives, and cheese. He drinks a quart of milk at a sitting. John rarely snacks between meals, but he eats large meals. A dinner without meat leaves him feeling unsatisfied. John's cholesterol and triglyceride levels clearly put him in the High Risk category.

John and Adriene have different family histories, different medical profiles, and different health concerns. To give them the same dietary recommendations without taking their differences into consideration makes virtually no sense.

John appears to be Profactor-H free; the high fat levels in his blood appear to come mainly from his body's inability to process the fats that he is eating. Adriene, on the other hand, shows many signs of being Profactor-H Positive; her body appears to produce too much insulin and is likely to turn the extra food she eats, *any food,* into fat.

Low-fat recommendations may make a great deal of sense for John, but Adriene's story is not that simple. Telling the Profactor-H Positive person to cut down on dietary fats may push them into eating more carbohydrates more frequently, including foods like pasta, bread, rice, potatoes, and fruit. While these foods are nutritious and low-fat in themselves, if you are Profactor-H Positive, your body may turn them into the very fats you are seeking to avoid.

Finding the right nutritional balance for you is, in some ways, like fitting yourself with a new outfit of clothes. It does not matter how attractive the suit or dress is, what matters is how well it fits you. In the same way, it does not matter how low in fat the foods you eat are, what matters is *how your body responds* to these foods, and how much fat it produces when you eat them.

What matters is *how your body responds* to certain foods, and how much fat it produces when you eat those foods.

The most common type of blood fat problem in the United States today is caused by carbohydrates in the diet, not fats. That's right, carbohydrates. Though physicians may refer to it as *Type IV hyperlipemia,* your laboratory reports will probably give exact counts of your various blood fat levels—describing the symptoms rather than identifying the cause.

Few medical professionals are aware that textbooks refer to this most common blood fat problem as "carbohydrate-induced"—meaning that the high blood fat levels are the result of eating carbohydrates, not high-fat foods.

If you are Profactor-H Positive, eating carbohydrates frequently may be as harmful to you as—or worse than, in terms of your blood fat levels—eating high-fat food may be.

Putting It All Together

One of the great myths that is currently being spread is that "food does not make fat, fat makes fat." This statement is simply untrue. The human body does not work that way. The fat you eat is not the same as the fat inside of you.

The fat you eat is called *exogenous* fat, meaning *fat that comes from the outside*. The fat inside your body is called *endogenous*, meaning *fat that comes from inside*. The fat you eat makes up only about one quarter of the fat inside your body. The rest of the fat in your body, the other three quarters, is fat that your body makes up on its own—from *all* the extra food you eat: the fat, the protein, *and* the carbohydrates.

Your body is wonderfully adaptive. It can take things apart and put them together at will. If you have too much of this or too little of that, your body will simply improvise, adding a bit of this or removing some of that, in order to make what it needs to survive. If you think you can fool your body into producing less fat, think about this. If you eat too little fat, you body will simply make extra fat from the other food you eat and the fat that your body makes may be far worse for your health than the fat you eat. There are, however, simple ways to slow down your body's fat-making machinery, and the secret lies in understanding how your particular body responds to food.

> Your body is a fat-making machine.
> If you eat too little fat, your body will simply
> make extra fat from the other food you eat.
> The fat that your body makes may be
> far worse for your health than the fat you eat.

First, let's get a few terms straight. Your total cholesterol level is made up of different components. Basically, your LDL (low-density lipoproteins) is often referred to as the "bad" cholesterol, because, for Americans, it has been linked to a higher incidence of coronary heart disease. HDL (high-density lipoproteins) is often called the "good" cholesterol, because its main function is to move excess LDL cholesterol out of your bloodstream and into your bile.

When the total cholesterol level in your blood is low, you do not need as much HDL to get rid of the LDL, but as your total cholesterol levels rise, you need more HDL to keep the LDL from doing harm. Your body stores fat in the form of *triglycerides*. For some people, high triglyceride levels have also been linked to an increased risk for coronary heart disease.

**If you are Profactor-H Positive,
eating a low-fat diet
may not bring down your blood fat levels.**

If you are Profactor-H Positive, eating a low-fat diet may not bring down (or keep down) your triglyceride or LDL-cholesterol levels. Your Profactor-H levels work hard at helping your body turn *all* of the extra food you eat—protein, carbohydrate, and fats—into fat so that it can be stored in your fat cells for future use. When your Profactor-H levels remain high, however, your body resists taking the blood fat into the fat cells and, with no place to go, much of the fat gets "caught" in the bloodstream. The result: high blood fat levels, which seem to forecast disaster.

Eating carbohydrates frequently, alone or in combination with high-fat foods, may be *your* particular problem, and if so, following a low-fat diet alone may do you little or no real good. In 1993, *Tufts University Diet and Nutrition Letter* noted that some individuals' "genetic makeup" does not allow them to respond to low-fat diets. If your genetic makeup includes being Profactor-H Positive, a low-fat diet alone is almost certainly not the answer to your blood fat problems.

Scientists are finding that for many of us, in particular those of us who are Profactor-H positive, low-fat diets have been disappointing in their ability to reduce our blood fat levels. Researchers at the Heart Disease Prevention Clinic in Minneapolis found that, contrary to expectations of great decreases in blood fat levels, their subjects on low-fat diets reduced their cholesterol levels by only 5 percent.

According to those figures, if you have a blood cholesterol of 260, you could expect that sticking to a low-fat diet would be rewarded by a reduction in your blood cholesterol of 13 points—from 260 to only 247.

If a change that small seems discouraging, the news gets worse. These same scientists report that the 5 percent decrease in cholesterol takes its form in a reduction of both "good" as well as "bad" blood fats, so that there is some real question as to whether you have reaped any benefit whatsoever from your low-fat diet. According to studies such as these, low-fat diets cannot be counted on to reduce blood fat levels or necessarily prolong life.

Profactor-H, which now appears to be responsible for high blood fat levels in many of us, has too long gone unnoticed while the high cholesterol and triglyceride levels that may be *the result* of Profactor-H have been wrongly identified as the problem.

Scientists are now referring to Profactor-H as the invisible, or pathogenic, link. Many scientists are finding that Profactor-H provides the missing connection that explains why only about one person in five who goes on a low-fat diet is able to effectively reduce blood fat levels. If you try to remove the symptom, not the cause, you cannot expect success. Now, over and over, Profactor-H is being reported as the causal factor in undesirable blood fat levels.

In 1990, Dr. Robert W. Stout, of the Queen's University of Belfast, Northern Ireland, reported that Profactor-H stimulates the production of fat in blood vessels. He went on to point out that Profactor-H is associated with raised levels of the "bad" blood fats (triglycerides) and decreased levels of the "good" cholesterol HDL. He concluded that the "multiple effects" of Profactor-H link it to a direct role in the development of atherosclerosis.

Where high blood fat levels are found, Profactor-H can usually be found as well, silently using your body's energy to build and store fats that, in turn, may clog the very arteries that feed your heart and other organs. In 1990, Dr. Henning Beck-Nielsen informed colleagues that Profactor-H may induce not only undesirable blood fat levels but diabetes and high blood pressure as well; "all variables," he added, "that add to the risk of coronary heart disease."

Scientists from around the world confirm: Profactor-H stimulates the body to produce and store fat and promotes the accumulation of fat in blood vessels, leading to a likelihood of heart disease.

One can only wonder why dietary fats are being too quickly—and, in many cases, falsely—identified as the blood fat villains. Certainly, business may play a role. It is far easier and more profitable to market so-called low-fat foods to a fear-filled public than to help individuals to understand what they need to do to help themselves. A fine rule of thumb that seems to apply says that when good common sense and irrefutable facts are *not* being used, look to economic gain as the underlying driving force.

For those of us who have reviewed the scientific reports one after another, for those of us who understand the importance of quickly getting this information to the general public, there is no time to waste. What matters to us now is helping those who need it most to break their Profactor-H–blood fat level link—before it's too late.

The Big Switch

When you change from a regular diet to a low-fat diet, you generally replace the fat with something else—usually carbohydrates. When you make dietary changes, then, it is important to look at not only what you are reducing (in this case, fat) but what you are increasing (carbohydrates) as well. Most of all, you should be aware of the ways in which your particular body responds to these substitutions.

> When you make dietary changes, it is important to look at not only what you are reducing but what you are increasing as well.

For many people, replacing a diet filled with high-fat foods with a supposedly more healthful low-fat, high-carbohydrate diet may fail to give them the positive effects they have been told to expect.

One of the major studies behind the current rage against fat was the Coronary Primary Prevention Trial. This study, and others similar to it, *did not* prove that lowering levels of dietary fat and cholesterol greatly decreased our chances of premature death. That's right—*they did not!* The study involved several thousand middle-aged men who had high blood cholesterol levels but did not have heart disease. Originally, one group was supposed to be given a cholesterol-lowering diet and the other a regular diet. Then both groups were to be checked after ten years to see the difference the diets had on how long they lived as well as the incidence of heart disease.

For some unexplained reason, the researchers did not follow their plan. Instead, they gave a cholesterol-lowering drug to the group on the cholesterol-lowering diet. Now the cholesterol-lowering group had two advantages over the other group: drugs and diet in combination. And, with both treatments in combination, they did succeed in lowering the group's blood cholesterol level. However, even that appears to have made a very small difference in life expectancy.

The men on the drugs and low-cholesterol diets had almost a 7 percent rate of heart attack; the men without drugs and on regular diets had an 8.6 percent rate—a difference of only 1.7 percent over a period of seven to ten years! What is more revealing is that when you looked at the rates of death from all causes combined, the two groups were nearly the same.

Though this study combined drug and diet together, which should make a strong and undeniable change, it still appears to show far less than impressive results. Yet based on this kind of evidence, low-fat and low-cholesterol diets are being widely recommended. To make matters worse, this study and others concentrate on limited age levels, one gender (usually male), and those with a specific level of blood cholesterol (in this case, the highest 5 percent). Even though the less than impressive findings relate to a very small segment of the population, the results, or rather the beliefs about the results, are generalized to everyone.

The truth is that researchers have *not* proved the long-term health benefit of low-fat diets. On the other hand, scientific studies comparing low-fat, high-carbohydrate diets with diets high in fats but low in carbohydrates have been conducted over the last twenty years and the results show that, contrary to what you might expect, diets that are low in fat and high in carbohydrates may actually raise blood sugar levels, raise "bad" cholesterol and triglyceride levels, and lower your "good" cholesterol levels—even more than diets that are high in fats.

The idea that a low-fat, high-carbohydrate diet may increase your risk factors may seem startling, especially after all you have read and heard on the news, but research scientists—not concerned with what the media thinks *should* be true—report quite a different story than does your local news reporter.

In the *American Journal of Clinical Nutrition,* Dr. Sam J. Bhathena and his team from the Carbohydrate Nutrition Laboratory and the Lipid Nutrition Laboratory of the U.S. Department of Agriculture and the National Cancer Institute reported that a low-fat, high-carbohydrate diet stimulated Profactor-H. In addition, they noted that, in women, these Profactor-H changes were increased at times, especially in relation to the phase of their menstrual cycle.

Looking at other important effects of the high-carbohydrate, low-fat diet, Dr. Ann M. Coulston and her fellow researchers at Stanford University School of Medicine studied the influence of diet on insulin and blood fat levels. Their results indicated that low-fat, high-carbohydrate diets (similar to those now generally recommended by most health agencies) led to increases in Profactor-H as well as to increases in triglycerides. This diet also resulted in reductions in "good" HDL-cholesterol concentrations. All of these low-fat, high-carbohydrate changes, these researchers concluded, "have been associated with an increase in incidence of coronary artery disease."

Time after time, scientists continue to find that for many of us, high-carbohydrate diets (rather than high-fat diets) lead to higher Profactor-H levels and to undesirable fat levels in the blood that signal an increased risk for heart disease.

Scientists reporting potentially harmful reactions to high-carbohydrate, low-fat diets may be saying things that differ from what "everyone" has told you. But these findings are important and they are real and they should not be dismissed simply because they are not in keeping with what is currently *believed* to be true.*

Remember that the beliefs of today were also once considered

---

*It is important to remember, as with any eating program, that you should check with your physician to determine the appropriate nutritional plan for you, especially in regard to fat and carbohydrate levels.

new and controversial. In its time, virtually every major medical breakthrough met with dispute from those who wanted to stay with the then-current way of seeing things. We would hope that, rather than judging a new approach on whether it agrees or disagrees with current practice, all of us would evaluate it simply on its merits and on how well the facts support it.

A Lasting Change—but Not One for the Better

When scientists first began reporting that blood fat levels were rising in response to low-fat, high-carbohydrate diets, some researchers thought that triglyceride levels would decrease over time. Since then, however, researchers have found that the negative effects of low-fat, high-carbohydrate diets seem to be long-lasting. In their report in *The New England Journal of Medicine,* Dr. Abhimanyu Garg and his associates at the Center for Human Nutrition at the University of Texas Southwestern Medical Center concluded that "increasing evidence" indicated that high triglyceride levels that had been triggered by high-carbohydrate diets were *not* temporary.

While some scientists were reporting undesirable blood fat level changes in normal healthy adults or those with high blood fat levels, other scientists began to look at changes in blood fat levels in diabetics on these same eating programs. Dr. Garg called on the scientific and medical communities to be aware that although current recommendations favored low-fat, high-carbohydrate diets for patients with adult-onset diabetes, "several previous studies in patients with diabetes pointed to the potentially harmful effects of high carbohydrate intakes" on blood fat levels. These diet-related effects included increasing levels of the "bad" triglycerides and very-low-density (VLDL) blood fats and decreasing levels of the "good" high-density lipoprotein (HDL) cholesterol.

What makes little sense is that the very same diet recommendations that brought about these potentially harmful effects are now being recommended for an entire population of diabetics—in an attempt to *better* their blood fat levels. These recommendations are very difficult to understand, especially when a Consensus Development Conference on Diet and Exercise in Adult-Onset Diabetes, sponsored by the National Institutes of Health, "raised doubts about the wisdom of recommending high-carbohydrate diets to all persons with diabetes."

Clearly, health agencies cannot keep issuing one-size-fits-all prescriptions for eating. Just as we would not recommend a single eyeglass prescription for everyone in the country, it does not make sense to recommend one eating prescription for everybody. Even as sweeping low-fat, high-carbohydrate dietary recommendations were first beginning to reach the general public, Dr. Sheldon Resier in his 1981 report in the *Journal of Nutrition* voiced the grave concerns that so many other scientists express. "One of the disadvantages in making specific dietary recommendations to a diverse population," he said, "is that these recommendations do not apply uniformly to individuals in that population." What is right for one person is *not* necessarily right for another. We are individuals in all ways, including nutritionally, and we must be treated as such.

> We are individuals in all ways, including nutritionally, and we must be treated as such.

If you are Profactor-H Positive, the research findings that we have included in this chapter are particularly important to you because *your* body is especially sensitive to carbohydrates. You need a special way of eating that will allow you to take in the carbohydrates you need, keep fats as low as your physician recommends, and keep your Profactor-H levels low as well. Fortunately, the Profactor-H Program will allow you to do just that, simply and without sacrifice or deprivation.

The Fiber Connection

If high-carbohydrate diets have been shown, in some cases, to be harmful, if they have been shown to increase risk factors for many people, why are they still being recommended for everyone?

Much of the confusion in current recommendations of high-carbohydrate diets came from early studies that, unfortunately, combined both high-carbohydrate foods and high-fiber foods in the diets they gave their subjects. When the results showed that these diets lowered blood fat levels, many people *assumed* it was the high-carbohydrate foods that were to credit, rather than the high fiber. It would be expected that high fiber would be beneficial; it may work well to slow the absorption of carbohydrates and, in doing so, may reduce Profactor-H surges.

Though current research now shows that fiber may have been the primary—or, often, the sole—reducer of blood fat levels, the beliefs and assumptions and often-inappropriate nutritional advice that came from those first studies, which included high-carbohydrate foods, lingers on.

A Working Plan for Life

As you have seen, Profactor-H can play a great role in carbohydrate metabolism and appears to have as great, or greater, an effect on blood fat levels as the amount of dietary fat you eat. Dietary recommendations are meant to be just that, recommendations that should be tailored to fit your own body and your own needs.

If you are Profactor-H Positive, an important part of your cardiovascular risk factor profile involves the impact that carbohydrates have on *your* body, and the diet you follow should be suited to *your* personal Profactor-H needs.

It is important to remember, as with any eating program, you should check with your physician to determine the appropriate nutritional plan for you, especially in regard to fat and carbohydrate levels. High fiber may be an important part of your program, so keep it in mind.

If you want additional information, and for a comparison of dietary fats, see the "Big Fat Lowdown" section in chapter 20, "Personalizing Your Program." If you would like additional information on incorporating health agency recommendations (in particular, those related to lowering dietary fat) into your Profactor-H Program, see "Health Agency Recommendations," page 345.

The Profactor-H Program guidelines are meant to help you and your doctor work together on an eating plan that will help you reduce your blood fat levels along with lowering their health-related risks.

"A Clear and Certain Miracle"
—Liz's Story

The woman who entered our offices was perfectly made up and expensively dressed. This, along with her confident manner, projected the appearance of a woman fully in control of her life, but, as Liz told us later, it was "all show." The woman within had quite a different story to tell.

> Liz projected the appearance of a woman
> fully in control of her life,
> but it was "all show."

By the time Liz M. came to see us she was convinced that she was "falling apart." And beyond the first appearance, although she was only fifty-one, Liz looked very tired and a bit worn. Her eyes seemed somewhat sad.

She sat down across from us and came right to the point. "My doctor recommended that I see you. He said he would call. I hope he did. He said he was very impressed with changes in two of his other patients who had worked with you, and he wanted to see if you could help me." She stopped suddenly and looked at us as if she expected an answer.

Liz's doctor had indeed called. We had listened with interest when, a few days earlier, he described how this bright, active woman had, in a matter of only a few years, started showing many risk factors connected with heart disease and stroke. When, at first, her blood pressure started to rise and her blood cholesterol levels increased, Liz's physician recommended a typical low-fat diet. In place of the fat, Liz was told to eat high-carbohydrate foods, especially complex carbohydrates such as pasta, whole-grain breads, fruit and juices, rice, legumes, and potatoes—all with very, very little fat.

Liz followed her low-fat diet with seriousness and commitment. Her father had died at fifty-two from a massive stroke, her mother had suffered several heart attacks and died in her early sixties. Both had high blood pressure and had been warned to lose some weight. Her father had been a borderline diabetic, as well. Though she knew little of her parents' attempts to control their diet, the fact remained that they had not been able to lose weight and keep it off, nor were they able to bring down their blood pressure levels.

Liz said that she was committed to taking better care of her health than her parents had, and she put a great deal of time and energy into "getting a handle" on her blood pressure and cholesterol levels by following her doctor's low-fat diet recommendations.

"A regular low-fat diet was not good enough for me," she told us. "I became a food fanatic. I ate no meat, not just red meat, but no meat whatsoever. I lived on fish and, for a special treat, I'd eat chicken or turkey without the skin. No dairy at all—I mean none," she added. "I had minuscule amounts of soy oil margarine on the heaviest, most fiber-rich bran muffins you can imagine. I ate fruit and vegetables all day long. It felt so restrictive and I felt so deprived, but I was determined. I craved a rich treat or even just a 'normal' meal, but I was committed to sticking to it. Sometimes I would think about letting go and eating anything I could get my hands on, but I told myself that I didn't want to end up like my parents, and I would hold out and stick to the diet, which, I must tell you, was not easy.

"When I went back to my doctor's office," she added more softly, as we could see the pain and frustration about to burst through, "after all that, after all that, I tried so hard, and then to find out . . ." She couldn't go on. But we knew the story.

> Liz's doctor told her to "try harder"
> (insinuating that she had been cheating).

After a few months of a dedicated attempt to follow her low-fat program, Liz returned to her doctor for a reevaluation. But she was in for an unwelcome surprise. Instead of being told that her hard work and sacrifice were paying off, Liz was told that her blood pressure was "skyrocketing" and that her triglyceride and cholesterol levels and ratios were getting worse—not at all what she expected! Her doctor told her to "try harder" (insinuating that she had been cheating). When she protested that she had stuck to the diet faithfully, she was asked if she had *ever* gone off the diet.

"Of course," she replied, "I'm only human. On rare occasions at a party, I might have something special. But surely"—she looked pleadingly at us as she had at her physician—"a few deviations couldn't have ruined all the hard work I put in. Does that mean I can *never* have anything to eat that I enjoy, ever again?" she asked.

Liz told us that her doctor had said something about a program being only as good as "how well you stick to it" and never responded to her questions. Then he recommended a diet *even lower in fat,* adding that if things didn't change "immediately" he was going to put her on blood pressure– and blood fat–reducing medications.

"The new lower-fat diet was insane. I felt like I was being punished. I couldn't eat anything I liked. I tried to convince myself that it wasn't so bad, but the truth was that I hated it. And I hated myself. And I hated my doctor. But just to show him, more out of spite than anything else, I stuck to it. This time, I didn't deviate—not once. Four weeks to the day, I remember the day because I was counting them, I returned for another blood test. And you know it, my blood fat levels and pressure had jumped once again; my triglycerides were "off the chart," my good fats were down, my bad fats were up. It was a mess. And this time, I was waiting for him."

Much to her surprise, her doctor did not accuse her of "cheating." We had, in the meantime, had two conversations with him and had sent him copies of some of the many research reports we had been reviewing. Combining the evidence with the failure of some of his other patients, much to his credit, he listened to Liz with an open mind and treated her problem with the assumption that she had been telling him the truth.

In a later conversation, he told us that though she had followed the very-low-fat diet, Liz's blood pressure had climbed so high that he had serious and immediate concerns for her well-being. He felt that if her blood pressure were to rise even a little more, he would be forced to hospitalize her. He said at that point, in his opinion, she would be in imminent danger of having a stroke. Her blood tests confirmed what he suspected, that Liz's fat levels were growing even worse. Something in the diet was working against, rather than toward, her health.

Not many of the people we have seen over the years show such quick and radical progressions as did Liz; most Profactor-H changes occur slowly over many years. It is, in fact, this slow, steady progression that can make it easy to disregard the problem. Still, the immediacy of Liz's difficulties brought her to our doorstep, and we were happy for that.

Liz took a breath and continued. "I'm afraid I'm going to die before anyone figures out what to do," she said. With that, the tears poured down her cheeks.

After a minute, she continued. "You know, I could understand it if I had been ignoring my doctor's orders, but it's not like I've been having a good ol' time, eating anything I want. I've been doing everything that I'm 'supposed to do' and it's just not doing any good." Her frustration and desperation filled the room.

> "I've been doing everything that I'm 'supposed to do' and it's just not doing any good."

We asked Liz about her hunger, weight, and tiredness, and her general personal and medical history. We explained that she showed several signs of Profactor-H. Her Profactor-H Evaluation Score placed her high into the High Risk range. You could see the relief spread across her face.

"Those questions, some of them looked like they were written for me. I know that means we are on the right track now. I feel better already." And with that, Liz agreed to begin a program that might have literally saved her life.

It is important to understand that not everyone follows the same pattern. Though it is the exception, some people show only one or two signs and never move on to additional symptoms and signs of Profactor-H or its related diseases. Some people may find they are tired and hungry in the afternoon and sluggish after dinner, yet they never develop blood pressure problems or any of the other signs of Profactor-H.

Some people may have only a few of the signs of Profactor-H for a long time before they show any progression. We have seen many overweight carbohydrate cravers who did not experience undesirable blood fat levels or high blood pressure for a long period of time. Depending on genetics and on an individual's body, lifestyle, and environment, one person's Profactor-H progression may be very different from anyone else's.

Liz, however, showed many of the classic signs of Profactor-H, and they increased in number and severity one after the other. Even without her blood test results, we would have been greatly concerned for her welfare; Profactor-H rarely stands still. By definition, Profactor-H can lead to greater and greater health problems and endangerment.

With her physician monitoring her progress, we began to familiarize Liz with the cause and correction of her blood fat and blood pressure problems. We explained to her that she had a hormonal imbalance caused by too much insulin in her blood and that we call this imbalance Profactor-H.

We told Liz that her doctor used to call this imbalance "hyperinsulinemia." Until recently he thought it was a rather unusual condition, but since he had been reading up on the research, he had started to learn how prevalent it is and how serious its effects can be. That was why, we added, he sent her to us.

We explained that, for Profactor-H-free people, low-fat diets and medications can be very helpful, but in general, the

Profactor-H Positive person must correct the *cause* of the problem. If the problem is due to high fat intake alone, then a low-fat diet makes sense. But if there are other problems, they must be eliminated.

We explained that there is a reason some people can eat high-fat diets and never have problems and why others, who try so hard to control their fat intake, cannot bring their blood fat levels down. Since, for Profactor-H Positive individuals, low-fat diets and medications treat only the symptoms and not the underlying cause, the underlying imbalance that caused the problem in the first place can continue to progress.

> Low-fat diets may work only on the *symptoms* of the problem; they don't always correct the *cause* of the problem.

We explained that sometimes we can see Profactor-H impact by the way that a person's body seems to be fighting a low-fat diet or medication, so that rather than responding to them in positive ways, blood pressure or blood fat levels stay the same or, over time, may get worse. Sometimes we can see the effect of Profactor-H as additional signs and symptoms start to appear over time. It would not be unexpected, we added, that her blood sugar levels might soon be found to be too high.

Liz looked startled. That was something she had not told anyone, she said. When she had visited her gynecologist recently, he had asked for the usual urine sample. This time, however, he found that Liz showed an unusually high level of sugar in her urine. He had recommended that she have some follow-up studies, but she had hoped it wasn't important and had not told her family doctor.

Our prediction of Profactor-H's next step was not surprising to us, we explained. It is simply a matter of understanding the way in which Profactor-H works and progresses. But just as we can predict how it can next endanger or harm you, we can also help you to stop and even reverse its progression.

> **The ravages of Profactor-H are not inevitable. You do not have to watch your parents' pattern of progressive ill health played out in your life.**

We explained that the ravages of Profactor-H are not inevitable and that you do not have to watch your parents' pattern of progressive ill health played out in your life as you grow sicker and sicker and old before your time. We told her we would try to help her correct what appeared to be the *cause* of her problems. We stopped and looked at Liz's face. She was crying again, but this time the pain and fear were gone; this time she was crying with relief and hope.

For the next three weeks, Liz familiarized herself with the Beginner's Program. She started by adding a salad to her evening meal and began walking for just about fifteen minutes each day. She felt better and had more energy. At the end of six weeks, she was well into the Intermediate Program, eating only Risk-Reducing Foods at lunch and for snacks as well as including salad and vegetables with her dinner. Her hunger, she reported, had dropped "incredibly" and she told us she rarely snacked at all anymore. "Not because I can't," she added. "It's just that I'm not hungry anymore"—quite a change from the Liz who once told us she could not go any longer than two hours without a piece of fruit or something "to keep my energy up." We explained that it was in fact those frequent snacks of fruit and fruit juice that, for Liz, were a major part of her problem; they had been priming her body with Profactor-H, wiping the blood sugar from her bloodstream, and converting the food energy to fat.

After being on the Program for ten weeks, Liz's blood pressure had dropped to a significantly safer level and her physician was becoming less concerned for her immediate health. Hospitalization was no longer looming in her future and she felt and looked like a new person. By three months into the Program, Liz's triglyceride levels had dropped to normal. She complemented her Risk-Reducing meals with an Essential Balance dinner that included many of the foods she so enjoyed. "I walk daily and really enjoy it. Just like they say, I've really changed my way of life. But I barely notice it. It's not a sacrifice and I still get to eat the foods I love so much." Her program was helping her lose weight and become healthier "by the day." "I have never felt so good," she told us at her six-month check-in. "I feel like this is the way I was meant to eat . . . and to live." We couldn't have agreed more.

Two and a half years have passed since that time. Liz's body is still slowly returning to normal. Her blood pressure tends to remain "a bit high," though now it is well within acceptable range, and her cholesterol is around 220, though much of the count is taken up by "good" cholesterol. Her triglycerides are excellent. Her doctor says that her progress is "amazing," but we know she could probably be doing even better. A difficult family situation has taken up a great deal of time that Liz might otherwise have given to herself. She is now working two jobs and suffering the stress of taking care of someone who is terminally ill. The wear and tear on her body, the stress, and the lack of time to fully utilize the Program are, most likely, taking their toll. But you wouldn't know it by speaking to Liz.

"If it weren't for this program," she told us at our most recent meeting, "I don't know what I would have done. I'm afraid to think of it. I would never have been able to deal with this. I can never thank you for what you have given me."

We looked down and there lay two lovely religious medals. "I'm not a very religious person," she said, "but I wanted you to have these."

Her eyes filled with tears and she added softly, "For me, this program has been a clear and certain miracle."

CHAPTER 8

Taking It to Heart

*Of all the ailments which may blow out life's little candle,
heart disease is the chief.*

When the heart is healthy, all else is possible.
—William Boyd

You will not find this chapter, nor any of the chapters that follow,
filled with dread forebodings about all of the diseases that are waiting to spring on you as time goes by.

Instead, you will find these pages filled with hope and joy, for the
success and progress we have seen and made are here to be shared.
We will tell you what *you* need to know—helpful information that
you can use and adapt to *your* needs and lifestyle.

> You will find these pages filled with hope and joy,
> for the success and progress
> we have seen and made are here to be shared.

In the coming chapters, we will explain terms that are often thrown
around all too casually or used incorrectly, and we will show you
how your body works and what we have discovered to help you
best put it into and keep it in fine working condition.

The Silent Process

Your heart is a muscle, about the size of your fist, that sits in the middle of your chest and points to the left. Like all muscles, it depends on a steady flow of blood for nourishment and oxygen.

When scientists and physicians talk about the heart, they are usually talking about the muscular wall of the heart. The blood that feeds that outside wall comes from the inside of the heart. In this way, the heart literally feeds itself, pumping blood into its own thick, muscular wall. The blood is pumped out from the internal chambers, then circles around through coronary arteries, and feeds back into the wall of heart muscle. It is within these pathways, the coronary arteries, that heart disease often begins.

> The heart pumps blood from inside its own chambers
> out and around, into its own thick, muscular wall.
> In this way, the heart literally feeds itself.

There are two main types of heart disease. The first, coronary *artery* disease, involves the arteries that lead out of the heart to the heart muscle. The second, coronary *heart* disease, involves damage to the heart muscle itself.

Coronary artery disease is the name given to several different diseases that narrow the coronary arteries or their branches. As the arteries narrow, they can decrease or prevent the flow of blood to the heart muscle. Without the appropriate amount of blood, the heart cannot get the nourishment or the oxygen it so vitally needs.

Until recently, the development of coronary artery disease had been a silent process. The arteries narrow slowly, over time. Changes to the arteries are most often caused by vessel injury and repair and the accumulation of cholesterol and other fats from the blood (contributing to the formation of plaque). These changes thicken the inside wall of the arteries so that the space through which blood can flow becomes narrowed. This is known as *atherosclerosis*.

Just imagine that you are drinking lemonade through a straw. As you drink, small pieces of lemon stick to the side of the straw. As lemon pieces continue to accumulate and stick, the space inside the straw becomes more and more narrow. Less lemonade is able to pass through until the straw becomes blocked; then no lemonade can pass through at all.

In a similar way, coronary artery disease can partially block or slowly reduce the blood supply to the heart. The heart will usually adjust and compensate by working harder, which, in turn, contributes to high blood pressure.

If coronary artery disease narrows the blood vessels enough, the reduced blood flow can result in a clot (embolism), which can greatly or completely block the blood flow to the heart. The heart may respond with a sharp onset of pain or irregular beat as the vital muscle suffers damage (heart attack). There may be nausea, loss of sensation in the arm or hand, as well as many other seemingly unrelated symptoms. In some cases, however, there appear to be no symptoms whatsoever (silent heart attack).

When a decrease in blood flow to the heart (partial or complete) causes damage to the heart muscle itself, coronary artery disease is said to have resulted in coronary heart disease. Blockage of blood flow to the heart can result in permanent damage to the heart, leaving its victim weakened and vulnerable to future heart problems.

Once damage is done to the heart, it cannot be undone, although other, healthier parts of the heart may take over. About half of the cases of heart attack result in sudden death. Coronary artery disease, on the other hand, is preventable and, in many cases, may be reversible.

The Heart of the Matter

You have probably heard that each year heart disease accounts for more deaths than any other disease or group of diseases. While this is true, we have to put this statistic into perspective. The category, death from heart disease, can include deaths from old age as well as many other natural or posttraumatic causes.

If a person is in a car accident, for instance, and sustains massive injuries followed by a prolonged hospitalization, the ultimate cause of death may be noted as heart failure (which may be categorized as heart disease). Though you and I might see clearly that it was the car accident that ultimately caused the death, the official cause of death may, still, have been a heart that failed to continue beating and might have been classified as such. In the same way, the elderly whose bodies simply can no longer function ultimately die from pneumonia or, in most cases, coronary heart disease. In these ways, statistics related to the incidence of heart disease may be greatly overstated.

The greatest overstatement related to death by heart disease comes from ignoring the *cause* of the heart disease. Diabetes, for instance, contributes to over 71,000 additional deaths per year, which are often then categorized as heart disease. Though these deaths may, in fact, be related to the diabetes that led to the problem, the final cause of death will, in most cases, be classified as "heart disease" rather than "diabetes."

Ignoring the underlying causes of death is no small point. It can be used to hide some very important and alarming trends. For instance, while we are always told that heart disease is the top cause of death in the United States, contributing factors may tell a very different story. The most recent report of the Surgeon General of the United States estimated that coronary heart disease accounted for 511,700 deaths. By comparison, cancers claimed the lives of 476,700. When the influence of diabetes is accounted for, however, coronary heart disease rates drop by over 71,000—placing it second to cancer as a cause of death in the United States.

> Statistics that report the incidence of heart disease
> or progress in prevention of heart disease
> may be far from accurate.

Statistics that report progress in the treatment and prevention of heart disease may likewise be far from accurate. Most recently, reports have emerged indicating that, in the United States, deaths from coronary heart disease are declining. This is, to put it mildly, a questionable statement. As you look over the reports, you begin to catch terms like recent "age-corrected" rates and the like, which allow statisticians to virtually discover all kinds of trends that may or may not be real.

Statistical manipulations of numbers may be used to make us feel better or worse, but to each of us, as an individual, population statistics may be meaningless. Understanding which factors increase our individual chances of getting heart disease and learning what we can realistically do to reduce our risk are, in fact, what really matters.

A Question of Risk

Heart disease is often called a "multifactorial" disorder—meaning that it comes from many factors. Traditionally, risk factors for heart disease have always included a family history of the disease, along with a personal history involving "the big three": smoking, high blood pressure, and elevated blood cholesterol levels. Additional risk factors for heart attack have included excess weight, inactivity, and stress.

The recent research findings, however, cast serious doubts on several of these risk factors. High blood cholesterol levels, for instance, so often cited as a major risk factor for heart disease, may not be as powerful a predictor of heart disease as previously thought. Although individuals with high blood cholesterol levels have heart attacks, so do people with low levels of cholesterol. Approximately one third of all heart attacks occur in people having a currently acceptable level of cholesterol in their blood—under 200 mg/dl, which puts in serious doubt the use of blood cholesterol as a risk factor measurement.

Risks related to your intake of dietary fat are also in question. In the past, a high intake of dietary fat has been reported to be a major risk factor in heart disease. All of us have been advised to cut down on our fat intake. Recently, however, many of these studies have been shown to be faulty or have been refuted and the conclusions that were drawn may not have been nearly as compelling as was first thought. Current research casts some doubt on the direct relationship of fat intake to heart disease, and in reality, lowering your fat intake alone may not significantly reduce your risk for heart disease.

Of greater importance, it now appears, is the fact that it is not the fat, per se, that causes an increased risk of heart disease but rather the way your particular body responds to the fat—that is, by an increase in insulin. As the insulin reaches and maintains Profactor-H levels, a whole chain of damage-causing events often begins.

In the Profactor-H Positive individual, eating high-fat foods may signal the Profactor-H process to begin. If you have already eaten high-carbohydrate foods earlier in the day, eating high-fat foods may signal the Profactor-H levels to rise further. It is your Profactor-H levels, which respond to the *frequent* intake of carbohydrates, *in combination* with the fats you eat, rather than eating high-fat foods *alone,* that appear to make you more vulnerable to heart disease. The combination of frequent carbohydrate intake along with a high fat intake may for some be the crucial coupling that leads to high blood fat levels.

This new insight explains why some Profactor-H-free individuals may eat high-fat diets with seemingly no ill effects and why Profactor-H Positive individuals may be far more vulnerable to the impact of high-fat foods. In both cases the diet may be the same, but there is a crucial difference in the way the two bodies respond to high-fat foods, especially when they are coupled with carbohydrates.

If your body does not respond to a high-fat diet with increased Profactor-H levels, you may never suffer heart-related consequences from eating these foods. If, on the other hand, your body does respond with Profactor-H, the stage may be set for future heart disease.

**The most recent research findings
may cast serious doubt on
traditional risk factors for heart disease.**

As you have seen in chapter 7, "Fats and Fiber: Fears, Facts, and Fallacies," the area of dietary fats and fats in the blood and their associated risks is filled with assumptions, overgeneralized conclusions, half-truths, myths, misunderstandings, and downright falsehoods.

Among the other risk factors being reexamined in relation to their role in heart disease is lack of exercise. While it is certainly not recommended that we sit around in bed all day, the benefits of a rigorous and demanding exercise regime may *not* be significantly greater than a simple, enjoyably active life, one that involves walking and moving at home or in the office.*

On a personal level, many of us have seen examples of the athlete, in his prime, looking like the model of health, cut down by a heart attack. Researchers are starting to recognize that being fit is not necessarily the same as being healthy.

Most important to each of us is the fact that statistics do not explain *why* risk factors such as high-fat diets and lack of exercise may increase your chance for heart disease. Statistics do not explain what risk factors actually do to the body to make heart disease more likely. Scientists and physicians know that although risk factors may occur before or at the same time as a disease, they do not necessarily *cause* the problem; they may simply co-exist.

Which leaves us to address a few vital questions: What causes heart disease? What actually happens to make us more vulnerable? Why do some of us eat all the fats we want and never have problems with high cholesterol or triglycerides, while others carefully watch our diets and are rewarded with only worsening levels of fats in our blood (or on our waistlines)?

Answers to these questions may spring from understanding that a single physical imbalance may, in fact, link heart disease to its many risk factors and that this imbalance may be preventable and, in many cases, reversible.

The first confirmation that a central, underlying, and causal factor of heart disease did indeed exist came by searching for a *single physical imbalance that heart disease risk factors held in common*— and that proved to be Profactor-H.

Long before Profactor-H's importance was fully acknowledged, physicians and researchers, each working without knowledge of the others' discoveries, were describing it and its relation to heart disease. In a monumental review published in 1990, Dr. Robert Stout of the Queen's University of Belfast, Northern Ireland, untangled and clarified many of the studies connecting Profactor-H to both heart disease and high blood pressure and emphasized that, though re-

---

*Always check with your personal physician when planning, beginning, or changing an exercise or activity regimen.

searchers in the last decade were actively investigating the blood pressure–Profactor-H link, the original connection had been established more than thirty years earlier.

For the decade and a half immediately following the landmark connection between high blood pressure and insulin, a serious lack in technological advances held back the discovery of Profactor-H. In the 1980s, new breakthroughs in science emerged and gave researchers the tools they needed to uncover the essential Profactor-H connection to many heart disease risk factors, including high blood pressure, high triglycerides, and other undesirable levels of fats in the blood, as well as excess weight.

In the last few years, however, as technology continues to hand us newer and better research tools, we have witnessed a virtual explosion in the scientific reports identifying Profactor-H as heart disease's essential link. As the 1990s approached, research scientists such as Dr. D. C. Simonson began to inform fellow scientists that it is well recognized that Profactor-H is "characteristic of a number of common human disease states including obesity, adult-onset diabetes, high blood pressure, and atherosclerotic heart disease." He explained that although the first investigations into insulin and insulin resistance took place in the 1930s, it is only during the past decade that the disease-causing importance of Profactor-H has begun to be understood. These discoveries have lead researchers to declare that Profactor-H is "now recognized to be the hallmark of several common disease states."

In the last few years, the relationship of Profactor-H to heart disease has been reported repeatedly by some of the finest researchers in the field. Numerous studies have suggested, wrote Dr. M. W. Stolar of Northwestern University Medical School, that Profactor-H "accelerates the development of atherosclerosis." Dr. A. Garg, at the same time, also reported that Profactor-H has been found to be "an independent risk factor for coronary heart disease."

An independent risk factor is one that is so strong that it stands alone; it does not depend on other risk factors to raise the probability of your getting a certain disease or disorder. In other words, Profactor-H is so powerful a risk factor for heart disease that, if you have it, even though you may not have high blood pressure or undesirable blood fat levels or be overweight, just having Profactor-H greatly increases your chances for heart disease. And the research findings testify to its independent power.

In his 1990 report, Dr. A. Grimaldi explained that Profactor-H seemed to encourage the narrowing of arteries, even when blood sugar levels were normal, and in his report, Dr. Robert Stout concluded that Profactor-H had an "independent" and "predictive" relationship to coronary heart disease.

As the research studies increase in number and grow in depth and complexity, the single consistent, common thread among heart disease risk factors proves to be Profactor-H.

For all of us, especially those who bear the burden of inheriting heart disease risk factors, the discovery of Profactor-H brings welcome news. Until now, the area of health risk was clouded and confusing. Now we have come to understand that many heart disease risk factors such as high blood pressure, undesirable blood fat levels, and excess weight may simply be symptoms of the same underlying problem: Profactor-H. In addition, we can see that reducing our risk for Profactor-H may help us reduce our risk for high blood pressure, undesirable blood fat levels, and excess weight, as well as for heart disease itself, all at the same time.

For those with a family or personal history of heart disease or those who love someone at risk, the many scientists whose research appears throughout this book may have provided answers to our most fervent prayers. They have helped us isolate and identify what appears to be the singular and most powerful life-threatening culprit in the area of heart disease—Profactor-H.

For all of us, especially those who bear the
burden of inheriting heart disease risk factors,
the discovery of Profactor-H
brings welcome news.

Profactor-H and Heart Disease: Reducing Your Risk

Profactor-H has a powerful ability to encourage and stimulate growth. It has been shown to play a crucial role in all three critical changes that can lead to the development of heart disease. The development of heart disease is not a simple, stepwise progression. Each of the changes may occur in varying order over time, but with each change, Profactor-H appears to play an important and preventable role.

> Profactor-H plays three crucial roles
> in the development of heart disease.

Critical Change 1

The all-important first step in the development of heart disease is the thickening of the inside walls of coronary arteries, which, in turn, causes a narrowing of space in the arteries through which blood flows to the heart. By stimulating the growth of the smooth muscle cells that line artery walls, Profactor-H directly activates and quickens the narrowing of these arteries. When Profactor-H is present, there is a continual bathing of the walls of these blood vessels with excess insulin, which encourages the cells to grow. As the cells increase in number, they reduce the space through which blood can flow to the heart.

Critical Change 2

In the second critical change, Profactor-H stimulates cholesterol production in the liver. Three times the amount of cholesterol comes from your body as from your diet, and the cholesterol that your body produces (endogenous cholesterol) is far more dangerous to your heart's health than that which comes from your diet. The Profactor-H–prompted cholesterol flows through your bloodstream and can accumulate, forming plaque, in blood vessels. As the plaque grows, the blood flow through the already-narrowed arteries is reduced even more.

Critical Change 3

In its third heart-damaging role, Profactor-H reduces the destruction of a substance called *fibrin*. Fibrin acts like glue, holding the plaque together. Fibrin is essential to the development of plaque buildup on artery walls. Less fibrin, less plaque.

When Profactor-H reduces the amount of fibrin that is destroyed, extra fibrin is available to aid in the formation and deposit of plaque. Again, artery space is narrowed and blood flow through the arteries to the heart decreases.

With blood vessels being narrowed by the combination of three different Profactor-H actions, the heart's blood supply can be sharply decreased or, worse, cut off. Profactor-H can leave its painful mark in narrowed, blocked arteries or in a diseased and damaged heart.

Along with the discovery of Profactor-H
came an understanding of how
to prevent it and how to correct it.

Disabling Profactor-H's Power

The Profactor-H Program was designed to help lower your risk of coronary artery disease and coronary heart disease by eliminating the *cause* of these critical changes. Disabling Profactor-H's powerful and dangerous "triple play" of artery damage depends on eliminating or greatly reducing an important cause: Profactor-H.

Fortunately, for all of us, along with the discovery of Profactor-H and its connection to heart disease came an understanding of how to prevent it and how to correct it.

As Profactor-H levels decline, signs of atherosclerosis often decline: cholesterol and triglyceride levels drop; lower density lipids

(LDL—the "bad" fats in the blood) go down; and higher density lipids (HDL—the "good" cholesterol) rise.

Our research has shown that within three months of being on the Profactor-H Program, many indicators of heart disease can drop dramatically and, in some cases, begin to disappear. As they continue on the Program, many people find that their blood pressure levels greatly improve and their total cholesterol may go down by as much as 20 percent—or, in some cases, more. For many people, decreases in triglyceride levels can average from about 15 to 25 percent, with the greatest decrease in those with the highest blood fat levels. In some rarer cases, total triglycerides have been shown to decrease by as much as 150 points. In addition, significant, steady, and easy weight losses are often reported.

The Profactor-H Program is easy and simple. It requires little time or sacrifice. Most important, the Profactor-H Program may be crucial in reducing your Profactor-H link to heart disease. For those of us who carry the heart disease risk factor burden, this can be the real miracle.

The Profactor-H Program may be crucial
in reducing your Profactor-H
link to heart disease.
For those of us who carry the
heart disease risk factor burden,
this can be the real miracle.

THE PROFACTOR-H TRIPLE-PLAY CAN LEAD TO PROGRESSIVE ATHEROSCLEROSIS

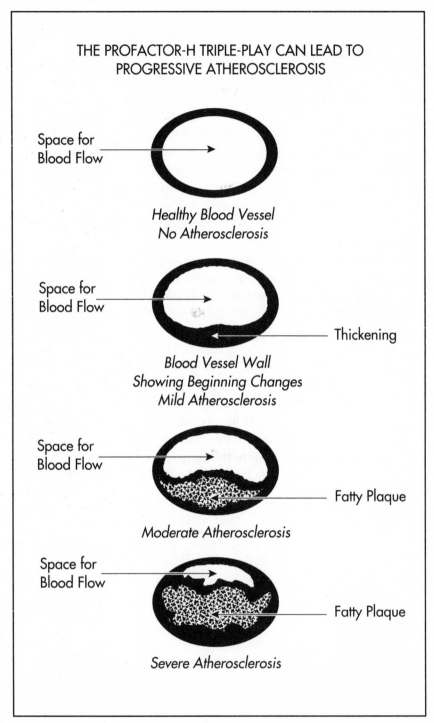

Space for Blood Flow

Healthy Blood Vessel
No Atherosclerosis

Space for Blood Flow

Thickening

Blood Vessel Wall
Showing Beginning Changes
Mild Atherosclerosis

Space for Blood Flow

Fatty Plaque

Moderate Atherosclerosis

Space for Blood Flow

Fatty Plaque

Severe Atherosclerosis

Not Too Young to Be at Risk: Jackie's Story

Jackie D. came to our office with three four-year-olds. The scene was amusing and quite unusual. We were not sure how to handle the three crawling tykes and we were about to reschedule the appointment when two of our research assistants offered to take the matter, and all three children, in hand.

"That's what my days are like," Jackie told us as the children were herded out of the waiting area. "I run a small day-care group out of my house and I'm always 'on.' Sometimes I get someone to help me out, but I'm never sure if I'm going to be able to count on them. I really only have myself to rely on. And I can be stuck in the house all day. I mean really stuck.

"With five or six babies to be responsible for there's no break, no matter how badly I need it. It's nonstop from the moment I wake up till the last one leaves. And at night, after their parents pick them up, I take my daughter out for dinner. I have to get out. I'm a single mother and I don't want to spend what little time I have with my daughter cooking and cleaning up. Besides, by the time the evening comes around, if I don't get out, I'll go nuts. Then I come home, clean up the mess that's accumulated during the day, go to sleep, and when I wake up the whole thing starts again."

A shadow of a thought crossed Jackie's face and she looked down, slightly embarrassed. "I'm not saying it's so terrible, it's just that I think I'm starting to feel the strain.

"I don't feel right," she went on. "I can't explain it, I just don't feel well and I even look old. I always looked young for my age, but not anymore. I'm not being hysterical, but sometimes I look in the mirror and for a moment I look like my own mother."

Though she was only in her late thirties, Jackie did indeed give the impression of being eight to ten years older. And she looked tired.

The combination of being cooped up with the children, the

responsibility of their care, no adults to talk to, and lack of stimulation took its toll on Jackie in terms of mental and physical stress.

Jackie's eating habits were deteriorating. "I eat when I'm not hungry. I don't know why I'm doing it. I've gained weight, but I just don't seem to care anymore. At home, I don't even get on the scale." At times she felt angry and "trapped," she admitted, but more often than not "felt nothing."

Jackie's last visit to the doctor awakened her from what she described as "a kind of sleepwalk." "My doctor went crazy," she said. "I had put on fifteen pounds and my blood pressure had jumped by forty points. He couldn't believe the blood tests. He made me come in and get them again and he told me frankly that I was beginning to look like an old woman."

Her doctor was an old family friend and had seen Jackie through a bad and abusive marriage and a difficult divorce, but the stress she was now experiencing seemed to be worse than any she had experienced before.

Until her last checkup, Jackie had tried to control her tendency toward high blood pressure and overweight by following a low-fat diet. She admitted to "slipping" once in a while and eating foods that were not on her eating plan, but explained that at times the plan was "next to impossible to follow." "Still," she added, "considering all I've given up, if a low-fat diet was going to help, I don't think things should be going downhill." She took a deep breath and her face grew sad. "I thought I was too young to have these kinds of physical problems," she added quietly.

Jackie did *not* have a strong family history for heart disease, although, with her parents still rather young, it was difficult to be sure. Her mother had been prescribed blood pressure–lowering medication only the year before, but no one else in the family seemed to have many of the classic heart disease risk factors.

Jackie told us what was on her mind. "It's hard enough to be a single mother, that's one strike against you. And I'm barely making it financially. I don't have a career, and child care is basically all I can do. Strike two. And now with me showing signs of the stress, it's strike three, and I can almost hear someone saying 'You're out!'

"I'm really concerned for my daughter," she added solemnly. "I'm afraid of what will happen to her if something happens to me. I'm all she has. I have no disability insurance, no one pays for my sick days, and my parents, well, I really don't want to have to ask them for any more.

"The worst thing is, I even worry about my worrying. You know, am I making myself sick worrying about getting sick? I'm really a pretty stable person," she added, "though you probably couldn't tell that from this conversation."

Jackie was wrong about only one thing. We could clearly see the rational, sane, but worried woman who sat before us. She had every right to be concerned—it only showed that she was clearly seeing the important changes of increased risk for heart disease that she was showing.

We gave Jackie the Profactor-H Evaluation and she scored at Moderate Risk. We explained that though her family history was not high in terms of heart disease risk, her soaring stress levels in combination with a low-fat diet that involved frequent carbohydrate intake was apparently greatly boosting her Profactor-H levels.

On her second visit, we looked over a food diary that Jackie had kept for us and we found two more culprits: artificially sweetened diet sodas and lots of refined sugars and fast foods. Jackie reacted with concern. "Please don't take my 'goodies' away," she begged. "I really need them. They keep me going."

We explained that within the Profactor-H Program, as long as her doctor agreed, Jackie could have all of the foods she loved and needed—and if she enjoyed her "goodies" within the timing guidelines of the Program, she would still be able to decrease her Profactor-H risk as well.

"All I could think of was what I was going to have to give up," she admitted. "You know, I came here because I heard that I could still eat the food I loved and get healthier at the same time. I really need a treat once in a while and I don't want to feel guilty, but I don't want to drop dead, either."

Her first week into the Program looked like a breeze. Jackie had no problem in choosing Risk-Reducing lunchtime foods, especially when she could still enjoy her "wonderful dinners." Clearly, the Nutritional Options in the Program were proving easy. Activity Options were also not a problem. "In the afternoons, I only take care of three kids, so I pile the kids into a special stroller and take them for a walk every day," she said. "I have been wanting to do it regularly anyway, and it fits easily into my schedule."

The third Option, which called for time away from a stressful situation, proved to be the most difficult. "I can't just walk away from the kids," she explained convincingly. "And there is no way I can emotionally separate myself from them. There is never a time when all of them are sleeping, so I can't do that Option." We explained that the Program worked as a whole, reducing all three levels of risk, and that, in her case, the Stress-Reducing Option was the most important. We asked her to continue her first two Options for another week or two and think of ways she could combine them with a Stress-Reducing Option.

The phone call we received the following week sounded as if it came from a different woman. She was full of energy, excited, and happy. "The idea came to me on the way back from your office," she told us. "I was thinking how much better I was feeling already and that I didn't want to give up on it. I knew that I was beginning to feel better than I had in a long time. Anyway, I remembered that there was this woman in the playground who asked if I could take care of her daughter for two hours a day. I told her no. I generally don't find that it's worth my time to have a child for such a short time—by the time they get settled, it's time for them to go, and, quite honestly, it's not worth the money. But then I started thinking about it. The baby is a sweet little girl, quiet and easygoing. Her mother really needs a break—she has to take her special-needs son for medical treatments in the mornings and she doesn't have much money for child-care. Her mother picks up the boy after his treatments, so after this woman takes him there and gets him settled, she's free for the rest of the morning. Then it came to me. I could exchange child-care responsibility with her. Take care of her daughter for two hours if she would take care of all my kids for a little while. That way, I could get out and get away. I called her up and she was at my doorstep in an hour. We worked out the details and we've been doing it ever since.

"I feel like a new woman," she announced. "I never knew how important it was for me to get away from some of the pressure. The Option that seemed the most challenging was the one I need most . . . and you knew it!"

In the weeks that followed, Jackie added the Chromium Bonus Option: "Taking a simple supplement that I need anyway seems like something I can handle," she told us with a sparkle in her eye, and added that she was ready to move to the Intermediate Program. "Now that I know I can still have my 'goodies' and feel wonderful as well, I'm ready to tackle the next level."

Six months later a very happy woman bounced into our offices. "Look," she cried, throwing the papers on our desk. "Read 'em and smile." There lay Jackie's newest laboratory reports. All of her heart disease risk factors were changing for the better—every single one. Her triglycerides had dropped by 50 points, putting her in the normal range, her cholesterol was down by about 40 points, and, in addition, her "good" cholesterol had increased while her "bad" cholesterol had decreased. Her blood pressure was "terrific," she reported, and "to top it off"—she smiled—"I've taken off ten pounds—officially." She said that her doctor was pleased and she was "ecstatic."

It has been a long, hard road for Jackie. She trades child care a few hours each week so that she can go to night school or come to see us. She told us at her last visit that she wanted to get a job in an office but that it was difficult to even think about it, given her busy and demanding schedule.

But she has maintained her program faithfully. "It's so easy; it's a way of life. I can barely remember what it was like before.

I eat the foods I love and have peace of mind as well." After two years, Jackie's laboratory and clinical signs continue to place her at very low risk for heart disease.

"Now that I look good and feel good, I want to get out of the house. I want to be like other people, going off to work each morning. I just want to be with adults. I know it's not going to be easy, but I also know I can do it."

We knew she was right then, but we know it now even more. The phone call we got right after Jackie left let us in on something that she was about to learn. Jackie's daughter's pediatrician's office called, hoping to catch her before she left. They told us that they would try her at home later, then added that they wanted to offer her a job as receptionist in the office. "She'd be just great here," the secretary added. "She is so young and full of energy; she's great with kids and she's got a good heart."

"Well put," we thought. "Very well put."

$$\vee$$

The Cancer Tie-in

While there are several chronic diseases more destructive to life than cancer, none is more feared.

—Charles Mayo

Cancer: Even the word frightens us. The media may tell us about improvements in outcome and increased chances for survival, but their assurances have little or no impact on the terror that may wait within. Cancer: Its definition is familiar, its cause somewhat obscure, and its power immense. Most of us would rather be told that almost anything else was wrong with us; we could handle almost anything except cancer.

Many of the fears surrounding cancer are quite appropriate; some are not. The confusion, which lies somewhere in the middle, can be deadly. If you do not understand what causes cancer and what you can do to help prevent it, you can spend your whole life needlessly giving up pleasures in the vain hope of lowering your risk, only to find out, when it's too late, that you were very wrong.

> You can spend your whole life
> needlessly giving up pleasures
> in the vain hope of lowering your risk
> only to find out, when it's too late,
> that you were very wrong.

Even worse, while trying to avoid false cancer culprits, you may unknowingly be exposing yourself to the real villains. Just as a child trying to avoid a barking dog may back into a busy street and put himself at greater risk, in the same way you may unknowingly be adding risk factors for cancer to your life by unthinkingly trying to avoid others.

> **While trying to avoid false cancer culprits,**
> **you may unknowingly be exposing yourself to the real villains.**

Most of us, for instance, try to lower our blood cholesterol levels without considering whether this is an appropriate action for us to take. We rarely, if ever, question if this is right, for *us,* given our family and medical history and our personal set of risk factors. Instead, we take the "it couldn't hurt" standpoint, assuming that there are general risk-reducing actions we should take that cannot hurt us and, most important, will make us feel better.

The "it can't hurt" philosophy can be wrong, dead wrong. Each action we take, even those we assume "can't hurt," can have an impact on our bodies, our health, and our future. Lower cholesterol levels, for instance, have been shown to go along with an *increase* in risk for colon cancer. As you lower your levels of blood cholesterol (below 180 mg/dl) your chance for colon cancer rises.

> **The "it can't hurt" philosophy can be wrong, dead wrong.**

This does not mean that you should intentionally go out and try to increase your cholesterol in order to try to reduce your risk for colon cancer or that a low cholesterol level itself causes colon cancer; the impact of high cholesterol levels can have serious effects on many other disorders. It is important to understand, however, that risk-reducing actions should not be taken lightly and should be chosen carefully, with *your* personal health risks in mind.

Any risk-reducing information you read or hear, therefore, includ-

You're already lugging a backpack and a gym bag—you certainly don't need five extra pounds. If you're fed up with carrying the weight around (and gaining it back every time you lose), then you need a diet that takes off five pounds for *good*.

A strict plan is not the way to go. When you drastically cut back on food, your body slips into starvation mode, burning fewer calories in an effort to preserve fat it thinks it needs. As a result, weight loss quickly tapers off—and hunger makes you tired and cranky.

What to do instead? Go slow. On our plan, you won't feel hungry and you'll consume enough calories to stay out of the starvation zone. You should lose at the steady rate of about a pound a week—and research suggests that pounds lost gradually are more likely to stay off. Plus, you'll be eating lots of fruits, vegetables and fiber. If you need to lose ten pounds, you can stay on the plan for up to three months; if you want to lose more, ask your doctor about a long-term method.

It Doesn't Even Feel Like a Diet

Here's the deal: No more counting calories or fat grams. Instead, mix and match choices from six food groups and indulge in unlimited amounts of "freebies." Combine the foods any way you like. The only rules are: (1) Eat all of the recommended servings from each food group every day, and (2) watch portion sizes carefully. (For example, a bagel is two grain servings even though it's only one bagel.)

The Fitness Factor

Of course, your exercise routine (or lack of one) has a lot to do with how much you can eat. If you exercise lightly–walking for a few minutes each day or taking aerobics once or twice a week–follow the basic plan. But if you're working out for half an hour or more three times a week (sweating out a step class, walking, running or lifting light weights), you need more calories. So treat yourself to all of the supplemental portions (listed as "add 1," "add 2," etc.) on the eating plan. Now, that's a real incentive to exercise.

Asparagus, 4 spears
Beans, green, ½ cup
Broccoli, ½ cup
Cabbage, ½ cup
Carrot, 1 medium
Cauliflower, ½ cup
Corn, ½ cup
Eggplant, cooked, ½ cup
Green pepper, ½ cup
Potato, white or
sweet, 1 small
Spinach, raw, 1 cup
Tomato, 1 medium
Tomato juice, 6 oz.
Zucchini, ½ cup

GRAINS 5 per day/add 2

Bagel, ½ medium
Bread, any kind, 1 slice
Cereal, wheat or corn flakes,
1 cup
Cereal, hot, 1 cup
Corn tortilla, 1
English muffin, ½
Grains, couscous or bulgur,
½ cup cooked
Muffin, bran or corn, 1 small
Pancake, 1 medium
Pasta, ½ cup cooked
Pita bread, ½ medium
or 1 mini pita
(continued)

DAIRY 2 per day (take a 600-mg calcium supplement daily while on the diet to make sure you get enough)

Buttermilk, 1 cup

Frozen yogurt, fat free, 1 cup

Hot cocoa, artificially sweetened and made with 1% milk, 1 cup

Milk, low fat (skim or 1%), 1 cup

Pudding, artificially sweetened, made with skim milk, 1 cup

Yogurt, plain nonfat, 1 cup

Yogurt, artificially sweetened nonfat, 1 cup

EXTRAS 4 per day/add 1

Apple butter, 2 Tbs.

Avocado, 2 Tbs.

Beer, one 12-oz. light beer

Chocolate-chip cookie, 1 small

Crackers, 4

Cream cheese, 1 Tbs.

Croutons, ¼ cup

Fig bar cookie, 1

Ginger snap, 1

Honey, 2 tsp.

Jam, 2 tsp.

Salsa

Sprouts, alfalfa or bean

Radishes

Vinegar, any flavor

low-fat dressing = **1 extra**

1 orange = **1 fruit**

How your favorite meals fit in To use this plan effectively, you'll need to start thinking about how many portions of vegetables, protein, grains, etc., the meals you normally eat contain. (Don't worry—it's easier than counting calories!) Here, we've analyzed three meals:

1 freebie

2 grains, 2 extras

1 fruit

∧ **Basic Breakfast:** A bagel with cream cheese, coffee and juice

2 veggies, 2 extras

∨ **Take-out Lunch:** Turkey on whole wheat with mustard, lettuce, tomato; coleslaw, nonfat frozen yogurt

2 grains, 4 proteins, 2 freebies

1 veggie, 2 extras

1 dairy

1 grain

∧ **Vegetarian Lasagna Dinner:** Made with spinach and zucchini, low-fat mozzarella and part-skim ricotta cheese; plus a salad and roll on the side

3 freebies, 1 veggie, 1 ex

2 grains, 3 veggies, 4 proteins

ing that which is presented in this book, should be incorporated with the help of your personal physician so that you can choose what is right for *you* as an individual.

If, for instance, you are a Profactor-H Positive woman, you may have special cancer-related risks. We will help you understand them and what you can do to help reduce your risk for them, but, in the end, you must consider your own history, needs, and lifestyle factors in making your own choices.

If you are a Profactor-H Positive woman, you may have special cancer-related risks.

What you are afraid of most may not be most important. Try to look rationally at your own risks and individualize the Profactor-H Program in order to best provide yourself with the health and long life and peace of mind that we all seek.

When Cancer Is a Matter of Opinion

In his 1988 *The Surgeon General's Report on Nutrition and Health,* Dr. C. Everett Koop defined cancer as "a group of conditions of uncontrolled growth of cells originating from almost any tissue of the body." Yet the determination of cancer is not always that simple.

A diagnosis as to whether or not a sample of tissue is *malignant* (cancerous) or *benign* (not cancerous) is usually made by a pathologist—a specialist in determining the nature and cause of disease. The diagnosis of cancer often depends on the pathologist's opinion. The pathologist examines a section of tissue or a smear of body fluid and looks for certain telltale signs. Yet the diagnosis of cancer is not always clear-cut. Some indicators for cancer may be present, while others may not. The sample may not necessarily represent the entire area that is in question, or there may be unusual characteristics to the sample.

Imagine for a moment that you are a pathologist and the diagnosis is up to you. You look at a slide through your microscope in order to determine whether or not there are cancerous cells in the tissue sample you have been given. Let us say that you have been taught that, in general, three important changes occur in cancers of the type you are looking for. You look through your microscope and see only two of the three signs. The tissue does not qualify as cancerous, though it is not "normal" either.

The patient from whom this sample was taken is going to expect a yes-or-no determination, and this diagnosis will help decide whether surgery and chemotherapy or radiation will take place or whether no action at all will be taken. Even if the material is classified as "atypical," "suspicious," or "precancerous," the patient's attending physician, using the pathology report, will have to make the decision whether or not, at this time, to treat the patient as if he or she has cancer. Different pathologists and attending physicians may have different opinions and may render different diagnoses. Based on different diagnoses, different choices could be made that could ultimately mean the difference between life and death for the patient.

> **It is important to understand that the diagnosis of cancer is often simply that: a diagnosis, an opinion, an evaluation, a judgment, a conclusion.**

It is important to understand that the diagnosis of cancer is often simply that: a diagnosis, an opinion, an evaluation, a judgment, a conclusion. In the same way, a diagnosis that a specimen is benign, not cancerous, is often likewise an opinion.

Since the choices that are made regarding any future treatment or nontreatment are often based in part on the pathologist's diagnosis, it is important to communicate with your doctor. You might want to understand whether the biopsy or sample provided the pathologist with enough information for a clear-cut diagnosis and how sure the pathologist was of the diagnosis that he or she made. Second and even third opinions can be very valuable. Some physicians may choose to use the same slide or sample or require a new one. At each step you should have a primary physician with whom you can communicate and who will help you to coordinate all of the information and will assist you in making these most important decisions.

With this in mind, let us look at what scientists know about the causes of the abnormal growth patterns we call cancer.

Cancer is defined as the abnormal growth and multiplication of cells. In time, if they are not contained, cancer cells usually invade, interfere with, or destroy surrounding tissue. When cancer spreads to other parts of the body it is said to have *metastasized.*

Tumors are abnormal masses that perform no life-benefiting function. Some tumors are benign; they do not contain cancer cells. Some tumors are malignant; they do contain cancer cells. The location of a tumor, its size, and its rate of growth can be as important to a patient's health as the diagnosis of cancer versus not cancer.

The location of a tumor, its size,
and its rate of growth
can be as important to a patient's health
as the diagnosis of cancer versus not cancer.

A benign tumor that is pressing against a critical blood supply to the brain, for instance, can be more threatening than a slow-growing malignant tumor that is neither spreading nor impacting on any other part of the body. The patient who listens only long enough to hear a determination of "cancer" or "benign" may be missing essential information. The diagnosis is important, but it is far from all that must be known and understood.

Playing by the Numbers

The incidence of cancer, in general, appears to be on the rise, yet the statistics and the ways in which they are being manipulated make it almost impossible to gain any meaningful overview.

According to *The Surgeon General's Report on Nutrition and Health,* cancer accounted for a little over 22 percent of all deaths in the United States in 1984, and an American born in 1985 has approximately a 30 percent chance of eventually dying of cancer. At the same time, we are told that cancer rates based on "age-adjusted totals" have remained stable over the last thirty to forty years. Clearly, these statements appear to be contradictory.

How can cancer rates be stable and our chances for cancer be rising? The answer to this question may lie in the ever-changing categories that are being established by statisticians for their tables and presentations. "Age-adjusted totals" allow for statistics to be molded and folded for legitimate and not-so-legitimate purposes. Current cancer statistics delete respiratory cancer rates from their counts. Respiratory cancer statistics were deleted, supposedly, because they included cancers due to cigarette smoking. We believe that removing respiratory cancer rates from statistical counts provides an artificially low cancer rate by not including cancers that are the result of air pollution and radon exposure as well. We are not even sure why cancers due to smoking, firsthand or secondhand, should be removed from the statistics.

While the statistical tables make it appear that cancer rates are stable, these numbers may reflect reality or they may, instead, reflect statistical manipulations that may be legitimate or may, in fact, have been designed to make us feel a bit more secure.

When it comes to cancer, not all of us are created equal. The incidence in rates of cancer can change depending on, among other things, age, race, gender, lifestyle, and economic level. In some cases, rates for specific cancers can differ by as much as 100 times, or 10,000 percent, depending on these factors. In men, the most frequent locations of cancer are in the lung, prostate, and digestive tract. In women, the most frequent locations are in the breast, uterus, and digestive tract. Age and lifestyle choices can strongly affect the incidence and death rates associated with these cancers.

The chance of getting cancer is higher in blacks than in members of other minority groups or in whites. The higher rate of cancer is particularly pronounced in black males. When blacks do get cancer, in general, they also have the lowest survival rates. The differences in black versus white cancer rates may be due in great part to social and environmental, rather than biological, differences. Overall cancer rates are the lowest in Native Americans, though there are strong variations in the types of cancer and the specific tribal group.

Given the impact of social and economic factors and recent changes in statistical categories, it can be virtually impossible to make sense out of population cancer statistics. By understanding what causes cancer you can, however, find out which risk factors are most relevant to you and what you can do about them.

A Double Standard of Risk

What has been shown to increase your risk for cancer? The list seems virtually endless. Food, food additives, alcohol, level of activity, genetic factors, weight level, environmental factors, stress, personal loss, hormonal levels, medications, and many other influences have, at one time or another, been linked to a higher incidence of cancer. The scientific conclusions are questionable, to say the least, and in many cases they are in complete conflict, one with the other.

In some scientific journals, for instance, you will find articles that link dietary fat intake to a higher incidence of breast cancer. At the same time, in other journals, you will find reports that indicate that no relationship between dietary fat and breast cancer was found. You might even find reports that certain kinds of fat decrease the risk for cancer. The same conflicts that have been found in the breast cancer–dietary fat controversy remain true for other risk factors for cancer as well.

In some cases, scientists are reporting opposite findings about the same risk factor for the same kind of cancer. What do you do? To whom do you listen?

In some cases, scientists are reporting opposite findings about the same risk factor for the same kind of cancer. If, in addition, you look at risk factors related to the incidence of cancer as a whole, you are probably going to find that almost any risk factor has completely contradictory findings and opinions being published at the same time.

What do you do? To whom do you listen? The first step is to learn which cancers may hold greater risk *for you* as an individual and what you can do to reduce these risks.

For the Profactor-H Positive woman, the risk for breast cancer and for benign and malignant tumors of the ovary and uterus (*endometrial neoplasms*) may be greater than for other women.

Groundbreaking research is uncovering Profactor-H as a key stimulator of growth in these hormone-dependent types of tumors. In 1990, in the journal *Onkologie,* Dr. P. Unterberger and his colleagues studied breast cancer in 752 patients. They found that individuals' weight and blood fat levels, age, and menopausal status had no relationship to the spread of cancer to other parts of the body. They did, however, find a strong relationship of Profactor-H to the spread of cancer.

Two years later, in 1992, Dr. B. A. Stoll and Dr. G. Secreto, two London cancer specialists, informed the medical and scientific communities of the discovery of new markers for increased risk for breast cancer. Profactor-H, they reported, can cause hormonal imbalances that stimulate the growth of abnormal cells in the breast, in particular cancerous cells.

But breast cancer growth appears to be only one of several cancers that scientists are linking to Profactor-H. In 1990, Dr. Yoichi Sugiyama, a specialist in gynecological cancers, reported that in addition to Profactor-H's being linked to excess weight, polycystic ovary disease, diabetes mellitus, and high blood pressure, it may also be linked to growth of cancers of the ovary and uterus. Only three years earlier, Dr. J. F. Randolph and his research team had uncovered the same connection, linking Profactor-H to an increase in both benign and malignant tumors of the uterus and ovary.

Cancer-Enhancing Foods?

In some cases, Profactor-H's cancer-producing potential appears to be strongly related to the types of foods we choose. When a Profactor-H Positive person consumes simple sugars such as table sugar, high fructose sweeteners, corn syrup, glucose (a typical ingredient in high fructose sweeteners), and even fruit or fruit juices, the Profactor-H response can have a powerful and deadly effect on cancer growth. In the December 1991 issue of *The British Journal of Cancer,* Dr. D. Yam and his research team described their examination of growth of cancer cells in animals fed fructose (fruit sugar) and glucose. Malignant tumors increased 83 percent and 57 percent in size, respectively, they reported. Summing up their findings, these scientists reported that though Profactor-H has already been well established as a cancer growth enhancer, it may, in addition, for those who enjoy fruit and fruit juices, lead to the development of these tumors.

Dr. Faiz Kakar and his prestigious research team, reporting in *Clinical Nutrition,* documented similar increases in cancer growth in Profactor-H Positive animals that had been fed simple sugars. Scientific findings such as these led *The Natural Healing Newsletter* to conclude that Profactor-H ". . . acts like a powerful fertilizer to tumor cells, greatly speeding up the growth of the harmful cells."

Profactor-H ". . . acts like a
powerful fertilizer to tumor cells,
greatly speeding up the growth of the harmful cells."

Weighing the Risks

For more than thirty years researchers have been reporting that, in addition to what you eat, how much you weigh is a major risk factor for breast cancer. Recently, however, it was discovered that most people who are overweight are also Profactor-H Positive. It became essential to distinguish which was the "true" risk factor, excess weight or Profactor-H, and several scientists set about to do just that.

In 1991, Dr. D. M. Klurfeld and colleagues of the Wistar Institute of Anatomy and Biology in Philadelphia informed physicians and scientists alike that, as a result of their research, they found that body fatness was *not* directly associated with risk of the development of cancer. Instead, they reported, Profactor-H, and its capacity to stimulate growth, rather than an individual's body fatness, appeared to determine tumor development. Dr. P. F. Bruning in his 1992 report, published in the *International Journal of Cancer,* concluded that in over 750 women studied, Profactor-H was the significant risk factor for breast cancer rather than weight or body fat distribution.

Like high sugar intake and excess weight, many other risk factors for cancer, including smoking, diabetes, high dietary fat, stress, and others, are all linked by a common connection: Profactor-H. This research is still in its infancy, but it appears that Profactor-H, with its growth-promoting ability, not only links these risk factors but may soon help to reveal what goes amiss in the many processes we call cancer.

Smoking, diabetes, high dietary fat, high sugar intake, and stress are all risk factors for cancer and are all linked by a common connection to Profactor-H.

For women, Profactor-H already appears to provide an important understanding in the prevention and treatment of breast, ovarian, and uterine cancers. For men, the research is just beginning, but the connection of Profactor-H to many already identified risk factors is clear and strong.

Profactor-H and Cancer: Reducing Your Risk

In the body as a whole, insulin, as the saving hormone, signals you to eat and take in more energy. On a microscopic level, it tells your cells to take in food energy, and as they do, many cells grow larger or multiply. In balance with glucagon, insulin's signals work perfectly.

When insulin is present in excess or remains in the blood for long periods of time, however, you become Profactor-H Positive. Your high levels of insulin can turn against you, working as a profactor (a first factor, a connecting cause) for many diseases. The excessive growth-promoting qualities of Profactor-H can now destroy the very balance that insulin was designed to create.

When Profactor-H overstimulates your cells to grow and store energy, it may lead to carbohydrate cravings, easy weight gain, diabetes, plaque formation and atherosclerosis, heart disease, stroke, high blood pressure, and many other diseases and risk factors. In the same way, in the right environment, Profactor-H may activate the waiting genetic signals that tell cancer cells to grow and divide abnormally. Profactor-H may help turn on a dormant cancer gene and then supply the new tumors with the energy they need to thrive . . . and to spread.

Profactor-H may help turn on a dormant cancer gene
and then supply the new tumors
with the energy they need to thrive . . . and to spread.

In the medical and scientific journal studies presented here, you have seen reports of research linking Profactor-H to several forms of cancer, as well as to the growth of tumors in general. In some cases, as in breast cancer, the cancer-causing effect of Profactor-H may be linked to other substances (such as simple sugars). In some cases, Profactor-H may make the body more susceptible to the impact of *carcinogenic* (cancer-producing) substances in our food, in our bodies, or in the environment. In other cases, Profactor-H stands alone, for scientists are now reporting its ability to stimulate tumor cell growth.*

In all of these cases, ridding yourself of Profactor-H may be a vital step in reducing your risk for several forms of cancer. The Profactor-H Program will help you begin.

The Profactor-H Program was designed to help lower your risk of

---

*K. G. Mountjoy and I. M. Holdaway, *Cancer Biochemistry and Biophysiology,* 1991.

breast cancer and cancer of the uterus and ovaries (endometrial cancer) by eliminating an important link to these problems. Disabling Profactor-H's powerful ability to stimulate tumor cells to grow depends on stopping Profactor-H—dead in its tracks.

Disabling Profactor-H's powerful ability to stimulate tumor cells to grow depends on stopping Profactor-H—dead in its tracks.

For over nine years, both our research and our lives have been dedicated to understanding how Profactor-H works and, most of all, to developing methods to prevent and reverse it. The Profactor-H Program is the product of all of our research. The simple, livable guidelines of the Program will help stop Cofactor-p from producing and releasing too much insulin into your bloodstream. They will help insure that Cofactor-r allows your body to freely move insulin out of your bloodstream. The result is a well-balanced and Profactor-H free body.

You may never know to what extent the Profactor-H Program has helped you to prevent or reverse cancer. You may never realize how critical this Program was to your health and well-being. And that is our wish. As you travel through life, healthy and worry-free, may you never realize how well-timed and vital this choice really was.

You may never realize how crucial this Program
was to your health and well-being.
And that is our wish.

Always Fighting: Melissa's Story

"When I signed up to be part of your research program three years ago," Melissa announced, "my only concern was my weight. Now"—her voice trailed off—"I wish that was the only thing on my mind." Pretty and pert, rounded but well-proportioned, Melissa C. sat facing us with an open, honest, and very vulnerable face.

Her short dark hair curled around her face and capped off a typical "Campbell's Soup Kid" look. Though in her late forties, Melissa looked more like a girl than a woman, and the directness and power of her next statement echoed in the room.

"I have cancer," she said. "Breast cancer."

"Could you tell us more?" we ventured.

"I'm afraid it's related to something I'm doing or eating. I'm afraid I am making it worse and no one can tell me what to do. Nobody seems to know what is going on. I'll change anything I need to, I just don't want to die."

So began a long and difficult meeting. Like so many of us, Melissa's feelings and the facts were so entwined that it was almost impossible, at times, to separate them.

After some discussion, we learned that two of Melissa's aunts had died of breast cancer. Both had been overweight and she connected their weight and their illness in a cause-effect manner. "I told myself that if I could keep my weight down, I would not get cancer too, but I couldn't and now, you could say, I got what I deserved."

In the hope of breaking what she thought was a weight–breast cancer connection, Melissa tried to bring her weight down in the usual ways. "I tried to eat sensibly," she sighed. "Each day I would promise myself I would eat like a normal person and I'd try, I'd really try, but sooner or later I'd lose control. I tried low-fat diets a few times, but I just can't seem to stick with them. Not totally. I mean I'll eat margarine instead of butter, though I think they're the same in terms of fat, and I'll eat only a little and I'll always choose 2 percent milk instead of regular, but I don't know if it makes any real difference in the end."

We asked her about the cancer treatment itself. "They did a lumpectomy and removed the glands under my arm, and after the chemotherapy they told me I have a good chance of cure. But here is the point." She moved forward in her chair. "If they don't know what caused it in the first place, if it's something I'm doing, then I'll just keep doing it and I'll just get it again.

"The way things stand I'm always fighting—fighting to keep my weight down, fighting to eat right, fighting to eat healthy foods, fighting to stay alive. And no matter what I do, I feel like I'm doing something that could be contributing to the cancer in some way. Don't you see, whatever I do is wrong. I even wonder if all this worrying itself could be contributing to the cancer coming back in some way."

Melissa's concerns were real and her feelings and fears needed to be addressed. Though her assumption of cause and effect of weight on breast cancer was not exactly on target, it was easy to see why she would make the connection.

We explained that the link between excess weight and breast cancer seemed to be through a third factor, Profactor-H, which may lead to hunger, weight gain, *and* breast cancer growth. And the foods you eat, we told her, may affect your chances of cancer growth but not in the way you think.

> The foods you eat may affect your chances of cancer
> growth but not in the way you think.

We gave Melissa a Profactor-H Evaluation and found her to be at High Risk for Profactor-H. "In the Profactor-H Positive person like you," we explained, "carbohydrate-rich foods, especially when eaten frequently or in the form of simple sugars, greatly increase your chances of Profactor-H and the disease and risk factors associated with it. The insulin levels that are the hallmark of Profactor-H have been referred to as fertilizer for cancer growth, and while there's no guarantee that reducing your Profactor-H risk will assure you of never getting cancer again, it would make a great deal of sense to do all that you can to increase your likelihood of living cancer-free."

We cautioned Melissa to remember that there may be many causes of breast and other cancers but added that, with her personal physician's approval, it really did make sense to begin the Profactor-H Program as soon as possible.

Melissa's motivation was outstanding. She flew through the Options, adding a new one almost every week. "I feel great," she told us after one month. "My energy is high, my weight is dropping, and I feel better than I have for as long as I can remember. I know this is right for me. I can feel it. Nothing has ever felt this good."

Within a few months Melissa had progressed to the Advanced Program. "It's so easy; I can't believe it. I never had much discipline—so I guess I just had to find a program that didn't require it. It's wonderful."

A little while ago, Melissa passed her five-year anniversary—cancer-free. "This is the day I've been waiting for," she said. "I knew I could do it." Without the hunger that used to be part and parcel of Melissa's day, her weight dropped to normal without effort. "I love it. People look at me and tell me that I'm getting too skinny." She laughed. "I'm not. I'm right on target but it's fun anyway. And I'm still eating the food I love. My Risk-Reducing Options take so little effort I never notice them. Best of all, now I enjoy every day."

If all goes well, we will never know how much the Program has done for Melissa. Neither will she. She will simply continue to enjoy each day for a very, very, very long time.

CHAPTER 10

The Blood Sugar Seesaw: Diabetes and Hypoglycemia

Man may be captain of his fate, but he is also the victim of his blood sugar. —Wilfrid G. Oakely, M.D.

With experience and confidence you slip into the driver's seat, start the car, and head down the road. As you continue to steer, you seem to take on an observer's role, watching your body do a job far more complicated than your mind could ever consciously control. You move the steering wheel this way and that, adjusting to curves, traffic, changes in speed, and the feel of the road. In order to handle this commonplace but incredibly complex task, you coordinate sensation and perception and then respond, all without thought. Even if you do not know how to drive, the procedure is familiar and predictable.

Every day, your body adjusts to the requirements of many such familiar tasks and you respond, effortlessly and often without awareness, to unexpected changes or interruptions. And, most of the time, all works as it should.

In the area of blood sugar regulation too, when everything goes right, your body maintains ideal levels without an awareness on your part.

As you begin to eat, in anticipation of the food energy you are about to receive, your body releases insulin into your bloodstream. The insulin waits there until the food that you take in is turned into a simple sugar that your body can use. This simple sugar, *glucose,* is your body's main source of energy. As the sugar enters your blood-stream, insulin helps to move it to different parts of your body where it enters cells and is used immediately or stored away for future use. Insulin helps open doors to the cells so that the blood sugar can freely enter.

Insulin's ability to help maintain an ideal balance between available blood sugar for immediate use and the blood sugar that is stored away is vital to your health and well-being.

If you are Profactor-H free, your insulin level remains in balance and a portion of the sugar in your blood is ushered to the cells that need it, a portion of the sugar is stored away for future use (in the liver and fat cells), and the remaining sugar stays in the blood-stream, available for use in the near future.

But sometimes things go wrong.

If you are Profactor-H Positive, your excess insulin may be leading you, step by step, to hypoglycemia or diabetes. Profactor-H acts like the typical playground bully, running this way and that, upsetting the insulin-sugar balance, tipping the blood sugar seesaw first in one direction, then in the other.

> Profactor-H acts like the typical playground bully,
> upsetting the insulin-glucose balance,
> tipping the blood sugar seesaw in this direction or that.

There are many causes of hypoglycemia. In some situations, blood sugar levels decrease slowly during a period without food (*fasting hypoglycemia*). Under other circumstances, in particular after eating, your body may move too much sugar out of your bloodstream and too little blood sugar is left to meet your body's immediate needs. The condition is called *reactive hypoglycemia*.

As the far-too-thrifty man who puts all of his paycheck in the bank may find himself with too little money to live on, in reactive hypoglycemia your overly frugal metabolism may channel too much of the sugar out of your bloodstream, often into waiting fat cells, and leave you without enough energy to carry on your daily activities. In reactive hypoglycemia, some people report that their blood sugar levels drop within a short time after eating, but, more often, the drop in blood sugar occurs after about two hours.

In reactive hypoglycemia, Profactor-H is often the reason that too much sugar is swept out of your bloodstream too quickly. Blood sugar is channeled into your liver and fat cells for future use while other cells that need it immediately, or will need it in the near future, may be robbed of their vital source of energy. They, and you, may no longer be able to function well.

You may begin to feel light-headed and weak, anxious or irritable, dizzy or confused, lose concentration, have heart palpitations, or feel intensely hungry. You may feel weak or start to perspire profusely. Through these symptoms, your body is telling you that it is not getting the energy it needs.* Like some mad miser, Profactor-H has taken the energy you need now and put it out of your reach.

In reactive hypoglycemia, Profactor-H may sweep too much of your sugar out of your bloodstream too quickly and you are left literally starving for the food you ate a few hours ago.

Diabetes: Caught Behind Closed Doors

In the early stages some diabetics may suffer from hypoglycemia. Over time, however, the body may attempt to protect itself from Profactor-H by reducing the number of doors through which sugar can leave the bloodstream and enter the cells. With fewer exits, much of the blood sugar literally has no place to go and so builds up (or rather backs up) in the bloodstream. While the kidneys may

---

*Similar symptoms can often signal several different disorders. Consult with your physician to determine if low blood sugar due to Profactor-H is the only source of your symptoms.

You may feel better for the moment after eating, but insulin levels will quickly rise too high once again, beginning the insulin-dominated cycle all over again. As the Profactor-H cycle repeats, blood sugar levels rarely ever get a chance to rise and fall in a normal and healthful balance.

remove some of the excess blood sugar and empty it into the urine, if diabetes is not treated, high levels of sugar and insulin remain in the blood, unable to supply the cells of the body with the energy they so desperately need.

Diabetes mainly affects two different age groups. Children below the age of fifteen are more likely to get Type I diabetes (commonly called *juvenile-onset diabetes* or IDDM*) and adults are more likely to get Type II (often called *adult-onset diabetes* or NIDDM*). Both types of diabetes are the result of having more sugar in your bloodstream than your body can handle, and both types of diabetes, if not well controlled, can lead to serious physical problems.

In diabetes, Profactor-H may help cause cells to shut their doors—doorways that are used to allow sugar to leave the bloodstream. If too much sugar remains in your bloodstream, your body cannot function well.

In general, unless we indicate otherwise in this book, when we use the term *diabetes* we will be referring to adult-onset (Type II, NIDDM) diabetes only. The research on which this Program is based supports its use for adult-onset diabetics only.**

Hypoglycemia: The Unfair Disadvantage

Statistics about hypoglycemia appear to be virtually useless. The American Diabetes Association and the Endocrine Society have is-

---

*IDDM (insulin-dependent diabetes mellitus) and NIDDM (noninsulin-dependent diabetes mellitus) are alternative names given, respectively, to Type I and Type II classes of diabetes. IDDM usually requires the injection of insulin to sustain life, while NIDDM may or may not require insulin for correction of high blood sugar levels.

**While Type I (juvenile-onset) diabetics have been known to become hyperinsulinemic because of the insulin they inject, their underlying problem stems from lack of insulin rather than an excess of it and the Profactor-H Program was not designed with them in mind. While anyone beginning a new health-promoting program should always consult with a physician, if you are a Type I diabetic, your physician will certainly have to determine whether this Program is appropriate for you given your special needs and, if this Program is recommended, may want to adapt the Program to fit your personal requirements.

sued a joint statement to the effect that hypgolycemia is probably often overdiagnosed. Indeed, some reports are questioning the very existence of hypoglycemia. This is due to the fact that several studies found that 25 to 30 percent of apparently healthy individuals had no hypoglycemic symptoms at the same time they had low blood sugar levels.

To us, as scientists, questioning the existence of a disorder because some people do not experience the symptoms is illogical, to say the least. In addition, this thinking is not typical of other areas of medical diagnosis.

Some people who have high blood pressure, for example, may have headaches or feel light-headed or experience warm flushes, while others may never know their pressure is high until they are told by their physician. For the person without symptoms, the only indicator that something is wrong with their blood pressure is the measurement taken by the physician. The fact that one patient out of four, let us say, does not have any symptoms does not mean that there is no such thing as high blood pressure or that the person without symptoms does not have it. It may simply mean that, among the many people with high blood pressure, bodies and sensitivities may differ.

To us, this new standard for diagnosing hypoglycemia is illogical, to say the least. In addition, it often puts the patient in the position of defending his or her symptoms. According to this standard, a patient who has a blood sugar level that is one half normal or who has hypoglycemic symptoms after eating may no longer be diagnosed as hypoglycemic. Now, in order to be given an "official" diagnosis of hypoglycemia, you must undergo a lengthy laboratory test in which you are given glucose to drink and then have your blood sampled at periodic intervals for the next five hours. Only when blood sugar levels of about half normal fasting levels are noted by laboratory technicians, *at exactly the same time* as the typical sweating, tremors, weakness, and other signs of hypoglycemia are experienced, will an official diagnosis of hypoglycemia be made. Given the convoluted and demanding requirements for a diagnosis of hypoglycemia, it is no wonder that meaningful statistics on how many of us have hypoglycemia are virtually unobtainable.

> The burden of proof of hypoglycemia
> now seems to have been placed on the patient.

The thinking behind this rigid procedure certainly seems flawed. In part, it is the fact that so many people have reported hypoglycemic symptoms that has led to the overly rigorous placement of proof on the patient. The logic behind the new requirement is this: (1) if so many people have it, it can't be real; and (2) if some people do not experience these symptoms when their blood sugar level is low, it can't be real either. But we know that reactive hypoglycemia is real, and for those whose hypoglycemia comes from Profactor-H, we understand why it happens and have designed this Program to help correct the Profactor-H that lies at the base of their low blood sugar levels.

> Every year, diabetes claims 6 percent
> more people than the year before;
> and things are getting worse.

Diabetes: The Other End of the Seesaw

For those concerned with the other end of the blood sugar seesaw, the statistics related to diabetes and its complications can be alarming beyond question. Since 1935, the incidence of diabetes in the United States has increased between sixfold and tenfold—that's between 600 and 1,000 percent. Every year, diabetes claims 6 percent more people than the year before; and things are getting worse. It is not coincidental that the increase in consumption of table sugar is about 700 percent for the same period of time, but we will talk more about that later. For now, it is enough to know that current recommendations appear to be failing at helping people prevent or effectively treat and control their diabetes.

Dr. Lawrence Power, Professor of Medicine at Wayne State University and director of the Metabolic Center in Southfield, Michigan, measured the effects of high-tech advances in diabetic care. His studies showed that the improvement in blood sugar concentrations in a group of diabetic patients over a ten-year period was only 1 percent—hardly measurable!

Adult-onset diabetes affects at least ten million Americans and outnumbers Type I diabetes (IDDM or juvenile-onset) by nine to one. Adult-onset diabetes usually appears late in life. It has a strong genetic component, which means that it tends to run in families.

But today, heredity is no longer destiny.
While we cannot change our genes,
we can change the way those genes affect our bodies.

But today, heredity is no longer destiny. While we cannot change our genes, we can change the way those genes affect our bodies. Each guideline in the Profactor-H Program has been designed to break your genetic connection to Profactor-H and, with it, to hypoglycemia and diabetes.

Essential Differences

If you have been told that you have diabetes, chances are your physician found one of the following: (1) that you had a very high blood sugar level together with some of the classic symptoms of diabetes, such as thirst, frequent urination, increase in food intake, change in weight level, etc.; (2) your fasting blood sugar level was high on more than one occasion; or (3) you had more than one high blood sugar level during a glucose tolerance test. In the past, urine testing for abnormal sugar levels was used to determine whether or not you had diabetes. While urine testing may alert a physician to a possible blood sugar imbalance, it is now used in combination with blood sugar testing in diagnosing diabetes.

The sugar level in your blood can be influenced by different daily activities. If you are having your blood sugar tested, be sure to tell your physician if you have been:

- Taking *any* medications
- Confined to bed
- On a restricted or low-carbohydrate diet
- Consuming large quantities of alcoholic beverages
- Involved in an exceptionally rigorous exercise regime

Gestational (pregnancy) diabetes is a special classification of diabetes. Gestational diabetes differs from adult-onset diabetes, and if you are pregnant or think that you might be pregnant, you should inform your physician before, or at the time of, testing.*

> **Adult-onset diabetes and juvenile-onset diabetes are very different. In some ways, they are almost opposite.**

Adult-onset diabetes and juvenile-onset diabetes are very different disorders. Though both adult-onset diabetes and juvenile-onset diabetes lead to high levels of sugar in the blood, in some ways the causes of these two disorders are almost opposite.

> **In juvenile-onset diabetes the body does not produce enough insulin to remove sugar from the blood and take it to cells.**

In juvenile-onset diabetes the body does not produce enough insulin to help remove the sugar from the blood and take it to cells for use or storage. In adult-onset diabetes, the body produces too much insulin or insulin is unable to leave the bloodstream or both. As it reaches Profactor-H levels, insulin causes cells to shut their doors and both insulin and sugar remain trapped in the bloodstream. As blood sugar levels rise and interfere with the normal workings of the body, a person is said to have adult-onset diabetes mellitus. In time, the pancreas, which produces insulin, may become exhausted and may stop making insulin altogether or the insulin it makes may be unusable.

---

*In addition, this Program may not be suitable for pregnant or nursing women because of their special needs. Check with your physician.

> In adult-onset diabetes, sugar is trapped in the bloodstream;
> cells do not get the nourishment they need to function normally.

In both adult-onset and juvenile-onset diabetes, the body's cells may not be able to get to the excess sugar that remains in the bloodstream, but in juvenile-onset diabetes the cause is a *lack* of insulin, while in adult-onset diabetes the cause is often the *excess* insulin levels we call Profactor-H.

Hypoglycemics: Twice Wronged

You may have heard that hypoglycemia is just "psychological" or that hypoglycemia is an overemphasized problem that seems to be in fashion these days. You may have heard that diabetes comes from not having enough insulin or comes from being overweight. And you may have heard very wrong.

> If you have hypoglycemia,
> you may have been wronged twice (at least).

If you have hypoglycemia, you may have been wronged twice (at least). First, your body's insulin imbalance may result in unexpected and powerful physical reactions, and second, there may have been times when people minimized or disregarded your symptoms. But hypoglycemia can be a real and serious problem.

In most medical dictionaries you will find a definition of hypoglycemia similar to this:

> Hypoglycemia—a deficiency in glucose in the bloodstream, causing muscular weakness and incoordination, mental confusion, and sweating.
>
> —*Bantam Medical Dictionary,* 1982

But scientists have connected low blood sugar to a far wider variety of symptoms than those described above, including headache, hunger, rapid heartbeat, anxiety, light-headedness, fatigue, tiredness or drowsiness, restlessness, a sense of uneasiness or irritability, altered awareness, and, for some, a lack of motivation.

Hypoglycemia should not be taken lightly; it is an important and powerful disorder that can affect an untold number of lives. Though there are many causes for hypoglycemia, we have found that when there is no other obvious disorder or disease, hypoglycemia may have an easily identifiable physical root: Profactor-H.

The impressive power of Profactor-H on blood sugar levels has led countless research scientists to investigate its workings and impact. Their words and accounts document their findings. Profactor-H's ability to lower blood sugar levels is potent, and scientists have found it is, by far, the most frequent *cause* of low blood sugar.

Some people experience the signs of Profactor-H–related hypoglycemia on a fairly regular basis—getting tired most days in the mid-afternoon, for instance, or getting hungry in the mid-morning, before lunch. This regular pattern of hypoglycemia often occurs about two hours after eating carbohydrate-rich foods, including breads and other starches, cereals, fruit and fruit juices, snack foods, or sweets.

Though you may never have been told officially that you are hypoglycemic, you may still have experienced its power. In *The Journal of Clinical Psychiatry,* Dr. Bonnie Spring and her colleagues reported their study of women who had no record of psychiatric hospitalizations, eating or weight problems, substance abuse, or any known blood sugar problems such as diabetes or hypoglycemia. Even these women reported noticeable tiredness and showed impaired performance on tests of concentration and speed approximately two hours after eating carbohydrate-rich meals. Even more impressive was the fact that the levels of tiredness experienced were greater after eating a carbohydrate-rich meal than after skipping lunch altogether. Dr. Spring and her research team concluded what so many of us already know: "A high-carbohydrate, low-protein meal eaten as lunch caused fatigue in healthy women two hours after eating." Profactor-H, of course, lies at the base, causing blood sugar levels to drop sharply in the hours following the high-carbohydrate meals.

Some people tell us that they do not experience low blood sugar symptoms after eating on a regular basis but find that, only on occasion, eating carbohydrates in the form of simple sugars brings on hypoglycemic symptoms. Whether regularly or on occasion, whether you respond to complex or simple carbohydrates, or both, Profactor-H may be the low blood sugar connection that can lead to hunger, cravings, and overeating as well as to the weakness, tiredness, and shakiness of hypoglycemia. Dr. Paula J. Geiselman of the Department of Psychology of the University of California reviewed many studies linking Profactor-H to low blood sugar and concluded that the Profactor-H–low blood sugar response can lead to hunger and sugar-induced overeating based on the body's own physical responses.

In some people, hypoglycemia never progresses to more serious imbalances, but in many, especially those with a family history for diabetes, hypoglycemia and the Profactor-H that may be causing it may be the first step toward adult-onset diabetes. In his 1988 *The Surgeon General's Report on Nutrition and Health,* Dr. C. Everett Koop advised that a diagnosis of hypoglycemia "may indicate the early presence of a disease such as diabetes." Dr. Maria C. Linder, in her distinguished book *Nutritional Biochemistry and Metabolism,* reported that rises and falls in blood sugar levels (which are often the hallmark of Profactor-H) "are the hallmarks of 'hypoglycemia' and may precede the development of some forms of diabetes."

Diabetes: Adding Injury to Insult

Some scientists have emphasized the role that excess weight plays in diabetes, repeating the fact that so many researchers have noted, namely that the excessively overweight are at increased risk for development of diabetes mellitus, as are relatives of diabetics. These researchers have even proposed a special blood sugar level classification for those falling into this category, one that might allow physicians and scientists to monitor their progress and health. This warning classification may be of special significance given that, as Dr. James W. Anderson notes, approximately 80 percent of those with adult-onset diabetes are extremely overweight.

It is very important, however, to understand that the fact that many people who get diabetes are overweight *does not* mean that being overweight *causes* diabetes. Many people who are overweight never get diabetes and some diabetics are of normal weight. Therefore, being overweight is not necessarily the cause of diabetes but may simply be connected to it, and the connection appears, once again, to be Profactor-H.

You see, diabetes has a strong genetic component, which means that it tends to run in families, as does being overweight. In laboratory animals, scientists have found genes that, for some, link excess weight and diabetes. So, while in the past it has been assumed that being overweight increased your likelihood of getting diabetes, it now appears that excess weight and diabetes may both be due to a single inherited genetic irregularity that causes them both.

As you will see in chapter 11, "Winning at the Losing Game," excess weight and easy weight gain are often symptoms of Profactor-H, and the same Profactor-H that causes cravings and weight gain can also cause the changes that can lead to diabetes. Excess weight may be a symptom of Profactor-H rather than the cause of diabetes. Assuming that being overweight causes diabetes can be a matter of blaming the symptom (and the victim) rather than looking for the cause. Profactor-H appears to be the common cause of both.

In addition to weight and hereditary factors, research has shown that age, stress level, smoking, alcohol consumption, blood fat levels, activity levels, fat intake, sugar intake, and many other factors may all increase your risk for diabetes and so its complications. With so many factors connected to diabetes, it is hard to avoid all of them and, in the case of age and genetic factors, impossible to escape at all.

To make matters worse, diabetes has been repeatedly shown to lead to serious and even life-threatening diseases. In the United States alone, 5.5 million persons are known to have diabetes and an estimated 5 million have the disease though, for them, it remains undetected. As Dr. James Anderson notes in the notable medical textbook *Modern Nutrition in Health and Disease*: "Diabetes is not a benign disease. It causes 50% of all amputations of the lower extremities in adults and 25% of all kidney failure, and is the leading cause of blindness in adults in the United States. Diabetes ranks sixth as a primary cause of death in the United States; when its complications are considered, it ranks third."

In recent decades the incidence of adult-onset diabetes mellitus has increased enormously, and no one can deny the fact that it has become a major health concern for many more individuals than it was in previous years. Adult-onset diabetes is often associated not only with an increased risk of blindness and kidney failure but with impaired circulation and coronary heart disease as well. "Deaths due to atherosclerosis are two- to threefold more common in diabetic than nondiabetic individuals," notes Dr. Anderson.

But diabetes' impact does not stop there. Hypertension is approximately twice as common in patients with diabetes mellitus as it is in those without. Approximately 30 to 55 percent of those with adult-onset diabetes develop high blood pressure. Stroke is up to six times more common in diabetic than nondiabetic subjects. Furthermore, those diabetic patients who have high blood pressure are twice as likely to have a stroke as are diabetics with normal blood pressure.

**At first, these statements may seem overwhelming.
But all is not what it seems.**

At first, these statements may seem overwhelming. Diabetes may look like a sentence to future illness or early death. But all is not what it seems. When you look closely, you notice that something is missing in the statistical reports. In each report, there is no inquiry as to *why* diabetes leads to so many health-threatening diseases.

This seemingly innocent question—"Why does diabetes increase your chances of developing a life-threatening illness?"—and the scientists who have sought its answer now appear to have led to the discovery of a common connection that, when corrected, may greatly reduce the risk of getting diabetes and may have changed the face of diabetes treatment forever. That common connection, the link between diabetes and these many risk factors and other diseases, is Profactor-H.

"Why does diabetes increase your chances
of developing a life-threatening illness?"
This seemingly innocent question may have changed
the face of diabetes prevention and treatment forever.

Eminent researchers such as Dr. Richard Anderson of the U.S. Department of Agriculture's Human Nutrition Research Center, as well as many others, have identified Profactor-H as the link between diabetes and cardiovascular disease, diabetes and high blood pressure, and diabetes and excess weight. Researchers such as Dr. H. R. Black of the Preventive Cardiology Program of Yale University School of Medicine and Dr. D. C. Simonson of the Harvard Medical School have identified Profactor-H as the link between diabetes and high blood pressure, heart disease, excess weight, atherosclerosis, and undesirable blood fat levels.

This country's major medical disorders—
high blood pressure, heart disease, excess weight,
atherosclerosis, undesirable blood fat levels, and diabetes—
have a common link: Profactor-H.

The reports continue to come in, almost by the day. Scientists are finding Profactor-H to be the link, the common denominator, a crucial connection to diabetes and the many diseases and risk factors associated with it.

If you already have diabetes, the Profactor-H link can be of vital importance and you should bring the Profactor-H Program to your physician immediately. Together, the two of you should work out an individualized program that is best for you.

If you are at risk for diabetes, the information you find in this book can, likewise, be crucial. Recognizing that you may be on a path leading to diabetes is particularly important now, while your blood sugar levels are normal or only somewhat above normal (impaired glucose tolerance). You, too, should take this book to your physician. The information in this chapter and in the chapters containing the Profactor-H Program itself has been written in order to help you, with your physician's guidance, to make intelligent and positive choices for the rest of your life.

Who Is at Risk for Diabetes?

If you have relatives with adult-onset diabetes or if you have reactive hypoglycemia, you are at greater risk for diabetes. If you have been told that you have impaired glucose tolerance, you are also at greater risk for diabetes. A diagnosis of impaired glucose tolerance means that you have a blood sugar level higher than normal but not high enough to be diagnosed as diabetes yet. According to criteria set by the World Health Organization, impaired glucose tolerance affects a little over 11 percent of this country's population (between the ages of twenty and seventy-four years).

If you are overweight or have cravings for carbohydrate-rich foods, if you struggle to maintain a normal weight, because all of these may simply reflect Profactor-H impact, you too may be at risk for diabetes.

Hypoglycemia and Diabetes: Reducing Your Risk

Whether you have hypoglycemia or diabetes, or want to reduce your risk for either or both, the correction of any imbalance should begin by eliminating the *cause* of the imbalance. As the Surgeon General declared in his 1988 report, control of hypoglycemia depends on finding "the cause of hypoglycemia in each individual."

If you have reactive hypoglycemia, Profactor-H has probably been sweeping too much sugar out of your blood. When blood sugar levels drop, you may feel weak or tired, hungry, or you get headaches. In order to eliminate the ups and downs of hypoglycemia, look first to the underlying cause of your hypoglycemia: If you are Profactor-H Positive, you may be eating yourself into the blood sugar blues. But the good news is that you can eat yourself out of them as well.

Scientists are discovering that, if you are Profactor-H Positive, several daily meals and snacks containing high-carbohydrate foods may trigger high insulin levels that, in turn, bring on the low blood sugar cycle.

Changing the kinds of foods you eat at some of your meals each day can correct the cause of your tiredness and hunger and can help stop your hypoglycemic symptoms. Drs. John T. Devlin and Edward S. Horton offer evidence that "when a carbohydrate-free protein meal is ingested, insulin concentrations increase slightly." With only a slight increase in insulin, rather than an extreme increase, the protein meal helps eliminate Cofactor-p. In addition, the protein meal helps correct the body's resistance to insulin (Cofactor-r) so that the body is free to build up protein in skeletal muscle rather than store the energy in the fat cells. The result is a Profactor-H free balance that prevents hypoglycemia.

Lifestyle factors such as stress, medications, illness, fever, trauma, smoking, alcohol, exercise or the lack of it, lack of sleep, even seasonal changes, may impact on your insulin and on your blood sugar levels. In the face of everyday stresses, challenges, and foods, the Profactor-H Program has been designed to help you keep your insulin levels balanced and your blood sugar levels ideal.

In 1990, scientists concluded that adult-onset diabetes is preceded by a long period, perhaps several decades, of being Profactor-H Positive.

In 1990, Dr. Steven Haffner and his colleagues reported that their own work as well as the research of other scientists led them to conclude that adult-onset diabetes is preceded by a *long period, perhaps several decades,* of being Profactor-H Positive. In addition, they note that Profactor-H may contribute to heart disease risk as well, both by virtue of its direct effects on the arterial wall and because it contributes to undesirable levels of fat in the blood and to high blood pressure.

Clearly, the time to act is now. The Profactor-H Program has been designed specifically to help you to reduce your insulin levels so that you can lower your risk for diabetes and the disease and risk factors that so often go along with it.

Whether you have hypoglycemia or diabetes or are at risk for either, any risk-reducing program should be aimed at breaking the Profactor-H connecting link. The Profactor-H Program is designed to cut the Profactor-H link . . . for life.

Long Before You Know It

It is now becoming obvious that it is the Profactor-H link between risk factors rather than diabetes itself that appears to contribute to the high incidence of heart disease, high blood pressure, and undesirable blood fat levels in diabetics. It is essential to understand that the Profactor-H link is present *before* diabetes actually appears, which means that those at high risk for diabetes no longer have the luxury of a "wait-and-see" attitude.

A Special Note: Blaming the Symptom

The average person holds a far different view of diabetes than does the physician. Most people think that if diabetics simply keep their sugar intake low, they will be just fine. Physicians, on the other hand, recognize diabetes as a serious, and sometimes uncontrollable, disease that can be health- as well as life-threatening. Unfortunately, some physicians may view diabetes as a freestanding disease. The research that you have seen here has shown you that diabetes should be regarded and treated as an important signal of a much larger imbalance.

Diabetes is not a disease that stands alone. Diabetes has been associated with so many different risk factors and diseases that, in combination with some of these disorders, it has been described as a "cluster" of diseases, all leading to higher rates of illness or early death. In the past, diabetes was believed to be the *cause* of the cluster. Recent research, however, sheds light on the probability that diabetes is, itself, simply one of the cluster of diseases, all of which spring from a central underlying problem—Profactor-H. (For more information on cluster diseases, see chapter 13.)

SIGNS OF PROFACTOR-H REACTIVE HYPOGLYCEMIA

An "official" diagnosis of Profactor-H reactive hypoglycemia calls for a five-hour laboratory sampling of blood, but here are some simple signs to help you see if you may have this blood sugar imbalance.

Within approximately two hours after eating a full meal:
 Do you feel weak?
 Do you feel uncoordinated or somewhat confused?
 Do you perspire without reason?
 Do you get hungry or have strong cravings?
 If you eat, do you eat rapidly or consume great amounts of food?
 Does your heart beat rapidly or start to pound?
 Do you feel anxious, fearful without reason?
 Do you feel irritable?
 Do you feel restless or uneasy?
 Do you lose energy, feel very tired and fatigued, find yourself without motivation?
 Do you get a headache?
 Do you feel faint?
 Do you feel drowsy?
 Do you have a strange sense of altered awareness, almost a feeling of observing your own behavior?

If you sometimes have one or more of these signs after eating, you may have Profactor-H reactive hypoglycemia.

THESE DRUGS CAN AFFECT YOUR DIABETES TEST RESULTS

Each of the following medications may have a strong impact on your blood sugar level. If, at the time they draw your blood, you are taking any medications, tell your physician.

These drugs and others can affect your blood test results for diabetes:
Acetaminophen (Tylenol and other brands)
Antismoking drugs
Antidepressant drugs
Antihypertensives (blood pressure drugs)
Aspirin
Beta blockers
Birth control pills
Chemotherapeutic drugs
Corticosteroids (steroids)
Diuretics
Female hormone replacement drugs
Heparin (blood thinner)
Morphine
Tetracycline (antibiotic drugs)
Thyroid hormones

Definitely a Win: Audrey's Story

In her brief phone call, Audrey T. had come straight to the point. Our research assistant had taken the call and relayed the urgency of the message. "I need your help. I'm an O.R. [operating room] nurse and I'm getting the low blood sugar shakes during surgery. *Please* call!"

We set up an appointment and Audrey arrived right on time. "I need your help with this before it gets out of hand."

The "this" Audrey was referring to was a mid-morning shakiness that some people experience when their blood sugar levels dip. "I've tried everything: eating 'better' breakfasts, eliminating simple sugars, even going without coffee—which I really missed—but nothing seems to help.

"The funny thing," she added, "is that the only time it didn't happen was last week when I had nothing for breakfast, but I'm sure it was just a coincidence."

We did not think it was a coincidence at all, but we spent some time learning more about Audrey's eating habits and history and the other signs she had of low blood sugar, some of which she did not know.

Audrey described her "incidents": periods of light-headedness and shakiness that came on around 11:00 A.M. "I'll be in the middle of an operation. I can't just say, 'Excuse me but I think I need to lie down' or reach in and pull a candy bar out of my pocket.

"Candy makes me feel better fast," she added, "but it almost makes me feel sick too. I can't explain it, and besides, I don't want to have to snack on candy all the time."

We asked her about other symptoms and found she showed the classic signs and patterns of low blood sugar. "I feel better when I eat, almost immediately, especially fruit or candy. But two hours later, I want to eat again. So, I go to lunch and feel fine. Then around three o'clock, I feel exhausted. All I want to do is lie down. Sometimes I'll grab a snack and that will make me feel a little better until dinner. Then after dinner, sometimes I feel like I'm dead to the world.

"I don't understand what's happening. I never used to feel like this—or, at least, only once in a while. Now it seems like I'm stuck in a rut and I can't get out."

What had "happened" to Audrey happens to a great many of us. She had upset a delicately balanced biology and ended up in a severe Profactor-H Positive state. Before this low blood sugar cycle began, Audrey had been eating well-balanced meals that, though they were high in carbohydrates, were complemented with salads and protein. Much of the carbohydrate-rich foods that she did eat were complex, foods such as whole-grain breads and pasta. ("I adore pasta and bread," she told us. "I could never get enough.") Though she was already

Profactor-H Positive, her body was still able to somewhat balance her blood sugar levels.

Then she decided that saving time and effort was more important than her own good health. She began to substitute a diet liquid formula drink for some of her meals—in particular, breakfast and lunch.

"It wasn't that I had to lose weight so much," she explained, "though it wouldn't kill me." she added. "It's just that it seemed like a great way to save time and money. I'd grab a cold can of the drink for breakfast and I'd be on my way. No muss, no fuss."

When the hospital at which she worked offered a new flexible time option, Audrey realized that by cutting out lunch she could leave an hour early. "I just selected the latest lunch option on the schedule and left then. It was great. I'd grab a carton or can of drink between operations and it would keep me going and I'd get home an hour early."

But it wasn't keeping her going. While she had no problems for the first few days or so, within a short time her blood sugar levels were rising and dropping like a roller coaster.

By the time she got home in the afternoon she was tired and irritable. Everything seemed like a chore and she began to eat ravenously.

"Everything tasted wonderful and made me feel better. I ended up gaining four pounds in less than a month—and on the very diet drinks that are supposed to help you lose weight!

"The worst thing was, when I stopped using the diet liquid formulas because somewhere inside I thought they might be the problem, the weakness and hunger and tiredness and irritability didn't go away. I had started the whole thing because I thought I could save time. I go to school two nights a week and I wanted a little extra time between work and school for myself. But after I was on it for a little while, I got so tired that I couldn't even get myself to leave the house to go to class.

"But the worst thing is the shakiness at work. It's really getting bad and I don't want to wait until something goes really wrong before . . ." She never finished her sentence. She didn't have to.

Audrey had just had her yearly physical at the hospital and there were no other obvious reasons that her physician could find for her problem.

We explained that the diet liquid formula she had been drinking was filled with simple sugars, sucrose (simple table sugar is usually the first or second ingredient), and that, combined with the other sweeteners and corn syrups they contained, these sugars were throwing her whole system off balance. Her Profactor-H levels were probably going through the ceiling and her blood sugar levels through the floor.

We asked her to try the Program for two weeks and come back, stressing that she begin by choosing Nutrition Option C— eating vegetables, salad, and protein only at lunch, so as to break the low blood sugar cycle immediately.

Audrey didn't wait for our next appointment to let us know how she was doing. A note in our hospital mailbox was waiting for us a few days later.

"The afternoon tiredness and hunger are gone. Not better, gone! The evening exhaustion is gone. Gone! What did you do and where do we go from here?"

What we "did" was to help Audrey's body remove the Profactor-H burden it had acquired so that blood sugar levels could remain adequate for her body's needs. Her next steps involved moving to Intermediate and Advanced levels of the Program, stabilizing her blood sugar for the entire day.

Five years later, Audrey still writes us notes of "Updates, News and Thanks" as she puts them. "I'm still happy and healthy and doing well," her latest note read. "I never get the shakes and I find that I'm hungry only when I haven't eaten for a while—rather than a few hours after I have eaten. I feel like I did before the whole thing started, and you know, that feels *so* good!"

"Only one problem," she added, teasingly. "When I'm cranky, I can't blame my blood sugar levels anymore. Oh, well, you win some, you lose some."

For Audrey, we knew, it was definitely a win.

$\vee$

Winning at the Losing Game

*The physician who is attending a patient has to know the
cause of the ailment before he can cure it.*
—Mo-tze (fifth–fourth century B.C.)

Weight loss. In few other areas of health care does there exist such
a lack of clear and logical thinking. Physicians may prescribe without nutritional education, scientists make discoveries that often go
unheeded, dieticians and nutritionists may make recommendations
without knowing the cause of the problems they intend to correct,
patients self-prescribe, and big business grows fat on the failures.
And the failures go on and on and on.

Currently, approximately 95 to 98 percent of people who diet and
lose weight will eventually gain it all back (or more). Still, with these
abysmal statistics known, health professionals and commercial programs recommend the same tried-and-untrue strategies for weight loss.
Or, as is the latest fad, they tell you not to diet at all, recommending
that you just eat sensibly (as if you had not tried that before).

A Simple Way Out

Imagine that you go to your doctor with a fever. Without asking
you anything about the fever, he gives you a medication that is

rather unpleasant. You take the medicine, determined that you will get rid of the fever, and though it seems to go away, it returns again. Let us say you go back to the doctor and he reprimands you or makes fun of you or doubts that you took the medicine as recommended. You might be hurt or confused or angry, to say the least. Now imagine that you find out that he recommends the same medication for all his patients with fever, no matter what the cause, and that almost all of his patients have their fever return. We will bet you would not go back to see that doctor again.

Yet, when it comes to weight loss, this is exactly what so many seem to do. People continue to use the same methods that let them down in the past, though they know they will, most likely, fail them in the future as well. They try the same diets and programs over and over again, blaming themselves for their failures and never stopping to question *why* these attempts do not keep off the weight. Like being caught in some disappointing movie that we have seen before, we keep hoping this time the story will end happily.

When it comes to weight loss, many people continue to use the same methods that let them down in the past. And when they fail, they blame themselves. The way out is simple and obvious.

The way out is simple and obvious, though most of us are so anxious to lose weight at any cost that we never stop and think about what we are doing. In order to correct a problem, you have to eliminate or correct the cause. That is it. Find out what is causing the problem, then correct it.

The Truth, the Whole Truth, and Nothing But

If you are overweight,* the unspoken assumption is that you eat "too much." Chances are, every diet you go on tries to make you lose weight by making you eat less. The assumption is that you were eating too much to begin with. Nothing could be further from the truth. The overweight have been shown to eat *no more,* and in many cases much less, then normal-weight individuals.

Though the belief that overeating causes overweight is not necessarily true, we hear these accusations repeated until we may begin to believe them. If you have some seconds at dinner or a treat or two between meals, chances are you blame yourself for overeating, forgetting that there are "naturally thin" people who eat just as much as you do, and perhaps a good deal more.

> Some overweight people have been shown to eat *no more,* and in many cases much less, than normal-weight individuals.

If you think that your weight is simply a reflection of how much you eat, you are in for a big surprise.

As far back as 1967, scientists found that what you ate did *not* necessarily determine what you weighed. Some people seemed to be "naturally thin" and have the ability to overeat without gaining weight.

---

*Obesity has been officially defined by some as 20 percent or more above one's ideal weight. This cutoff point, however, is greatly in question. Ideal weights themselves differ according to the chart that is being consulted, the year it was published, and the policies of the moment. Using a 20 percent definition of obesity, a woman who should ideally weigh 120 pounds would be considered to be obese at 144 pounds. For this reason, in paraphrased or direct quotes, the term *overweight* shall be used in place of the term *obesity* or to designate excess weight of any level.

> ## As far back as 1967, scientists found that what you ate did *not* necessarily determine what you weighed.

As far back as 1967, in the journal *American Clinical Nutrition,* Drs. D. S. Miller and P. Mumford documented the fact that some people are able to consume an additional 8,000 to 10,000 calories per week and still lose weight. One year later, the prestigious researcher Dr. E. A. H. Sims and his colleagues tested the "you are what you eat" hypothesis by overfeeding their subjects by up to 3,000 calories per day. Though the goal of the experiment was to increase these subjects' weight by 25 percent, even 3,000 extra calories per day did not bring about that level of weight gain. For those subjects, the extra calories they took in did not become excess weight; yet some of us seem to magically take in pounds from the air around us.

Contrary to what people believe—and, in some cases, want to believe—your weight may not reflect how much you eat. In 1982, Dr. J. B. Morgan and his fellow researchers found that large eaters weighed less and had a lower percentage of body fat than did small eaters. Even more amazing than his first discovery was a second finding—that these large eaters, who weighed less than small eaters, consumed almost double the number of calories of small eaters! Clearly something else, other than just food intake, was influencing the weights of these individuals. Many of us have suspected as much from our own personal experience, but it was important, just the same, to have this fact documented by reputable scientific research.

Scientists have shown that people who are overweight may not lose weight even though their food intake is greatly restricted. In 1978, Dr. J. V. Durnin reported that even under severe instances of caloric restriction, the overweight tended to maintain their excess weight levels.

> ## Scientists repeatedly show that some people are "naturally slender" and some are not.

In a fascinating study in 1984, Dr. R. Leibel of the Rockefeller In-stitute reported that normal and obese women who had been kept in similar in-patient conditions provided some startling results. He found that though both groups of women took in the same number of calories, each group maintained its original obese or normal weights, respectively. When both groups ate the *same food,* the nor-mal-weight women stayed at normal weight and the obese stayed a hundred pounds overweight. In order to lose weight, the obese women had to eat far *less* than the normal-weight women.

Despite the fact that, in general, scientists have found that a pat-tern of overeating does not necessarily go along with being over-weight, many health professionals, the media, and most of the public have a hard time believing that the excess weight you may carry may not be due to overeating.

The newest trend is to claim that the overweight eat the "wrong" types of foods. This is but another way of blaming the victim. Scien-tists know that when animals that are genetically predisposed to be obese are fed the same foods as normal-weight animals and exer-cised the same amount and in the same ways, the genetically obese animals become fat and the lean ones stay lean.

Sweeping generalities about food consumption simply do not ap-ply to the overweight. Some may crave carbohydrates and have trouble controlling their eating. Others may fight their cravings and suffer and deprive themselves. Others may say they "just like to eat." Others may swear they do not eat enough to be as overweight as they are. And they are all right.

If you are Profactor-H Positive and are overweight or tend to gain weight easily, it is essential to understand that it is not what you eat or how much you eat that may be keeping you in your weight-gain struggle but rather how *your particular* body reacts to certain foods. You are no more to blame for your weight than for the color of your eyes, but because you are Profactor-H Positive, there is a great deal you can do about it.

The Essential Element

Researchers continue to find, time and time again, that the slender person has a body that resists putting on weight and the overweight person has trouble taking weight off and keeping it off. We know these facts intuitively and we know them scientifically. Yet we still tend to blame ourselves and others for gaining weight (or not taking it off). This "blame the victim" thinking is irrational and illogical, but when answers do not come readily, we often look for a handy scapegoat—ourselves or others. Still, easy assumptions of blame crumble in the face of obvious questions:

Why are some people naturally heavier than others, even though they do not seem to overeat?

Why do some people get intense and recurring food cravings?

Why, when some people diet, do they gain the weight back almost as soon as they take it off?

Why do we eat when we feel stressed?

As we grow older, why do some of us gain weight on the same food that used to keep us at a normal, or near-normal, weight?

Why do many women have trouble losing their pregnancy-related weight gain?

Why do some women get premenstrual cravings?

Why do so many people gain weight when they stop smoking?

The answer to all these questions is usually the vague response "Metabolism." But the term *metabolism* has a meaning that is so indistinct, yet so complex, and involves so many different processes and chemicals, that to say something is due to "a slow metabolism" has no practical meaning.

Suppose, for a moment, that you found a single physical imbalance involved in the process we call metabolism and that this imbalance occurred in those people who put weight on easily or crave carbohydrates as well as in those who are stressed, in those who are pregnant or premenstrual, and in those who stop smoking. This imbalance also increases, naturally, as we grow older. You might be tempted to say that you found the essential element that repeatedly forces some of us into the battle of the bulge.

The imbalance that you would have discovered, of course, is Pro-factor-H, and in experiment after experiment, scientists are now heralding its importance.

Profactor-H has been shown to cause food to taste especially good or to cause recurring carbohydrate cravings.

In 1982, Dr. Paula Geiselman and Dr. David Novin found that in some individuals the sight, smell, taste, and eating of carbohydrate-rich foods can lead to high Profactor-H levels culminating in weight gain. Dr. D. C. Simonson of Harvard Medical School has confirmed the importance that Profactor-H plays in a hunger–weight gain cy-cle, and Dr. Judith Rodin of Yale University, Drs. T. Silverstone and E. Goodall, and many others confirm the Profactor-H–carbohydrate connection to hunger, cravings, and weight gain. Since, however, we cannot eliminate carbohydrates such as starches, snack foods, or sweets from our diets (nor do most of us want to), reducing your risk for Profactor-H can, in itself, easily break your weight-gain struggle.

In 1993 and 1994, at the American Institute of Nutrition's annual meeting, we presented our research documenting that subjects with Profactor-H Positive carbohydrate cravings experienced fewer and less intense cravings and, in addition, lost weight without struggle by changing not *what* they ate or *how much* they ate but rather the pattern of their food intake. This corrected way of eating allowed our subjects to enjoy all the foods they needed and wanted but without the hunger and cravings and weight gain that had plagued them for so long.

The vicious cycle of hunger and cravings
followed by increased energy storage (into fat cells)
is controlled by Profactor-H.
But even if you never overate,
your body may have a much stronger tendency to
put weight on easily and to keep it on.

If you are overweight, your weight, the amount of food you consume, the kinds of foods you desire, and the way your body metabolizes your food may be directly linked to Profactor-H. The vicious cycle of hunger and cravings followed by enhanced energy storage (into fat cells) may well be caused by the fact that you are Profactor-H Positive. If you have a family history of weight or eating problems, the impact of frequent high-carbohydrate meals on your particular system can be devastating, or worse, dangerous.

**If you are overweight,
your weight, the amount of food you consume,
the kinds of foods you desire,
and the way your body metabolizes your food
may be directly linked to Profactor-H.**

The Easy Scapegoat

Many different diseases are associated with obesity and, in general, excess weight is blamed as the causal factor in almost all of them. In the case of osteoarthritis, the weight connection does seem to be warranted. We can understand that being overweight may put increased demands on joints and that the pressure may, in time, lead to physical deterioration. This attribution of excess weight as a cause of disease is, however, the exception.

Most weight-related illness and associated risk factors *cannot* be logically traced back to weight as their direct cause. The media, health professionals, our families and friends, and we ourselves tend to blame or punish that which is most obvious; and underneath you may even feel that you should be blamed for your extra pounds. It is a simple and easy answer—but it is not true.

**You may blame your ill health on your weight.
It is a simple, neat, and easy answer—but it is not true.**

We, and many other scientists, have seen repeatedly that it is not excess weight itself that causes so many diseases and risk factors, but rather it can be Profactor-H's powerful and silent influence.

Many people gain weight over time, or put it on quickly during periods of stress, pregnancy, or change, only to find they cannot easily take it off. But weight gain is the most obvious symptom of Profactor-H and usually the first to appear.

Over time, additional risk factors and chronic illnesses such as high blood pressure, undesirable fat levels in the blood, diabetes, atherosclerosis, heart disease, and others may begin to appear. We will talk more about their connection in chapter 13, "The Profactor-H Cluster," when we discuss cluster diseases, but for now, we want to dispel the myth that excess weight causes so many health problems and let you see that scientists are discovering Profactor-H as the underlying connection to all of these disorders and of weight gain as well.

In 1991, Dr. G. M. Reaven of Stanford University School of Medicine reported that his research indicated that Profactor-H is commonly associated with high blood pressure in the overweight. Three years earlier, the Surgeon General of the United States noted that Profactor-H can occur in all types of obesity and may be a link connecting high blood pressure, excess weight, and high blood sugar levels. Harvard's Dr. L. Landsberg agreed, reporting that weight-related high blood pressure is the "unfortunate by-product" of a Profactor-H Positive body.

At Harvard's Obesity Conference of 1991, Dr. D. Heber told his fellow researchers that besides the fact that Profactor-H appears to be involved in excess weight gain, it appears also to be involved in weight-related adult-onset diabetes as well. Other scientists have repeatedly voiced the same findings, yet the assumption that excess weight is the cause of all medical problems is a hard belief to shake.

In 1990, Dr. R. J. Mahler's research findings seemed to sum it all up when he reported to fellow scientists that excess weight appears to be unconnected to high blood pressure and adult-onset diabetes, with the common link, instead, being Profactor-H.

Profactor-H and Weight: Correcting the Cause and Reducing Your Risk

If, in caveman times, you had extra insulin coursing through your bloodstream, you were lucky indeed. When you smelled or saw food, insulin pushed you to eat more than others. You could eat your fill and then some. If food was not available, your high levels of insulin spurred you to find food and eat well and heartily. With food in your belly, your extra insulin stored the food energy in your fat cells so that you had energy to stay alive when food was scarce.

Your ability to keep extra insulin in your bloodstream may have meant the difference between life and death. Now it means the same thing but often in the opposite direction.

Extra insulin does little harm when it occurs only on occasion. If you are Profactor-H Positive, however, your body is thrown out of balance and the regularly high levels of insulin can lead to excess weight, diabetes, high blood pressure, atherosclerosis, heart disease, and more.

Any treatment program aimed at having you lose weight without correcting the cause of your weight gain in the first place is bound for failure.

Any treatment program aimed at having you lose weight without correcting the cause of your weight gain in the first place is bound for failure.

Remember, if a weight-reducing program does nothing to correct your Profactor-H levels, it probably will not help you permanently reduce your risk factors for the many diseases associated with being overweight or help reduce your weight permanently.

The Profactor-H Program
does away with deprivation and sacrifice
because it has been designed to correct
the underlying *cause* of your cravings and weight gain.

The good news is that the Profactor-H Program can help you lose your cravings, lose weight and keep it off, and, at the same time, reduce your risk for weight-related diseases. The Profactor-H Program does away with the deprivation and sacrifice that are the hallmarks of so many diets. It is easy and struggle-free because it has been designed to correct the underlying *cause* of your cravings and weight gain.

Our Personal Victory

We have a personal, as well as a professional, interest in "Winning at the Losing Game." Together we have lost over 200 pounds (Rachael, 165 pounds, and Richard, over 35 pounds) and have maintained our normal weights for over eleven and nine years, respectively. We tell our stories in chapter 1, "New Bodies, New Hopes, New Lives."

Now that our weight is no longer a concern or struggle for us, it is still important to us to share our good fortune, our weight-loss victory, and our good health with you. That is why we have continued our research and our writing, and have brought you this Program.

Dozens of Dieting Disasters: Anna's Story

When Anna C. came to see us she was "desperate." She was getting married in six months, but she was gaining weight and her eating was "out of control." Anna was likable and her pretty face was alive and engaging. Her humor was contagious. She told her story amusingly and made us smile even while she spoke of her fear and embarrassment. Deep down, we understood the worry she could only express in jokes.

> Anna was getting married in six months, but she was gaining weight and her eating was "out of control."

Her wedding dress had had to be refitted twice already and she knew it would again be too small. She couldn't bring herself to hire a photographer, and when her father suggested that a friend might videotape the wedding, she had refused to discuss it.

Anna had started gaining weight "from the day I got engaged. So help me, I swear he put that ring on my finger and I gained five pounds. Since then I've been gaining on an average of about a pound or a pound and a half a month. But it adds up. I'm twenty pounds heavier than when I got engaged and I was about twenty pounds overweight then. I'm going crazy. I registered for one of those commercial programs where you buy the packaged meals from them. I tried it for a couple of weeks. I lost weight the first two weeks but I was starving all the time. Still I stuck to it anyway. When I didn't keep losing weight the third and fourth week I dropped it. Then I gained all the weight back in a week or so. Now I'm having more trouble than I did before I started with them."

> "All I think about is food.
> This is supposed to be the happiest time of my life and I'm miserable."

"All I think about is food. I don't know what's the matter with me. Ron is understanding about it, but I think he's worried. I think he's afraid he's going to end up with a blimp." We cringed at the term. "I can't stand it. This is supposed to be the happiest time of my life and I'm miserable. I've thought about having my jaw wired, if they're still doing that. I have this picture of me walking down the aisle, slender and beautiful, Ron slowly lifts my veil, I smile, and . . . my jaws are wired shut." It was hard not to laugh. Her image was so vivid. But beneath the image was a very frightened young woman.

Anna's Profactor-H Evaluation placed her on the border between the Mild and Moderate Risk range. Anna explained that she wasn't feeling as energetic or particularly well lately. "My doctor says I'm fine, but I feel lethargic and weepy. I don't know if it's the weight or that I just can't control myself anymore.

"When I really get going," she added, "I have to do everything except lock myself in a closet in order to hold myself in check. Something's getting worse and I'm not sure what it is."

Anna had very little family history of weight or eating problems, but from her personal history it appeared that she had dieted so drastically and so many times in the past that it looked like she had dieted herself into being Profactor-H Positive.

Anna had dieted so drastically and so many times in the past that it looked like she had dieted herself into being Profactor-H Positive.

We explained that some people appeared to upset their natural "set-point" or metabolic regulators by repeated and severe dieting. Normal in weight in the beginning, some of the people we had worked with had dieted in order to become "extra-skinny." In doing so, they took in so few calories that their bodies responded by entering "efficiency modes." If they then tried to go back to eating normal amounts of food, they found that they gained weight.

Such was Anna's history. Of normal weight in her teens, she had continuously dieted. "It was almost a competition to see which girl could be the skinniest. My mother kept telling me that I was going to make myself sick, but I didn't care. All I wanted to be was skinny. Not anorectic or anything, just really skinny. Then when I hit twenty or so, I noticed that I was having a harder and harder time staying thin. I tried diet pills and those diets you see in women's magazines. I tried eating only fruit for a couple of weeks and fasting one day a week. I'd take off four or five pounds and put them back on. Then I'd gain a pound or two and try the whole thing over again.

"I was twenty-four when I met Ron; that was two years ago. I thought I was really overweight. My doctor said I was about ten pounds too heavy, I thought I was twenty pounds too heavy, and Ron thought I was just right. Anyway, I held my weight, more or less, until I got engaged and since then it's been non-stop eating. I have this friend who's in therapy and she keeps telling me it's psychological and that maybe I don't want to get married, but that's not true. I can't wait to get married. I think that it was just that all of those diets, one after another, caught up with me, like you said, coincidentally by the time I got engaged. Anyway, I want to get married and I want to lose weight and I really need help."

We explained the Profactor-H Program to Anna, telling her that we wanted her to begin with a Nutrition Option first. We explained that she should lose no more than about 1 percent of her weight each week, about one and a half pounds would be ideal, and that she would probably be able to reduce her risk for many diseases as well.

We told Anna that most people make the mistake of trying to lose weight too fast and find that they hit "efficiency plateaus"— times when you cannot lose weight no matter how hard you try. When you lose weight too fast, we explained, your body thinks that it is starving and Profactor-H levels rise to help store any energy that might make its way in. When you don't eat enough, we explained, your body will try to conserve energy and you will find it more and more difficult to lose weight. Anna said that she understood and would follow the Program as directed.

The next week found a very happy Anna waiting for her appointment. She had no trouble sticking with her Nutrition Options, she said. The food was satisfying and her experience of hunger was "almost completely nonexistent." "It's the same feeling of lack of hunger I had when I was fasting," she said, "except that I'm eating! And I've lost five pounds."

We were not as ecstatic as Anna. Her weight loss was far too fast and we were concerned—first, as to why she was losing so rapidly, and second, with such a fast weight loss, how to keep her from rebounding or hitting efficiency plateaus.

When we asked her about her week, we found that Anna was not following the Program. In her enthusiasm, rather than choosing one Option, Anna had added all three Nutrition Options in the Beginner's Program—all at once—and far too fast to allow her body to accommodate and move easily into a lifestyle routine.

"But it's easy," she said, "no problem at all. Besides," she added, "I have to take the weight off fast. I have less than six months to lose forty pounds."

We cautioned her to move slowly so that her body had time to adjust and explained that *permanent* weight loss was the goal rather than *quick* weight loss, but her excitement was hard to contain and she was, in fact, working with her family physician, so, against our better judgment, we allowed her to continue all three Beginner's Options. We warned her that she must add Activity and Stress-Reducing Options more slowly and told her that she should not move to the Intermediate Program until she had done so. She agreed.

But the next week was a repeat of the first. Four more pounds lost made a total of nine pounds for the first two weeks. We found that she had literally taken off on her own, adding food restrictions that were no part of our Program. She was eating low-fat, low-carbohydrate foods for all meals. At times she had almost nothing but salads. She was, she admitted, using some of the rules she had learned in her many diet programs.

We took more drastic action with Anna. First, we explained that she was not, in fact, following the eating plan that was part of our Program and that would be most likely to help her in the long run. She was, instead, taking parts of the Program and changing it to meet her goals. She had added no Stress-Reducing or Activity Options and was turning a program designed for weight loss *and* health into a quick-weight-loss scheme that would probably end in failure . . . or worse.

> Instead of trusting the Program to help her,
> Anna was using the same dieting techniques
> that had failed her in the past.

Her thinking made no sense. Instead of trusting the Program to help her, she was using the same dieting techniques that had failed her in the past . . . without ever giving this Program a chance. It had been our experience, we told her, that her kind of dieting was doomed to failure and, in good conscience, we could not continue to see her if she continued to disregard our recommendations. This brought Anna to near tears.

Although she had heard us tell her to lose weight more slowly, she thought that secretly we were pleased with her "success." She was confused and upset. Again we defined *success*. Success, we explained, is sticking to a program that will reduce the frequency of your carbohydrate intake and thereby reduce your Profactor-H response. That's all we wanted. "The weight will take care of itself," we added. "If we need to adjust the plan to make you lose weight more quickly or slowly we can do it, but it should never exceed one to two pounds each week. Your weight and your health are one. They are both related to the same problem. Give yourself and your body a chance."

This time Anna seemed to hear us. She told us that she didn't like the idea of losing weight so slowly and always took it off much more quickly in the past. "And put it right back on," we reminded her. She agreed to slow her weight loss in the coming weeks and, to a large extent, stuck by her word. She was always right on the brink, pushing over the two-pound weekly weight-loss limit every few weeks. Occasionally her body would respond by going into an efficiency mode and she would remain at an efficiency plateau for a few weeks.

> She looked beautiful in her size-eight wedding dress.

Still, in the end, Anna lost her weight in about the same time that she would have if she had not tried so hard to lose it fast. She looked beautiful in her size-eight wedding dress, and after nearly four years of marriage and a year after her new baby son was born, she's "two pounds lighter and just as happy" as the day she was married.

And, we added to ourselves, healthy as well.

CHAPTER 12

$\vartriangledown$

Defusing the Blood
Pressure Time Bomb

You may delay, but time will not.   —Benjamin Franklin

High blood pressure could be called "the disease most likely to be ignored." Though we may feel a vague sense of concern if our doctor tells us that our blood pressure is "too high," this news does not typically have the same impact as being told that we have a heart condition or cancer.

Though most of us know high blood pressure signifies something that is vaguely dangerous, we lack an understanding as to how important and compelling a diagnosis of high blood pressure should be to us.

High blood pressure, technically called *hypertension,* is a health problem of enormous magnitude, and although the estimates and definitions may vary, it now appears that as many as 58 million people have been told that they have high blood pressure.

Two readings make up your blood pressure level. The top reading is called your *systolic* reading. This reading reflects the pressure that is being exerted by the blood on the walls of your arteries as your heart contracts. This is the period of greatest pressure. The bottom reading is called your *diastolic* reading. This reading reflects the pressure that is being exerted by your blood on the walls of your arteries during the period of relaxation between your heart's contractions. This is the period of least pressure.

Each of the readings provides important information individually; taken together they provide additional vital facts. Lowering systolic pressure without lowering diastolic pressure is not always a good sign. The systolic (top number) is normally about 40 points greater than the diastolic (bottom). If you bring your systolic pressure down but find that this does not lower your diastolic in proportion, this can be an important sign of danger.

SAMPLE BLOOD PRESSURE READING

120 top number is systolic reading, pressure of heart in contraction
80 bottom number is diastolic reading, pressure of heart at "rest"

Normal difference between top and bottom numbers: about 40 points.

While there can be a great deal more involved in interpreting blood pressure levels than just the numbers, we have included Classification of Blood Pressure guidelines adapted from the *The Surgeon General's Report on Nutrition and Health* (1988).

CLASSIFICATION OF BLOOD PRESSURE IN ADULTS 18 YEARS OR OLDER

(Classifications may vary according to age)

Range, mm hg   **Category***

Systolic pressure**(top number)
   less than 140   Normal blood pressure
     140–159   Borderline isolated systolic hypertension
    160 or greater   Isolated systolic hypertension

Diastolic Pressure (bottom number)
   less than 85   Normal blood pressure
     85–89   High normal blood pressure
     90–104   Mild hypertension
    105–114   Moderate hypertension
    115 or greater   Severe hypertension

   *Based on average of two or more readings on two or more occasions. Precedence of diastolic or systolic readings in the same person vary depending on other classifications. Adapted from *The Surgeon General's Report* (1988). *Surgeon General's Report* source: 1988 Joint National Committee. Blood pressure levels should be adapted according to age.
   **Categories based on systolic reading when diastolic reading is less than 90.

The Unheeded Warning

Having high blood pressure has come to be accepted in our society and, in general, we have learned to live with it—we think. But finding out that you have high blood pressure is a very important event, one that gives a warning, a chance to correct a physical problem before it is too late. And it could be your last reprieve.

> Finding out that you have high blood pressure is a very
> important event. It is a warning, a chance to correct a problem
> before it is too late. It could be your last reprieve.

High blood pressure may be a clear sign that something is going wrong in your body. It can be a serious signal that, if heeded early enough, may help reduce your risk for heart attack or stroke.

Most of us never think what high blood pressure means and how grateful we should be for knowing its importance. Instead, we begrudgingly take our medication or try to avoid salty foods and hope that it will all go away.

Most of us do not have the same attitude when it comes to cancer. If, for instance, our physician were to tell us that we had a condition that, should it remain uncorrected, could lead to cancer, we would most likely do virtually anything we could to reverse it. When we are told, however, that blood pressure can be the first stage in a life- and health-threatening process leading to stroke or heart attack, most of us are inclined to push this fact to the back of our minds and try not to think about it.

> The illusion is that time is on your side;
> if nothing has happened *so far*, you are okay.
> Nothing could be farther from the truth.

When it comes to our blood pressure, our unwillingness to take our health into our own hands is due to two misconceptions. The first is that we have all the time in the world. When we are told, for the first time, that we have high blood pressure, chances are most of us figure it will be years before any real damage is done. On the other hand, if we have been told repeatedly that our blood pressure is above normal, we probably think that since it has not hurt us so far there is nothing for us to worry about. In either case, the illusion is that time is on our side and that if nothing has happened *so far,* we are okay.

Nothing could be farther from the truth. High blood pressure is not just a sign of a problem, it is often the result of something going wrong. There is a reason that your heart has to push hard in order to move the blood along its path. High blood pressure is not only a danger sign for the future, it is a sign that a health-endangering situation may exist *right now.*

> High blood pressure is not only a danger sign for the future, it is a sign that a health-endangering situation may exist *right now.*

The statistics are staggering. Because of a second and deadly misconception, many of the 58 million people with high blood pressure do not take their condition seriously. They hold the false belief that there is very little you can do about high blood pressure.

The most prevalent form of high blood pressure is called *essential hypertension,* which is high blood pressure without a clear and certain cause. If you have high blood pressure, the chances are nine to one that you have essential hypertension. Though the *cause* of their high blood pressure is unknown, patients with essential hypertension have been told to change their diet, increase their exercise, and make other lifestyle choices in the hope that these changes would bring down their high blood pressure levels. For years, patients have continued to take their medications, watched their salt and fat intake, exercised, and told themselves that they should be satisfied with mediocre, if any, reductions in their blood pressure. Often the sacrifices may not seem to be worth the results.

Though they tried to follow their physician's recommendations for a while, many found their blood pressure levels did not respond. Sooner or later, most patients went back to their old patterns and habits; and, like so many of us, they probably blamed themselves to boot.

From their side, physicians are confirming that these same efforts do not appear to be making much headway. "Despite our efforts to identify and to treat high blood pressure over the past fifteen years," reported Dr. Norman M. Kaplan in the *Archives of Internal Medicine,* "the average diastolic blood pressure for the population at large has changed little and, in fact, has risen among white males during this time."

These dismal results are not surprising. How can you expect to correct a problem if you are not even sure of the cause? Remember, by definition, essential hypertension means high blood pressure without a known cause—how can it be assumed, then, that all the standard remedies will work to correct a cause that isn't even known? The proof is there for all to see—in general, these standard treatments are simply not working.

Today, scientists are making astounding breakthroughs in the study of high blood pressure. This information, however, is not always filtering down to the public.

But today scientists are discovering that there *is* a reason why people get high blood pressure and, best of all, that this very reason may be easily correctable—well before it is too late. This information, however, is not always filtering down to the public.

Profactor-H is being uncovered as the underlying link to high blood pressure. In 1990, a French research team headed by Dr. E. Feraille pointed to Profactor-H as the most important cause of weight-related high blood pressure, and only one year later, in 1991, Drs. Landin, Tengborn, and Smith published their research findings in *The Journal of Internal Medicine*. In this important paper, they called for fellow scientists and physicians to be aware that Profactor-H may play an important role in the development of high blood pressure. In their research summary, these well-respected scientists noted that, in addition to their experiment demonstrating Profactor-H's link to high blood pressure, they also conclude that the Profactor-H connection to high blood pressure may open up a new field for the treatment of cardiovascular disease.

Two years before the Landin team published its findings, Dr. Norman Kaplan detailed four different ways in which Profactor-H can raise your blood pressure. Each of Dr. Kaplan's Profactor-H pathways could, in itself, lead to dangerously high blood pressure, and taken together, the changes, all the result of Profactor-H, can be deadly.

Bearing the Burden of Blame

High blood pressure has long been linked to excess weight, and because these two disorders often occur together it was often *assumed* that excess weight was the cause of the high blood pressure. Family physicians have often blamed the patient for his or her high blood pressure, falsely assuming that excess weight was the cause of the blood pressure problems. The discovery of the Profactor-H connection has hopefully corrected that false assumption.

Recent scientific findings repeatedly proclaim the importance of Profactor-H as a causal factor in both excess weight *and* high blood pressure. With Profactor-H lying at the base of both high blood pressure and overweight, the finger of blame for both disorders now points to Profactor-H.

In the overweight, reported Dr. G. M. Reaven in 1991, Profactor-H is commonly associated with high blood pressure. More important, this fine researcher did not stand alone in his observation. Scientists from around the world are, at the same time, uncovering the same Profactor-H link to high blood pressure.

> In the lean and overweight alike, it is Profactor-H that is linked to the development of high blood pressure.

In 1991, an excellent review of the work of many scientists, published by Dr. J. R. Sowers in the *American Heart Journal,* specifically linked Profactor-H to high blood pressure and detailed the ways in which Profactor-H may work its blood pressure–raising power. In his conclusion, Sowers cautions physicians to reconsider pharmaceutical recommendations and carefully choose blood pressure–lowering medications that will not worsen their patients' Profactor-H levels.

> Before the discovery of the Profactor-H connection,
> researchers assumed that
> excess weight made you guilty by association.

As further proof that obesity is *not* the underlying cause of high blood pressure, researchers have found that even though a person is *not* overweight, Profactor-H continues to provide a consistent link to high blood pressure. In his twenty-year perspective study, Dr. Robert W. Stout points out that although some patients with high blood pressure are overweight and/or have diabetes, other patients with high blood pressure are not, and that these normal-weight nondiabetic patients who have high blood pressure may also be Profactor-H Positive. Profactor-H levels and blood pressure, Dr. Stout continues, are "closely related." Dr. Sowers agrees, noting that many nonoverweight adults with high blood pressure are Profactor-H Positive.

The Symptom We Call High Blood Pressure

With a growing understanding of the Profactor-H connection, the link between many other risk factors and diseases to high blood pressure becomes obvious. In his prestigious 1990 research review, Dr. Stout concluded that Profactor-H is closely associated with a cluster of cardiovascular risk factors, including high blood pressure and undesirable blood fat levels, high levels of sugar in the blood, and excess weight.

One year later, Dr. H. R. Black of the Yale University School of Medicine confirmed Dr. Stout's views, adding that during the past several years it has become clear that Profactor-H constitutes the link between high blood pressure, excess weight, and adult-onset diabetes mellitus, three conditions in which the rate of coronary artery disease is very high. Dr. Black pointedly adds that other studies have shown that Profactor-H is a potent "cardiovascular risk factor," and like Dr. Sowers, he calls for physicians to reconsider their pharmacologic recommendations in view of the fact that some medications may worsen Profactor-H levels.*

---

*Remember, if you are taking any medication, you must discuss this matter with your physician before making any change. The information presented here simply reports current research that should be discussed with your physician.

High blood pressure, once strongly associated with stroke and heart disease, is now less often seen as the *cause* of these life-threatening diseases. Today it is being recognized as a *symptom* of the underlying imbalance, Profactor-H.

> Now, high blood pressure is seen less often
> as the *cause* of life-threatening diseases as it
> is being recognized as a *symptom*
> of the underlying imbalance, Profactor-H.

Three Roads

In the past few years, we have come to a great new understanding regarding the ways in which Profactor-H can bring on high blood pressure. Profactor-H can lead to high blood pressure in at least three different ways.

> Profactor-H can lead to high blood pressure in at least
> three different ways.

First, Profactor-H stimulates the sympathetic nervous system directly, causing the heart to beat faster, blood vessels to narrow, and blood pressure levels to rise. In this first way, for the person who has a history of high blood pressure, Profactor-H often leads to chronic (ongoing) high blood pressure.

Second, Profactor-H helps to regulate salt levels in the blood. The higher the Profactor-H level, the more salt is retained. The more salt, the more water is channeled into the blood. Soon you find that even though you may have been sacrificing some of the food you love in order to reduce your salt intake, Profactor-H has overpowered all of your efforts. Your blood pressure remains high because, now, more fluid is flowing through your arteries. It's a simple law of physics.

Forcing more fluid through the same space results in greater pressure or, in this case, high blood pressure.

The third way in which Profactor-H can lead to high blood pressure is by narrowing the arteries through which the blood flows. As you have seen in chapter 7, "Fats and Fiber: Fears, Facts, and Fallacies," as well as in "Taking It to Heart" (chapter 8), Profactor-H can stimulate the production of cholesterol and the buildup of plaque in walls of arteries. The space for blood flow is decreased, and as would be expected, blood pressure rises.

As blood pressure rises from Profactor-H's three effects, the heart must work harder, pumping against more and more resistance. The end result is a rise in blood pressure.

The Medication Maze

To make matters worse, some of the medications that you may be prescribed, which are aimed at lowering your blood pressure, may, as a side effect, increase your Profactor-H level. It is important to understand that if you are taking medication, you must discuss this matter with your physician before making any change. We simply want you to know that certain medications may be working for you and against you at the same time.

In the reference section at the end of this book, we list the sources for the research quotes we use. Should you and your physician wish, these articles can be pulled and reviewed in their entirety, in particular with regard to medication recommendations for the Profactor-H Positive individual.

A Cluster of Clues

As scientists continue to find strong connections in high blood pressure and heart disease, abnormal blood fat levels, excess weight, and diabetes to Profactor-H, they have given them a new name: *cluster diseases.*

Cluster diseases often show themselves, first, as a single risk factor or disease, such as excess weight. Over time, second and third risk factors develop, such as high blood pressure and/or abnormal blood fat levels. Each risk factor or disease puts you at greater risk for additional health problems. In the end, in combination, they are often thought to lead to heart disease, diabetes, or stroke. Until recently, little was understood regarding the cause, prevention, and treatment of cluster diseases, but now Profactor-H has given us the clues for which we have hoped for so long. You can find out a great deal more about the Profactor-H connection to cluster diseases in chapter 13, "The Profactor-H Cluster."

The Secret to Success

Traditional recommendations of exercise, quitting smoking, and weight loss sometimes result in lower blood pressure because, coincidentally, these are some of the many ways that you can also reduce Profactor-H levels. On the other hand, because these lifestyle changes do not correct the cause of high Profactor-H levels, and because they are not easily maintained, an increase in weight, a decrease in interest in exercise, and a rise in high blood pressure usually return over time. A successful lifestyle change must be a choice that you find simple, easy to maintain, and pleasurable, all at the same time as reducing the cause of your high blood pressure levels.

The Profactor-H Program has been designed to offer you realistic and enjoyable Options that can help you begin to bring your blood pressure down, to help you to reduce your risk for heart disease and stroke, and make the pro-health changes that you have always wanted to make.

A Not-So-Typical Tale: Peter's Story

Peter L. was in his mid-forties when we first met him. He entered our research program in order to "get a handle" on his weight. Peter had been gaining about four or five pounds a year, he said. "My story is probably pretty typical. I've been gaining weight slowly but it's been steady. I'm not so concerned about the weight—I mean, my wife loves me anyway, though I know she wishes that I'd lose weight—it's just that my father died young, and I don't want the same thing to happen to me."

> "It's just that my father died young," Peter told us, "and I don't want the same thing to happen to me."

Peter's first marriage had ended in divorce and his second now brought him as much joy as his first marriage had brought him unhappiness. He and his new wife had just had twins and the only things spoiling Peter's happiness were concerns about his health. "It's not so much for me," he confessed. "I don't think I would even be here if it were up to me, but Marcy, my wife, is really worried ... and now with the twins ..." His voice trailed off.

Peter's last physical exam added to their concerns. Peter had gained his typical five pounds during the past year and his laboratory tests showed the yearly rise in cholesterol and triglyceride levels that he had come to expect. It was not, by far, a terrible report. It might have been typical to Peter, but it showed a progression toward heart disease that Peter had also witnessed, year by year, in his own father and both of his uncles.

"My dad wouldn't go for regular checkups on his own," Peter told us. "But when I would plead with him and finally convince him to go, you could count on his weight creeping up, along with his blood pressure and cholesterol. It didn't happen overnight, just a little bit at a time. And each time the doctor would caution him to change his eating habits or get more exercise, and each time my dad would go right out and do the same thing. He didn't want to give up all the things he really loved, so he just kept doing what he had done all his life. I tried to make him do something. I pleaded with him after my second uncle died of a stroke, but it was impossible.

"I'd stop nagging him and for a while I'd let it go, then I'd try again but nothing ever really changed," Peter continued. "My dad's weight slowly climbed and then one day he turned to me and said he wasn't feeling good. I was living at home at the time, right after my divorce. He went in for a nap and that was the last time I ever saw him. My mother never got over it.

"I don't want that to happen to me . . . or to Marcy. But I'm so much like my father. I love to eat and I know, realistically, I'm not going to change my whole way of life. I'm following right in his footsteps—weightwise, healthwise, everything. And I'm scared where that is going to lead.

"I know heart disease is often inherited," Peter said, "and I thought if I could take some weight off, even if I can't change my whole life, I'd be better off." Peter stopped and waited for a reply.

We had a lot to say . . . all good. Yes, we confirmed, having a parent with heart disease could put you at greater risk than having no heart disease in your family whatsoever. Yes, we said, excess weight—even putting on a few pounds at a time—was a risk factor for heart disease as well.

But then we had something new and essential for Peter to hear: He did not have to change his "whole life" in order to avoid following in his father's footsteps.

> Peter did not have to change his "whole life" in order
> to avoid following in his father's footsteps.

The Profactor-H Program could help him lose weight—and keep it off—and it could, at the same time, help him reduce his

risk for heart disease as well. In addition, our Program was designed to help reduce his cholesterol and triglyceride levels and
help keep his blood pressure down. He could reap all of the
benefits at once, we explained, because all of these problems
were often related to the same underlying cause.

"It's really very logical," we told him. "When you eliminate
the cause, you eliminate the problem." And the Profactor-H
Program had been designed to eliminate that cause—without
changing his "whole life."

> "It's really very logical," we told Peter.
> "When you eliminate the cause, you eliminate the
> problem." After only three months, Peter's lab tests
> were well within normal limits.

We started Peter on the Profactor-H Program, and as we predicted, his risk indicators started dropping at a steady rate. His
weight, cholesterol, and triglyceride levels dropped at an even
pace.

After only three months, Peter's lab tests were well within
normal limits. A year on the Program and he had dropped to
the low-moderate range of cardiovascular risk. Two years to the
day of his first visit, Peter's laboratory test results placed him in
the lowest possible risk category for heart disease. He had been
at his goal weight for over a year and a half and he had maintained it without sacrifice or struggle.

> Instead of accepting his father's fate,
> Peter had literally taken his life into his own hands.

Still, any real change must stand the test of time. Peter
stopped by the other day to drop off a book that he had bor-
rowed quite a while ago. His sons, now four years old, were

with him. They were quite a handful and Peter, nearly fifty now, had just about all he could handle to keep them from running in all directions.

We smiled with pride as we watched Peter half carry, half drag his boys through the door. He had come to us four years ago, a worried, overweight, middle-aged man, beginning to show signs of following in his father's medical footsteps—a path that led to early and, we felt, unnecessary death. But instead of accepting that his father's fate would be his own, Peter had literally taken his life into his own hands. He had turned his rising risk factors into incentives to become healthier as he grew older. He had lost his excessive weight and kept it off and his blood fat levels were ideal. Peter voiced his appreciation, once again, and wrestled the boys out of the office.

After he left, we sat back in our chairs and talked about Peter's first visit. He told us, back then, in his unassuming way, that his was a pretty typical story. But in the years to follow, he had done what so many people want to do but never know how to accomplish. We may have shown him the way, and a way that he could live with, but Peter's commitment to his children and his wife made him willing to do what he might never have done for himself.

We smiled to ourselves. "Peter," we thought, "you may think you are typical, but you are quite special to us."

CHAPTER 13

The Profactor-H Cluster

Everything is clear if the cause be known.
—Louis Pasteur

The First, and Deadly, Mistake

The power of Profactor-H cannot be denied.

We know that Profactor-H can make our bodies save too well or promote too much growth. The result: buildup of plaque leading to atherosclerosis, coronary artery disease, and heart disease.

We know that Profactor-H encourages the body to retain water and salts. The result: high blood pressure and the possibility of stroke.

We know that Profactor-H can sweep too much sugar out of the bloodstream and signal fat cells to store more and more energy. The result: recurring hunger, then weight gain.

We know that if the body reacts to the Profactor-H overload, it may shut down the doors to many of its cells and, in protecting itself from an insulin insult, may withhold vital nourishment. Sugar, unable to move into the waiting cells, can back up in the bloodstream. The result: adult-onset diabetes.

Cravings and weight gain, narrowing of arteries, high blood pressure, heart disease, diabetes—Profactor-H can lead to a predictable set of diseases and disorders that do not always appear at the same time but rather one by one, over time.

Depending on your family history, your lifestyle, and your environment, you may be prone to excess weight gain or to diabetes or to high blood pressure. In addition, each disorder requires a different length of time to appear.

But rather than understanding that these disorders appear, one after the other, from a single underlying problem, we may mistakenly see them as separate disorders, one causing the other, giving us what we term the *Illusion of Sequence.*

The Illusion of Sequence is a misunderstanding about disease that comes from seeing different symptoms emerge at different times. It is a logical assumption but can be a deadly mistake.

The Illusion of Sequence is a misunderstanding about disease that comes from observing different symptoms of a disorder as they emerge at different times. In the Illusion of Sequence you assume that the first symptoms to appear *caused* the later symptoms or that the first of a set of diseases or disorders caused later ones to appear. It is a logical and human assumption, but it can lead to a deadly error in judgment.

If you assume that the first symptoms are causing the appearance of later symptoms, you may put your energy into trying to avoid or reverse the first symptoms rather than looking for a common cause of all the symptoms. Like the little Dutch boy running from hole to hole trying to plug up the leaks in the dike, you are bound for failure unless you can stop the cause of the onrushing tide of water.

It is easy to see the mistake that people make in the Illusion of Sequence when we look at diseases we understand. Even though fever often shows up before the telltale rash, we would never say that fever causes a child to get measles. We understand that the same microbe causes both the fever and the rash, and that the fever may simply show up before the rash.

In diseases with which we are not as knowledgeable, however, confusion about cause and result more easily occur. Not too many years ago, when antibiotics were still in their infancy, people were frightened when they or someone they loved caught a cold. It was thought that the cold could lead to pneumonia, a disease that was often associated with a high risk of death. People took many precautions to try to avoid a cold, hoping to reduce their chance for pneumonia.

Since that time, we have come to realize that the bacteria or virus that causes pneumonia may bring on some of the symptoms of a cold as an earlier stage of the development of the disease. A generation ago, however, the cold was seen as a causal risk factor for the pneumonia and the belief that naturally followed was that avoiding the cold would better your chances of avoiding pneumonia . . . and death.

Today we are battling the diseases of civilization, and if we are not careful, our illusions and assumptions may lead us up the same blind alleys that failed to help our parents and grandparents.

The Crucial Link

When we look at the major diseases affecting our health and longevity today, it becomes obvious that we are suffering from the same Illusion of Sequence. Just because a person gains weight, for instance, and then later becomes diabetic does not necessarily mean that the weight gain caused the diabetes. It is essential to look for a different single underlying cause that might be responsible for both conditions.

In the last few years scientists have been doing just that and the results are truly astonishing. Profactor-H is connected to so many of today's major diseases that these diseases are being grouped together as "clusters"—all connected by the same single crucial link: Profactor-H.

> Profactor-H is connected to so many of today's major diseases that these diseases are being grouped together as "clusters" —all connected by the same single crucial link: Profactor-H.

In their review of the work of 307 research scientists, Drs. R. De-Fronzo and E. Ferrannini concluded that Profactor-H appears to be a syndrome that is associated with a "clustering of metabolic disorders," including adult-onset diabetes, excess weight, high blood pressure, undesirable blood fat levels, and heart disease.

Most recently, this cluster of diseases, all related to Profactor-H and all of which have been viewed in the past as separate diseases, has been given a new name: Syndrome X. Dr. G. M. Reaven coined the term to describe a cluster of diseases that include high blood sugar levels, high blood pressure, increased levels of "bad" very-low-density lipoprotein (VLDL), triglycerides, and decreased levels of "good" high-density lipoprotein (HDL) cholesterol, adult-onset diabetes—and Profactor-H.

With this newest of breakthroughs in research comes an understanding that no single one of these diseases or risk factors causes the others to develop, but rather that Profactor-H is the connecting link to them all as they develop, each in its own time sequence.

For Women of All Ages

In women's health, scientists have known that Profactor-H is strongly related to the development of polycystic ovary disease. Recent research has clearly revealed Profactor-H's widespread health-endangering impact on women.

The Profactor-H link to polycystic ovarian disease has been reported in medical journals such as the *American Journal of Obstetrics and Gynecology* and *Hormone Research*. Profactor-H is now recognized as a characteristic feature of women with polycystic ovaries.

Profactor-H has been linked to excess testosterone production in women and can lead to excess facial hair, or *hirsutism*. Some

Profactor-H Positive women bearing heavy facial hair and excess weight may be prone to multiple ovarian cysts. Yet they never realize that Profactor-H may lie at the base of all of these problems.

In 1991, Dr. W. Urdl and his research team identified Profactor-H as the likely "trigger mechanism and therefore the key" to the genetic-determined cause of polycystic ovarian disease.

Even those of us who have no history of any of these diseases or risk factors, those of us who are healthy and disease-free, may not be free of Profactor-H's influence.

Healthy As Can Be? No Guarantee of Being Profactor-H Free

Today, researchers are finding that Profactor-H can be found in approximately one in four of us who show none of the generally recognized signs of being Profactor-H Positive.

In his article for the medical and research journal *Hormone and Metabolic Research,* Dr. D. C. Simonson concluded that Profactor-H is found in a "variety of disease entities" as well as in a "substantial portion of apparently healthy individuals." And Dr. H. Rupp, using the term *metabolic syndrome* to describe Profactor-H's effects, explained that, in recent years, Profactor-H has emerged "as an important health risk" that is present in approximately 25 percent of those showing absolutely no signs of high blood pressure, undesirable blood fat levels, excess weight, or the like.

It is important to understand that, when we talk about Profactor-H, we are *not* talking about a disorder that is rare or one that you would be sure to recognize if you had it. While Profactor-H is often present in those who are overweight or have high blood pressure or diabetes or undesirable blood fat levels, as Drs. DeFronzo and Ferrannini point out, Profactor-H is a "common disorder, which occurs with high frequency in the general population."

And though it is common, it can still be deadly. In their study published in *The New England Journal of Medicine,* Dr. Ivana Zavaroni and her colleagues concluded that healthy persons with Profactor-H and normal blood sugar levels still "have an increase in risk factors for heart disease" as compared with a well-matched group of subjects who are Profactor-H free.

And so, for those who do not yet show any outward sign of weight- or health-related problems, being Profactor-H Positive must still not be taken lightly. Dr. Rupp's warning reads loud and clear: If Profactor-H "persists over a prolonged period of time, detrimental influences" on the heart and blood vessel system become apparent, including adult-onset diabetes, high blood pressure, and athero-sclerosis.

A Gene Turned Mean

Scientists are now beginning to understand how Profactor-H orig-inated and what purpose it once served. According to Dr. M. Wen-dorf, the Thrifty Gene that the Profactor-H Positive person carries "may have once allowed founding populations to survive 'feast' and 'famine' conditions of several generations."

Profactor-H, once an essential means of survival to the caveman, has now become the metabolic plague of our affluent civilization.

But we have for you the best of all possible news: We know how to help you decrease your risk for this destroyer of health and short-ener of life; we can help you reduce your risk for the diseases that come under its mighty influence and increase your likelihood for a long and healthy life.

We have for you the best of all possible news:
We know how to help you increase
your likelihood for a long and healthy life.

The Ticking Clock

The Profactor-H Program that follows is the result of over nine years of work on our part and untold years of work by other research scientists. It is based on fact, not assumption; science, not speculation. It is easy to follow and enjoyable as well. It can be adapted to your needs and to your lifestyle. It can be incorporated in its entirety, all at once, or assimilated a little at a time.

Whatever your choice, we urge you to turn to the Program that follows without delay. The time to act is now, for "the clock has already begun to tick."

Second Chance: Larry's Story

Larry L. barely looked at us as he entered the office. He sat down, tight-lipped, and gazed out of the window, literally avoiding our eyes. His wife, Emily, came hurrying through the door and slipped into the chair next to him, speaking as she ran. "I'm sorry we're so late. We got caught in traffic. Nothing's moving out there and . . ." As she continued we watched Larry. He never looked at her or at us.

This was not Larry's first appointment. Two years earlier he and Emily had come to see us. Larry had taken control of the conversation then. He explained that he did not want to be there and that the appointment was his wife's idea—and, he added, he wanted us to know it. He had arrived almost a half hour late for his first appointment and about twenty minutes late for this meeting.

"My wife thinks that you are going to do something fantastic for me," he told us at that first meeting. "Something that all of the specialists that I have seen haven't been able to do. She thinks you know something that no one else knows. I'm a little bit more realistic," he added. Having said his piece, he looked away and essentially dismissed us.

Emily looked like she was going to cry. Her eyes had been red when she entered the office, and we wondered if they had been having an argument. We were pretty sure, now, that had been the case.

"I'm sorry," she explained. "It doesn't have anything to do with you. It's just that he's really tried a lot of things and he's pretty upset. He doesn't want to try one more thing. He just wants me to leave him alone. But I'm afraid that . . ." Her voice trailed off and she started to cry again. After a few moments, Emily went on to explain Larry's medical history and treatment experience.

Though he was about fifty-five years old at that first appointment and about fifty pounds overweight, his health problems began when he was in his late forties. He was only about ten or fifteen pounds overweight then. Slowly and subtly he began putting on weight. His cravings and hunger pushed him toward food and within a few years he had gained most of the weight we saw at that first visit. By fifty years of age, he was told that he had high blood pressure. His blood fat levels were above normal and his doctor recommended a low-fat diet. Within two more years, his blood pressure and blood fat levels were far worse and medication for the blood pressure seemed to do little more than keep it from going higher.

Larry tried to lose weight, but he would "cheat" on little things. Emily nagged him and he got angry with her. He would use the blow-up as an excuse to eat what he wanted. His weight continued to rise. He began to truly feel poorly and a lengthy blood test revealed that, like his grandfather and his father's brother, he had developed adult-onset diabetes.

The next few years were not good ones for Larry, or for his wife. He suffered a series of heart attacks, and though an angioplasty had been performed to open a blocked artery to his heart, his blood fat levels indicated that it was unlikely the artery would remain open.

During that whole first conversation, Larry's face remained motionless and his eyes looked out of the window—very much like this second meeting. The first meeting had ended as it had to with an explanation on our part that Larry did not appear to want to take part in the Program and that without his enthusiastic commitment to it we could not accept him as a participant.

We wondered why he had returned this second time, and in what we hoped were noninsulting words, asked him as much. He turned and looked at us full face. He explained that over the last two years his health had grown worse. Far worse. He went on to explain that he was slowly but surely going blind from the vascular changes that can result from diabetes. Laser surgery and medications had been useless. The increased pressure was slowly stealing his vision. He was showing signs of decreased blood circulation in his extremities as well. Unless something changed he could end up losing a toe or foot or leg. His health was clearly deteriorating.

"It's not that I necessarily believe in what you're doing," he said. "But after Emily convinced him, my doctor thought it might not be a bad idea to give it a try. After all, what do I have to lose at this point?" he added.

These were hardly words of eager excitement, but for Larry, they were probably as close to willing participation as we could ever expect.

We told Larry that we wanted to evaluate him for Profactor-H, to see if the many problems he was experiencing might have a single cause. When he realized we were not speaking of a series of blood tests or invasive procedures, but rather a simple questionnaire, his mood lightened a bit. He answered our questions readily and scored high in the Severe Risk range.

But his mood quickly reversed when we told him his score. "So what does that mean?" he asked. "What does that have to do with anything?"

What it had to do with, we explained, was a link, a single connection to his many problems. "You keep thinking you are 'falling apart,' as you put it," we explained—"or 'just getting old.' You see yourself acquiring one disease after another. We, on the other hand, see all of them as predictable symptoms of the same underlying problem. And we believe that we know how we can help you to correct that problem."

We gave Larry some research articles to take with him and to discuss with his physician, and made another appointment. "We want you to feel sure that this is the right program for you and to be certain that you really want it." Larry told us, "I said I'd give it a chance, didn't I?" but we stuck to our decision to begin after he had seen his physician one more time.

The next time we saw Larry, his manner was decidedly different. He was still the cynic and far from enthusiastic, but "the whole thing does make a lot of sense," he admitted. And, though he would not say how happy he was to have discovered what looked to be his only way out, as he left he shook our hands and thanked us.

Larry's road to health has been a bit bumpy. At first, his doubtfulness made him unwilling to fully commit to the Profactor-H Program. He chose whichever Option appealed to him at the moment, either from the Beginner or Intermediate or Advanced level, and he would follow the Option as long as he felt like it. When he didn't feel like eating a salad or taking his chromium supplement, he would just not do it. Still, even with his less than sparkling adherence, his body began to respond.

At first, subtle signs of vascular problems began to reverse. The coldness in his feet disappeared. Sensation returned to his toes. And he began to feel "better." His blood pressure started to go down, just a little at first, then more and more.

But the real change came when his eye doctor told him the pressure within his eyes was "significantly better." Blindness was Larry's deep-seated fear, and finding that there was noticeable improvement in the pressure in his eyes brought him out of his isolation. Emily called and told us the news, and said that "his whole attitude changed." "He seems like his old self," she told us in tears.

Larry's next appointment did indeed bring a somewhat different Larry to our office. He wanted to know more about the Program, and we encouraged him to follow the Program as it was written, explaining that all of its parts worked to complement each other and to bring the best results.

Though Larry is clearly not one to follow directions, he did try in his way to do his best. And the results continued to reward his efforts. His blood pressure and blood fat levels continued to improve. His diabetes was clearly under control and he was able to greatly decrease his medication. His eyes and legs continued to grow healthy once more and, slowly, his attitude became more positive and hopeful.

"It's better. I have to admit it. It does seem to be working," he told us after his doctor's second positive report. "But let's see if it keeps up," he added. We could swear he seemed to almost smile.

Two and a half years later, Emily and Larry made an appointment to ask if we could bring Larry's brother into the Program. We explained that the long waiting list would make it doubtful that we would see him for several years. Larry admitted that he'd thought that would be the case but had hoped to persuade us to let his brother enter earlier, given the results we had seen in him. We explained that this was research protocol and that we could not do that.

"Just as well," he said with a dramatic sigh and a sparkle in his eye. "He might not be as easy to work with as me."

PART TWO

THE PROFACTOR-H PROGRAM: REVERSING YOUR RISK

CHAPTER 14

The Profactor-H Program: How It Works

Plan the flight, fly the plan. —NASA

At this moment you hold your future health and well-being in the palm of your hand. The choices you make after reading the next few pages can help increase your chances for a long, happy, and healthy life.

The Profactor-H Program is different from any you have ever seen. We will not ask you to follow the difficult, unrealistic, and often unlivable guidelines that so many other programs require. Many recommendations from other programs are almost impossible to continue for life, and they often let you down in the end, either because they require great deprivation or sacrifice or, no matter how closely you follow them, they do not really seem to make much of an impact.

The Profactor-H Program, on the other hand, will invite you to enjoy foods you never thought could be included as part of your regular eating program, recommend that you be physically active (if you can), and will help you to reduce the stresses in your life in ways that will surprise, amuse, and intrigue you.

> This Program is different from any you have ever seen.
> We will not ask you to follow the difficult, unrealistic, and
> unlivable guidelines that so many other programs require.

We will *not* ask you to weigh or measure your food. We will *not* ask you to follow a demanding exercise regimen. We will *not* ask you to give up the foods you love. We will *not* ask you to add to your already overcommitted time and energy schedule. Real change can come only when a program comes to live with you, meets you on your ground, and can be easily incorporated into your life.

> Real change can come only when a program comes
> to live with you, meets you on your ground,
> and can be easily incorporated into your life.

Each of the guidelines in this Program comes from a scientific understanding of how your body works. Each Option is designed to help correct the hormonal imbalance that can rob you of your good health and long life. We do not need to resort to measuring and weighing, exchanges, restrictions, and limitations because each guideline within the Program has been chosen for its ability to correct the basic cause of the problem.

Making Your Mark

By choosing this Program you have taken an important step in helping to reduce your Profactor-H health risk factors. Read the chapters that follow carefully and take notes if you like. Write on the pages, underline important sentences, circle important points. Don't be afraid to make your mark. This is your book. This is your Program. This is your life. We want to be part of making it work best *for you*.

Write on these pages, underline important sentences, circle important points. Don't be afraid to make your mark. This is your book. This is your program. This is your life. We want to be part of making it work best *for you.*

ONE WORD OF CAUTION:

Do not mix and match guidelines from this Program with guidelines from other plans. The Profactor-H Program is different because it has been designed to do one thing and one thing only: to eliminate the Profactor-H link that ties so many diseases together and that may put you at risk for ill health or early death.

Certainly, you should be guided by your personal physician; let your doctor help you and make important suggestions. Bring this book to your physician's office. Have your physician read it and understand the Program so that you are not patching other recommendations into our well-balanced and focused plan.

This Program is not intended for pregnant or nursing women or for children or teens. Their needs are specialized and cannot be addressed here.

The Profactor-H Three-Step Program

Three progressive Steps make up your self-paced Profactor-H Program:

Step #1—The Beginner's Program
Step #2—The Intermediate Program
Step #3—The Advanced Program

Within each Step (Beginner's, Intermediate, and Advanced), you will be guided in choosing Risk-Reducing Options that are most appropriate *for you.* Risk-Reducing Options are small lifestyle changes. Most take only a little time and energy, but they can greatly decrease your risk for Profactor-H and increase your probability for health and long life.

Risk-Reducing Options are small lifestyle changes that take only a little time and energy.

You will learn more about Risk-Reducing Options as we take you, step by step, through the Profactor-H Program in the chapters that follow. At each of the three Steps (Beginner's, Intermediate, and Advanced), you will be asked to choose Risk-Reducing Options in the areas of Nutrition, Activity, or Stress Reduction, as well as additional Bonus Options.

Each Risk-Reducing Option carries a weighted value that is based on its relative ability to decrease your Profactor-H risk. As you look over each Option, you will be able to see how much change that Option is likely to have in reducing your risk for Profactor-H and bettering your health. You can choose Options that best fit your preferences, your needs, your time schedule, and your goals. We will offer several Options, but the choice will always be yours.

Each week, on the sheets we provide, you will be able to chart your progress in terms of the relative percentage of risk reduction that week's Option is likely to give you. Your Progress Chart and your Risk-Reducing Percentage Chart will help you stay both focused and motivated.

Risk-Reducing Options in each area (Nutrition, Activity, and Stress Reduction) are listed from the easiest (in terms of your time and energy) to the most challenging, and you will be able to choose Options that are realistic and appropriate to your needs, your preferences, your time constraints, and your lifestyle.

Progressive Benefits

Each of the three Steps has advantages and benefits unique to its level. The Beginner's Program is easy to learn. Risk-Reducing Options are simple and pleasant. Uncomplicated choices will make change easy. You will find that your health benefits begin to accrue without resistance or struggle.

The Intermediate Program requires additional changes, but they are natural consequences of the benefits and experience that come from the Beginner's Program. In the same way, the superior Risk-Reducing benefits that come from the Advanced Program flow naturally from the two previous Steps. With each Step you will gain the strength, energy, and encouragement you need to move to the next Step.

> Most of us try to take on too much, too fast.
> On the Profactor-H Program,
> you will learn to let the Program help you succeed.

Most of us try to take on too much, too fast. On the Profactor-H Program, you will learn to let the Program help you succeed. It is important that you move at your own pace, stay as long as you like at any Step, and when (and only when) you feel ready, move to the next Step.

Each Step of the Program is a natural and easy transition from the previous Step. Just as the Beginner's Program paves the way for Options in the Intermediate Program, the Intermediate Program's Options are designed to lower, even further, your Profactor-H levels, making the Advanced Program's Options far easier and more enjoyable than if they had been attempted from the start.

As you reduce your Profactor-H levels, you will probably notice an increase in energy, a sense of well-being, and a feeling of control. Each increase in energy and motivation will make new Options easier and more enjoyable. Options that would have, in the past, seemed like "too much trouble" will seem far more appealing.

> As you reduce your Profactor-H levels,
> you will notice an increase in energy,
> a sense of well-being, and a feeling of control.

Most important, these changes will come from your body, not your mind. You will not have to convince yourself to do things that you know are "good for you"; you will want to do them and you will be able to do them, successfully. We call these "progressive benefits" because they progress, or increase, as you continue the Program, because they stem easily and naturally from your body's becoming balanced, and because they allow you to move from level to level, step to step.

As you begin to feel the changes that each Option can bring, old thoughts and feelings of effort, sacrifice, deprivation, failure, and conflict give way to feelings of accomplishment, success, control, health, and victory.

Allison L. was a perfect example of the ease that progressive benefits can bring on the Profactor-H Program. When Allison started on the Program, she had little energy and "no incentive."

"I know I have to do something," she told us. "My blood pressure is going up and so is my weight, but I feel tired and unmotivated and, the truth is, I just don't have the time."

On the Beginner's Program, Allison began to eat only Risk-Reducing Foods at lunch. Her tiredness in the afternoon vanished and she "felt like a new person." She was able to get her work done without a struggle and had energy to go home and make an enjoyable dinner for herself. She no longer fell asleep after supper and, most of all, stopped blaming herself for her lack of motivation.

In the weeks to follow, additional Options such as walking for fifteen minutes each day became easy, and almost without noticing it, Allison progressed from the Beginner's Program to an Intermediate level. With each Option, she felt better and was more willing and able to take on other Options.

Several weeks into the Advanced Program, Allison made a comment that we never tire of hearing. "You know, it's funny," she said. "I'm doing now what I've always wanted to do. I'm taking care of myself, eating well, losing weight, and the change in my blood pressure is incredible. But what is most amazing is that I am doing things I never could see myself doing before.

"Before I began the Program I was just sort of resigned to the fact that I could never get it together to do this kind of thing. Now I understand that I kept taking on too much at once. I know now that it wasn't me. It wasn't my fault. I was trying to be someone else. I would take on too much all at once and I just didn't have the energy or the time to do it.

"But, on the Program, when I only had to take on one Option at a time, it was easy. As I started feeling better, I could handle more. And it was great knowing I didn't 'have' to do more if I didn't feel like it.

"With each change, I felt better. For me, that was what was important—no, actually it was essential. Nobody was making demands on me—or pushing me. With only one simple Option to do, I wasn't getting in deeper than I wanted to. One Option at a time was just perfect. 'That,' I told myself, 'that, I can handle.' And I did. And do."

Allison is like so many of us. When we look up at a steep, high staircase in front of us, we don't even feel like trying. If, on the other hand, we find that taking a single step makes us feel good, makes us feel healthier and more energetic, we are willing to take the next step . . . and the next. For some of us, a step or two is all that we will take, and that is still better than taking none. For some of us, one step will lead to another. In either case, we will no longer be able to tell ourselves that we "can't" help ourselves become healthier and happier. We can do it; but we must do it at our own pace and we must do it one step at a time.

Custom-made Changes

You may be twenty-five years of age—or younger. You may be slim and in perfect health—or not. You may be sixty or sixty-five. You may be somewhere in the middle. You may have chronic health problems or you may have just started to show changes in high blood pressure or blood fat levels so typical of being Profactor-H Positive.

You may be carrying an extra fifty pounds—or more. You may be a busy professional with multiple demands on your time and energy. You may have far fewer responsibilities. On the Profactor-H

Program you will move at your own pace. You will tailor your Options to fit your needs and preferences.

You will pace yourself by adding Options you choose, when *you* are ready. Each successive Option will often bring you increased feelings of energy and well-being and these, in turn, will help motivate and encourage you. This Three-Step Program has been designed to bring about healthful changes that can be maintained—without struggle or deprivation—for life.

On the Profactor-H Program you will pace yourself by adding the Options you choose, when *you* are ready, so that it can be maintained—without struggle or deprivation—for life.

INCLUDING HEALTH AGENCY RECOMMENDATIONS IN YOUR PROFACTOR-H PROGRAM

Reports coming from the U.S. Department of Agriculture, the Department of Health and Human Services, the American Heart Association, and the Surgeon General of the United States have contained dietary recommendations for Americans.

These well-respected agencies offer these guidelines to aid in the prevention of adult-onset diabetes, cardiovascular disease, cancer, chronic liver or kidney disease, obesity, high blood pressure, osteoporosis, and stroke.

Recommendations contained in health agency reports* are completely compatible with, and easily included in, the Profactor-H Program.

Suggestions for incorporating dietary guidelines into your program can be found in "Health Agency Recommendations" on pages 345 to 347.

It is important to remember that only your physician can determine which health agency dietary guidelines are appropriate for you. Before including any recommendation in your eating plan, be certain to consult with your doctor.

*The Surgeon General's Report on Nutrition and Health; the U.S. Department of Agriculture and the Department of Health and Human Services's Report on Dietary Guidelines for Americans; the American Heart Association's diet, Eating Plan for Healthy Americans; and the American Cancer Society's Eat to Live.

CHAPTER 15

Step #1—The Beginner's Program: Quick and Easy

The first step is one which makes the rest of our days.
—Voltaire

The job of a beginner is simply that, to begin. No one expects you to immediately master the Program or to do it perfectly. As in most things, we learn best by doing.

Some of the Options that follow may seem simple, but the changes they can produce are far from small. Each of the Risk-Reducing Options* has been chosen for its ability to lead to a lower Profactor-H risk and a greater probability of your good health and long life.

The Options in this chapter are just right for the beginner because they are uncomplicated, clear, and, most important, will immediately begin to reduce your risk for Profactor-H–related illnesses. Your Options are explained in more detail in chapter 16, "Options, Options, Options."

> Some of the Options that follow may seem simple,
> but the changes they can produce are far from small.

*Please select Options only if they do not conflict with your personal physician's recommendations.

We dislike hearing people falsely claim that you have to sacrifice your pleasure, freedom, or time in order to be healthy. We have found it is simply not true. Most people have had many experiences that disprove the "no pain, no gain" rule. Some of the best things that have happened to us may, at times, seem to fall into our laps or have come from little work. At other times, we have tried and tried and end up with very little to show for it. Not all changes require great sacrifice. Small steps *are* important, especially when you add them together. Small steps can make great change, and so can you.

HOW TO BEGIN YOUR BEGINNER'S PROGRAM

Beginner's Week #1: Nutrition

1. Look over Beginner's Nutrition Options A, B, and C, which follow.
2. Choose one Option as your first Nutrition selection. For one week, add that Option to your regular routine.

    If there is no Beginner's Nutrition Option that is appropriate for you or that you are willing to select, or if you find that there is a Nutrition Option that you are already doing on a regular basis, see the "Special Circumstances" section on page 207.

Beginner's Nutrition Options

A. Include a large Risk-Reducing salad (at least 2 cups) with your usual dinner.   **(1 point)**
    Continue eating any Essential Balance Foods and Risk-Reducing Foods you normally have at any meals and for any snacks you usually have. Risk-Reducing and Essential Balance Foods are listed on pages 220 to 223.

B. Include an average portion (about 1 cup) of a Risk-Reducing vegetable as part of your usual dinner.
    (2 points)
    Continue eating any Essential Balance Foods and Risk-Reducing Foods you normally have at any meals and

---

for any snacks you usually have. You can find a full list of Risk-Reducing and Essential Balance Foods on pages 220 to 223.

C. Every day at lunch, eat only Risk-Reducing Foods, including protein, vegetables, and/or salad. **(3 points)**

Continue eating any Essential Balance Foods and Risk-Reducing Foods you normally have at breakfast and dinner as well as for snacks, if you desire. See pages 220 to 223 for a full list of Risk-Reducing and Essential Balance Foods and page 303 for sample meals.

After one week of adding your new Option to your regular routine, if you like, you can chart your progress. For simple directions in charting your progress and using your Progress Chart, see the "Charting Your Progress" section later in this chapter.

3. When you are ready to select a new Option, read "Beginner's Week #2: Activity," which follows.

Beginner's Week #2: Activity

1. Look over Beginner's Activity Options A, B, and C, which follow.
2. Choose one Option as your first Beginner's Activity selection. Add it to your regular routine for the coming week, *while continuing* your Nutrition Option.

If there is no Beginner's Activity Option that is appropriate for you or that you are willing to select, or if you find that there is a Beginner's Activity Option that you are already doing on a regular basis, see the "Special Circumstances" section on page 207.

Beginner's Activity Options

A. Walk for 15 minutes, three times each week. **(1 point)**
Any Light Activity Option from the list on page 227 may be substituted.

B. Swim, jog lightly, or bike (on a regular or stationary bike) for 15 minutes, three times each week. **(2 points)**
Any Moderate Activity Option from the list on pages 227 to 228 may be substituted.

C. Play tennis, racquetball, jog briskly, or do step aerobics for 15 minutes, three times each week. **(3 points)**
Any Vigorous Activity Option from the list on page 228 may be substituted.

3. After one week of adding both the Nutritional and Activity Options to your regular routine, you may add a Beginner's Stress-Reducing Option to your routine. When you are ready to select your new Stress-Reducing Option, read "Beginner's Week #3: Stress Reduction," which follows.

Remember, at the end of each week, if you choose, you can continue to chart your progress by using your Beginner's Progress Chart. The "Charting Your Progress" section later in this chapter will guide you with simple directions.

Beginner's Week #3: Stress Reduction

1. Look over Beginner's Stress-Reducing Options A, B, and C, which follow.
2. Choose one Option as your first Stress-Reducing selection. Add your Stress-Reducing Option to your regular routine for the coming week, *while continuing* your other Options.
   NOTE ON STRESS-REDUCING OPTIONS: If you do not smoke or drink alcoholic beverages on a regular or semiregular basis, do not choose a Stress-Reducing Option that asks you to limit or eliminate these practices (Stress-Reducing Options B or C). If you do not regularly find yourself in a stressful situation at either home or at work, do not choose Stress-Reducing Option A.

After adding your Stress-Reducing Option to your previous Options and incorporating all three Options into your regular routine for one week, you can chart your progress to date.

Beginner's Stress-Reducing Options

A. At least three times each week, for at least 15 minutes each time, remove yourself from an environment (home, work, or other) that you find stressful. **(1 point)**

You may want to physically remove yourself by leaving the premises or you can close the door (and your eyes) and listen to some soothing music or to one of the many relaxation audiotapes available commercially. You might want to meditate or simply take a nap. You may want to take a book or audiotape and sit alone for a while in your car. Or, if no other private place is available, remove yourself to a bathroom stall.

B. Have no alcoholic beverages (wine, beer, mixed drinks, etc.) during lunch. (Select this Option only if you have one or more alcoholic drinks with your lunch on a somewhat regular basis. **(2 points)**

C. If you smoke (cigarette, cigar, or pipe), reduce your smoking by about one-half. **(3 points)**

Set a schedule, defining when you can and cannot smoke. Keep the schedule handy and stick to it.

3. When you are ready to select additional Options, read the "In the Weeks to Come" section on page 210.

Special Circumstances

There may come a time when you cannot find an appropriate Option from that week's choices or when you don't want to choose any of the Options offered. In either case you may choose a Bonus Option (see page 209) in its place. *When it is possible,* we have found it's best to choose from that week's Activity, Nutrition, or Stress-Reducing Options. If, however, you find that any week's Options are not appropriate for you or will not be easily maintained, simply select a Bonus Option in place of the regular selection for that week and add it to your routine. Then continue as usual.

There may also come a time when you find that you have, on your own, been following one of the Options offered as part of any particular week's selections. If so, consider that you have already fulfilled that week's Option. Continue that Option on a regular basis, and if you chart your progress, chart it as part of your progress total for the week and for all the weeks to come (just as if you had chosen it new, as a regular part of the Program).

Bonus Options: Flexible Alternatives

Bonus Options can be used in two ways. Each Bonus Option offers an easy and flexible substitute for any week's Nutrition, Activity, or Stress-Reducing Options. They also provide additional ways to maximize your Profactor-H risk reduction.

If, for any Beginner's Nutrition, Activity, or Stress-Reducing Option, you cannot select one that fits your needs, preferences, or time concerns, you can choose a Bonus Option in its place. Simply substitute your Bonus Option in place of the selection for that week and continue it and your other selections in the weeks to come.

In addition, after you have selected all of your Beginner's Nutrition, Activity, and Stress-Reducing Options, in order to increase your risk-reduction choices, add as many Bonus Options as possible to your regular weekly Options—but remember to add no more than one new Option each week.

Bonus Options provide easy substitutes as well as extra ways to increase your risk reduction.

Bonus Options*

A. Take 200 micrograms of Glucose Tolerance Factor (GTF) Chromium** with dinner every night. **(6 points)**

B. If you regularly chew gum or eat mints, refrain from all gum chewing or mint eating except immediately following meals. **(6 points)**

> This includes both regular and artificially sweetened varieties.

C. Avoid all monosodium glutamate (MSG). MSG may be included as an ingredient under these names: hydrolyzed food starch, hydrolyzed vegetable protein, flavor enhancer, or natural ingredients. **(6 points)**

> MSG is a natural ingredient in soy sauce and Teriyaki.

D. Avoid all caffeine. In addition to coffee and tea, caffeine may be found in *some* herbal teas, chocolate, soda (regular and diet varieties), and some over-the-counter medications. **(6 points)**

E. Avoid all artificial sweeteners. Artificial sweeteners can be found in soda, mints, flavored coffees, desserts and sweets, ice cream and ices, yogurt, and many other foods (even those sweetened with sugar). In addition, artificial sweeteners can be found in over-the-counter medications including, among others, cough drops and cold remedies. **(6 points)**

F. Avoid all between-meal snacks. Eat no more than three meals each day. Meals may be eaten at any time. **(6 points)**

*Please select Options only if they do not conflict with your personal physician's recommendations.

**More information on Glucose Tolerance Factor (GTF) Chromium can be found in chapter 19, "Chromium: The Missing Link."

In the Weeks to Come

Once you have added a Beginner's Nutrition, Activity, and Stress-Reducing Option (or Bonus Option alternatives) into your daily routine, by adding them one week at a time, all of the Options in this Step are open to you.

First, look over your Beginner's Nutrition Options and see if there are any new selections you wish to add. If so, add no more than one each week, while you continue your past selections. Do the same with Stress-Reducing Options. Again, add only one Option during any one-week period. Bonus Options should be added in the same way. Add them one at a time, while continuing your past selections.

Even though Options come from different categories—Nutrition and Stress-Reducing, for instance, or Bonus and Nutrition—add only one new Option during any one-week period.

Even though Options may come from different categories, add only one of them during any one-week period.

When it comes to Activity Options you may find that you do not want to add a new Activity Option to other Activity Options; instead, you will probably want to substitute one Activity Option in place of another. Activity Options are offered in mild, moderate, and vigorous levels (Options A through C, respectively). If you like, substitute any Activity Option for another Activity selection in this same Step. If, however, you feel so inclined, you may add more than one Activity Option to your weekly schedule.

Remember to try to match your Options to your Profactor-H Evaluation subscores in chapter 4, so that if your Nutrition subscore, for instance, proved to be at the higher end of the range for you, you would choose as many Options (or those with the highest points) as possible in this area. In the same way, try to suit the Options you choose in the areas of Activity and Stress Reduction to your subscores in each of those areas as well.

Making a Change

There may come a time when you want to exchange one of your Beginner's Options for another. You may have been overly optimistic regarding your time or energy, or both. On the other hand, you may have thought that a Mild Activity Option, for instance, was all that you could handle, but in doing it, found that you want to increase the vigorousness of your selection. In any case, exchanging one Option for another is easy.

There may come a time when you will change your mind and want to exchange one of your Options for another. Exchanging one Option for another is easy.

If you want to exchange one of this Step's Options for another, simply look over the Options in the *same category* as the one you wish to exchange; Nutrition, for instance.

Choose your new Option and exchange it for your previous same-category selection by adding it to your regular routine. Be sure to continue it for an entire week, in combination with the other Options you have been following (other than the one you exchanged) before moving on to your next Option choice.

If you cannot find a satisfactory substitute for your Option in the same category, choose a Bonus Option in its stead.

At Your Own Pace

The Profactor-H Program was designed to decrease your Profactor-H risk week by week. Each new Option brings new opportunities for improving your probability of good health and long life. For a program to be livable, however, it is important to recognize that we are, after all, only human.

Time crunches, deadlines, unexpected illness, unforeseen situations, holidays, vacations, and more may all slow or halt the addition of an Option each week. In some cases, you may just want to lay back and temporarily "glide" on your past good behavior. Or you may feel a bit lazy. You don't need an excuse.

This is your program. If you would like to stop adding Options at any place along the way, do it. For that week, or for several weeks to come, select no additional Options. Just try not to let too long a time go by without beginning, once again, to add new Options as you continue the Program.

And most important, during your "time out" continue to practice the Options you have already selected. If you stop the Options you have been following, it will be that much harder to begin again. Remember how good you feel, each step of the way, as you have begun to take your life and health into your own hands. Even if you do not choose additional Options, try to keep following the ones you have already selected.

Charting Your Progress

Each week, you can measure your progress and see the ways in which your Options can help you reduce your Profactor-H risk. Keeping track of your progress on a weekly basis is completely optional, though most people find it important and very motivating.

Here is how we do it. Simply add up the points for all of the Options that you have been following as part of your daily routine for that week (that includes Options you may have already been following when you began the Program). Points can be found to the right of each Option on the charts on pages 204 to 207 and 209, as well as in the Beginner's Progress Chart at the end of this chapter. Count up your total week's points and mark them on your Progress Chart.

Now turn to the Risk-Reducing Percentage Chart on page 502. The Risk-Reducing Percentage Chart will help you keep track of your progress week by week. Look across the top and find your week's Option total. Follow your Option point column down until it crosses the row that holds your Profactor-H Evaluation score (from the quiz you took in chapter 4). The box in which your week's Option points and your Evaluation score meet gives you your relative

Risk-Reducing Percentage for that week. Mark this number in the appropriate space in your Progress Chart (page 215).

Here's a real example:

Sonia T. was in her third week on the Program. When she added up all of the values for her Risk-Reducing Options for that one week, she got a total of 13.

She marked this number on her Progress Chart.

Turning to the Risk-Reducing Percentage Chart, Sonia located the number 13 (the total of that week's points) across the top of the Percentage Chart and followed the column down until it crossed her Profactor-H Evaluation score, 43, from the side.

Sonia found that if she continued to follow these Options, she could reduce her Profactor-H risk by as much as 30 percent. In the weeks to come, as her points increase she can continue to chart and compare her progress.

CHARTING YOUR PROGRESS IS SIMPLE

1. Each week add up your Risk-Reducing points for all of the Options you have been following. Points can be found to the right of each Option in the Beginner's Risk-Reducing Options charts as well as on the Beginner's Progress Chart, page 215.

2. Fill in the total of this week's Option points on your Progress Chart. Include points for all the Options that you have followed during that week, along with points for any additional Options you might have been doing before beginning the Program. Include Nutrition, Activity, and Stress-Reducing points as well as Bonus Options.

3. In order to see your Profactor-H risk reduction in terms of relative percentages, turn to the Risk-Reducing Percentage Chart on page 502. Across the top of the Risk-Reducing Percentage Chart, find the total of your Option points for that week. On the left, locate your Profactor-H Evaluation score (from chapter 4). The box in which these two lines meet will give you your risk reduction in terms of relative percentages.

Risk-Reduction Percentages are relative and are based on the assumption of the continuation and combination of your Risk-Reducing Options. Calculations have been based on interpretation of all of the scientific data we have found available to date.

In your first few weeks on the Profactor-H Program, your relative percentage of risk reduction may be modest, but week by week, almost without noticing it, as you add new Options, your percentage will steadily increase. After a few weeks, you will be happily surprised at your own progress.

The Next Step

After you have selected all of the Nutrition, Activity, and Stress-Reducing Options, and/or Bonus Options that you want to select from this Step, and have made them a part of your regular routine, if you like you can choose to move to Step #2, the Intermediate Program.

There is no upper limit as to the total number of Options in any Step you may choose, and the greater the number of Options you select, the greater your relative Profactor-H risk reduction.

Please remember that while you may choose as many Options as you wish from any Step, you must choose at *least* three Options—one each from Nutrition, Activity, and Stress Reduction (or substitute Bonus Options)—before you are ready to move to the Intermediate Program.

You may choose to stay at any Step for good.

You may decide to stay at any Step for a while, or you may choose to stay at a Step for good. That is truly your choice and one that you can make with your physician's guidance. In general, it is far better to remain indefinitely at a Step you find comfortable than to move to the next Step only to find its Options a bit too challenging.

If you find a Step's Options that are "right" for you, comfortable and do-able, stay with them. There may come a time in the future when you are naturally ready for a new Step, but for now you have found a comfortable and livable way to reduce your Profactor-H risk. Stay with your Step and relax; enjoy knowing that you have found the very basis of true lifestyle change.

To complement your new way of life we have added chapters 20 and 21. They provide important information that will help you tailor the Program to fit your needs and preferences, and they offer you strategies for success in remaining successful, healthy, and happy.

STEP #1: BEGINNER'S PROGRESS CHART GUIDE

Use this chart to count up your total Option points each week. Keep track of your progress on the chart that follows on the next page.

Beginner's Nutrition Options	Risk-Reducing Values for Each Week

A. Include mixed green salad with your usual dinner .... 1 point
B. Include Risk-Reducing vegetable as part of your
   usual dinner .... 2 points
C. Eat *only* Risk-Reducing Foods at lunch .... 3 points

Activity Options

A. Light activity, 15 minutes, three times each week............. 1 point
B. Moderate activity, 15 minutes, three times each week...... 2 points
C. Vigorous activity, 15 minutes, three times each week .... 3 points

Stress-Reducing Options

A. Leave stressful environment, 15 minutes, three times
   each week.. 1 point
B. Stop all alcoholic beverages at lunch .... 2 points
C. Reduce smoking, by approximately one half.................. 3 points

Bonus Options

Take 200 micrograms of GTF-Chromium with dinner
   every night.. 6 points
Refrain from gum chewing/mint eating
   (Regular or artificially sweetened) .... 6 points
Avoid all MSG (monosodium glutamate)............................ 6 points
Avoid all caffeine .... 6 points
Avoid all artificial sweeteners... 6 points
Avoid all between-meal snacks .... 6 points

STEP #1: BEGINNER'S PROGRESS CHART

Week Beginning (Date)	Total Points for Week (Nutritional, Activity, Stress-Reducing, and Bonus)	Profactor-H Risk-Reduction Percentage*

*See Risk-Reducing Percentage Chart on page 502. Risk-Reduction Percentages are relative and are based on the continuation and combination of Risk-Reducing Options. Calculations have been based on the scientific data we have found available.

CHAPTER 16

Options, Options, Options

When choosing, trust none but yourself.
—Henry David Thoreau

The Profactor-H Program is the blueprint, the step-by-step plan that will help you in building your "house of health." The Nutrition, Activity, and Stress-Reducing Options that you choose are the bricks that, one by one, will make that house a reality.*

Each brick should be chosen carefully so that it will last and help make your house permanent and strong. Before you select an Option, take a moment to think about it. Choose one that makes sense given your preferences and your lifestyle. Choose Options that will be pleasant additions to your daily routine. You are a unique individual. Do not fashion yourself after anyone else. Choose an Option because *you* want it, not because you think other people would approve.

The Best Personal Match

When possible, try to move to higher-point Options in those areas where your Profactor-H Evaluation showed higher risk for *you*. If,

*Please select Options only if they do not conflict with your personal physician's recommendations.

for instance, according to your Profactor-H Evaluation in chapter 4, your Nutrition subscore was in the high end of the range, choose the greatest number of Options possible, or the Option with the highest points, in the area of Nutrition. In the same way, try to suit the Options you choose in the areas of Activity and Stress Reduction to your subscores in those areas. If your risk was highest in those areas, choose Options with the highest number of points to best insure reducing that area of risk.

Most of all, whenever possible, select an Option because it looks like fun or it is interesting or it is something that you really would like to do. Also, be realistic. Choose an Option that can easily fit into your schedule. A program that asks for just a little of your time is one with which you can live. If you want to move to more challenging Options you can; if you do not, that is just fine. It is better to remain consistently successful with an easier Option than to give up on one that you find is simply too demanding.

Nutrition Options

On the Profactor-H Program, foods are divided into two basic categories: Risk-Reducing Foods and Essential Balance Foods.

Risk-Reducing Foods include foods that are high in fiber, low in fat, and low in carbohydrates. They include fowl, meats, fish and shellfish, tofu, many vegetables, and salads. Eating Risk-Reducing Foods has been shown to lower your risk for Profactor-H and is an essential part of the Profactor-H Program.

Man and woman cannot live on Risk-Reducing Foods alone. It is necessary to your good health and well-being, and enjoyable as well, to add Essential Balance Foods to your eating program. Essential Balance Foods are foods that are moderate or high in carbohydrates and include many of the foods we need and love: bread, pasta, rice, cereal, potatoes, fruit, juices, and more.

We call these foods Essential Balance Foods because it is essential to add them to your Risk-Reducing Foods in order to maintain a nutritional balance. Risk-Reducing Foods help reduce your risk for Profactor-H; Essential Balance Foods provide the nutritional complement and pleasure you need to maintain this program for life. The combination of Risk-Reducing Foods and Essential Balance Foods can help you find the ideal balance of Profactor-H risk reduction within an ideal nutritional framework.

Risk-Reducing Foods:

Are high in fiber, low in fat, low in carbohydrates

Do not increase your insulin levels

Help reduce your Profactor-H risk

Risk-Reducing Foods include, among others:

Lean meats, fowl, fish, tofu, eggs, and low-fat substitutes

Salads

Low-carbohydrate (nonstarchy) vegetables

Cheese, cream cheese, cottage cheese, sour cream, and low-fat substitutes

And many more foods on the Risk-Reducing Foods list that follows

Essential Balance Foods:

Are moderate or high in carbohydrates

When eaten frequently, may increase insulin levels

Most are essential to good health and to maintaining the Program for life

Essential Balance Foods include, among others:

Breads of all kinds, pasta, other starches

Potatoes and rice

Legumes (beans)

Starchy vegetables

Milk, cream, yogurt

Fruit, juices

Snack foods

Sweets, candy, and desserts

And many more foods on the Essential Balance Foods list that follows

---

Although Essential Balance Foods may cause your insulin levels to rise when eaten frequently, some—in particular, those that contain complex carbohydrates—are absolutely necessary to your good health. More than half of the calories you consume each day must come from Essential Balance Foods. Fortunately, we have discovered two ways to "fool" your body, allowing you to eat the Essential

Balance Foods you need and enjoy, every day, and at the same time reducing the insulin-releasing power of these foods.

Your body can be fooled into releasing less insulin because the amount of insulin you release depends on two factors: first, the concentration of Essential Balance Foods during any particular meal; and second, how often you eat Essential Balance Foods in any one day.

If you decrease one or both of these factors, either how concentrated a particular meal is in Essential Balance Foods or the number of times each day that you eat Essential Balance Foods, you will lessen their ability to stimulate your body to release insulin and, as a result, decrease your risk for Profactor-H.

The good news is that you don't have to figure out how to balance Risk-Reducing and Essential Balance Foods yourself. We have done it for you and we will guide you each step of the way in the chapters that follow.

RISK-REDUCING FOODS LIST

NOTE: Any food not listed below should be considered an Essential Balance Food.

Quantities depend on your individual needs. Unless your physician advises otherwise, choose "average-size" portions. There is no need to measure or weigh your food.

Meats

All regular and lean meats,
   including:
   Bacon
   Beef
   Corned beef
   Hot dogs (all meat)
   Lamb
   Pastrami
   Pork and ham
   Rabbit
   Sausages (no sugar added)

Veal
Venison

Fowl

Chicken
Cornish hen
Duck
Goose
Pheasant
Quail
Turkey

Fish and shellfish

All varieties, canned or fresh

Dairy and nonmeat alternatives

Regular or low-fat varieties of:

Eggs and egg substitutes

Cheese

Cream cheese

Cottage cheese

Sour cream

Tofu (soybean curd)

Vegetarian meat alternatives that contain 4 grams of carbohydrates or less per average serving

Oils, fats, and dressings

Butter or margarine, or low-fat substitutes

Oils—all varieties, including: Olive, sesame, safflower, soybean, corn, vegetable, sunflower, etc.

Salad dressings—all regular and low-fat varieties

Vegetables

Asparagus

Bamboo shoots

Bean sprouts, alfalfa sprouts

Broccoli

Brussels sprouts

Cabbage (all varieties)

Cauliflower

Celery

Cucumbers

Green beans (also wax and snap)

Green peppers

Greens (all varieties)

Kale

Kohlrabi

Lettuce, endive, arugula

Mushrooms

Okra

Onions (as seasoning only)

Parsley and watercress

Radishes

Scallions

Sorrel (sour grass)

Spinach

Swiss chard

Tomatoes (raw, about ¼ per meal)

Condiments

Olives (green and black)

Dill pickles

Herbs, spices, and wines for cooking (all varieties)

Horseradish

Garlic or onion, fresh or powder

Ketchup (about 1 to 2 tablespoons)

Mayonnaise (regular or low-fat)

Mustard

Salt and pepper

Soy sauce, Teriyaki

Wines and citrus juices, for cooking only

Beverages

Coffee, tea

Carbonated water, seltzer, club soda

ESSENTIAL BALANCE FOODS LIST

SPECIAL NOTE: Below find examples of *some* of the many Essential Balance Foods. All foods that are not specifically listed as Risk-Reducing Foods should be assumed to be Essential Balance Foods.

Quantities depend on your individual needs. Unless your physician advises otherwise, choose "average-size" portions. There is no need to measure or weigh your food. See page 294 for balance guidelines.

Remember: If a food is not listed in the companion Risk-Reducing Foods list, it should automatically be considered an Essential Balance Food.

Breads, grains, and cereals

All varieties, including regular, low-fat, whole-grain, low-sugar, and low-salt:
Bagels
Biscuits
Bread
Cereal (hot or cold)
Corn meal
Couscous
Croissants
Grits
Pancakes
Tabuli
Tahini
Tempura coating
Stuffing
Waffles

Dairy

Regular, frozen, and low-fat varieties of:
Milk, cream, yogurt
Ice cream and ice milk

Legumes, seeds, and nuts

Kidney beans, black beans and lima beans, garbanzos, peanuts, chestnuts, cashews, pistachios, pumpkin seeds, and all other varieties of beans, seeds, and nuts

Rice and pasta

All varieties

*Snack foods

All varieties

*Sweets, sugars, desserts, cakes, candies

All varieties; any food containing sugar or honey

Vegetables

All those not listed as Risk-Reducing vegetables, usually the starchier or root vegetables, such as:
Beets
Carrots
Corn, peas
Potatoes
Squash, zucchini
Tomatoes (when more than ¼ per meal)

Fruit and fruit juices
All varieties, including fresh,
dried, or cooked:
Apples
Bananas
Cantaloupe, honeydew
Dates, figs
Grapes, cherries
Grapefruit, pineapple
Oranges, tangerines, lemons,
limes
Mangoes, papaya, kiwi fruit
Peaches, pears, plums,
nectarines

Strawberries, blackberries,
blueberries
Watermelon

Beverages
All fruit juices and drinks
All beverages containing
alcohol
All naturally- and artificially-
sweetened drinks

*Luncheon meats with filler
All varieties

*Although it may seem odd to include these foods as Essential Balance Foods because they may not seem essential to good health, they must be included in this list because of their insulin, and Profactor-H, impact.

Two Choices to Risk-Reducing Nutrition

At each Step you will find two kinds of Nutrition Options. The first type of Nutrition Option will ask you to add Risk-Reducing Foods to one of your regular meals.

When you choose a Nutrition Option that asks you to add Risk-Reducing Foods to a meal, over time your body will "learn" that it no longer needs to stimulate the release of as much insulin as it has in the past. You will be able to steadily reduce your body's insulin response and, along with it, your Profactor-H risk as well. An example of the "addition" type of Nutrition Option is one that asks you to "add a salad to your dinner."

The second type of Nutrition Option involves eating *only* Risk-Reducing Foods at a particular meal; at lunch, for instance, or during snacks. When you eat only Risk-Reducing Foods at a meal, your body releases far less insulin. The result: an immediate drop in Profactor-H risk. In combination, these two Nutrition Options can work extremely well in reducing your Profactor-H risk.

In each of the Steps, we will offer you simple Nutrition Options that will tell you how you can reduce the Profactor-H impact of your normal diet and still enjoy the benefits and pleasure of moderate- and high-carbohydrate foods every day. Each Option carries a Risk-Reducing Value from 1 through 12; you will be able to compare different Options' risk-reducing impact as well as keep track of your progress.

For your use, if appropriate, we have also included guidelines for following low-fat, low-salt, and other recommendations of the American Heart Association, the U.S. Department of Agriculture, the Department of Health and Human Services, and the Surgeon General of the United States. They can be found on page 345.

Remember: Essential Balance Foods are moderate- or high-carbohydrate foods, such as breads, pasta, rice, cereal, and potatoes. Essential Balance Foods provide a satisfying, well-rounded balance to Risk-Reducing Foods such as protein, salads, and many vegetables. Each day, you will enjoy foods from both groups.

Do's and Don'ts

Please do not make up Options of your own. Do not eat *only* Risk-Reducing Foods for all meals in hopes of more quickly lowering your risk for Profactor-H. Risk-Reducing Foods do not, in themselves, provide fully balanced and adequate nutrition. They must be combined with Essential Balance Foods at the same or at other meals every day.

Balance is the key for good health and well-being. Each day your Nutrition Options will help you combine Risk-Reducing Foods and Essential Balance Foods, so that you can be sure of getting all of the foods you need and love.* The combination of Risk-Reducing Foods and Essential Balance Foods in each Step's Options offers you the best of all possible worlds: ideal nutrition and lowered risk for Profactor-H.

*Subject to your physician's recommendations.

RISK-REDUCING FOODS CAN HAVE A POWERFUL IMPACT

**Please . . . do not make up your own Options.
And never make Risk-Reducing Foods your entire diet.**

While it may be of great benefit to *combine* Risk-Reducing Foods with other foods, at the same or other meals, Risk-Reducing Foods cannot, and should not, make up the majority or the totality of the food you eat.

It is important to balance your Risk-Reducing Foods with Essential Balance Foods (foods moderate or high in carbohydrates, including pasta, cereal, breads and other starches, fruit and juices, and the like). We call moderate- or high-carbohydrate foods Essential Balance Foods because they provide an essential balance to Risk-Reducing Foods. Essential Balance Foods may be confined to one major meal each day, but in total they should make up 55 to 60 percent of your daily intake of calories.

Your Nutrition Options will guide you each Step of the way and, in addition, current "Health Agency Recommendations" can be found on pages 345 to 347.

Activity Options

After you have selected a Nutrition Option and incorporated it into your daily routine, you will select an Activity Option. For your Activity Option, you will be able to choose from a wide variety of activities, movements, and exercises that include walking, dancing, jogging, swimming, pool exercises, jumping rope, biking (stationary or regular), skiing, tennis, racquetball, free weights, aerobics, treadmill home exercisers, Stepmaster® and stair aerobics, NordicTrack® home exercisers, and any other similar activities and machines or workout systems.

As a beginner, you will select one Activity Option and engage in that activity for a period of fifteen minutes, three times each week. Intermediate and Advanced levels will include somewhat longer periods. To help you compare activities and to keep track of your progress, Activity Options have been assigned Risk-Reducing Values from 1 through 7. More details can be found in the chapters defining each Step of the Program.

You will see that, within any of the Steps, you will be able choose from a variety of activities that range from mild to vigorous. As you move to advancing Steps, however, Activity Options require a greater length of time. It may seem odd that we concentrate on the length of time of an activity rather than demanding an intense exercise program. The reason is simple.

Within a given Step, the purpose of any Option is to work with other Options to reduce your Profactor-H risk. For Activity Options, this risk-reducing "matching" can best be accomplished by either gentle or rigorous activity. While vigorous activity can bring about a significant change in insulin levels, the length of time of an activity seems to be most crucial in Profactor-H risk reduction.

So, in trying to reduce Profactor-H levels, do not concern yourself about choosing the most energetic or demanding activity. Choose the one that you are more likely to enjoy—walking, for instance—so that you will increase your chances of continuing it. Consistency and length of time, rather than the demands of the activity, are the two factors that are most likely to keep your Profactor-H levels low.

Choose the most pleasant activity, not the most demanding one. Select the activity—walking, for instance— that you are more likely to enjoy.

Some people have been told that the more demanding an activity, the more calories it will burn. For the Profactor-H Positive person, this is not always so. Your body is bent on saving energy. An important way to pull it out of its "saving" mode is to maintain an active lifestyle—rather than a demanding exercise regimen that cannot be maintained.

When you are active, your risk for Profactor-H decreases. By adding an Activity Option to your Nutrition and Risk-Reducing Options, you can begin to make a real change in your Profactor-H levels and in your health risk factors as well.

Aerobics or other formal exercise regimens do have their place in programs with other health- and fitness-related goals, but for purposes of Profactor-H reduction only, gentle and regular activity can bring about results similar to those of more rigorous workouts. In addition, an enjoyable easy walking, movement, or dancing routine may be an activity that you will be most likely to maintain and that, in the end, will bring about the best Profactor-H–reducing results possible.

Activity Options are grouped by energy expenditure: mild, moderate, or vigorous. At each Step, although the length of time of you engage in an activity will increase, you will always be able to choose whether you prefer an activity that is mild, moderate, or vigorous. Don't overdo it. Select an activity that you will find most enjoyable and easy to maintain.

ACTIVITY OPTIONS*

At Beginner, Intermediate, and Advanced Steps, choose from *any* of these categories (see the Activity Options for each Step):

Light activity

Walk: briskly
Dance: moderate pace
Pool exercises: a wide variety of light, easy activity
Biking (regular or stationary): easy, even pace
NordicTrack®, Stepmaster®, treadmills, and similar systems: very easy, even pace
Golf
Bowling

Moderate activity

Walk: very fast pace, without interruption
Dance: fast pace, without interruption
Pool exercises: brisk, intense exercises, without interruption
Jogging: light, brisk running
Swimming: moderate, even pace
Rope jumping: light to moderate pace
Roller skating: light to moderate pace
Biking (regular or stationary): moderate pace
Skiing (cross-country or downhill): light to moderate pace

Moderate activity *(cont.)*

Tennis, racquetball, volleyball: light, easy pace
NordicTrack®, Stepmaster®, treadmills, and similar systems: moderate, even pace
Free weights: moderate pace, some rest time included
Aerobics: light to moderate pace

Vigorous activity

Jogging: intense running
Swimming: fast pace
Rope jumping: fast, consistent
Roller skating: fast pace
Biking (regular or stationary): strong, fast pace
Skiing (cross-country or downhill): fast pace
Tennis, racquetball, volleyball: moderate to fast pace
NordicTrack®, Stepmaster®, treadmills, and similar systems: fast pace
Free weights: intense workout
Aerobics: intense, fast pace

*Please select Options only if they do not conflict with your personal physician's recommendations.

Stress-Reducing Options

When most people hear the word *stress* they think of emotional tension, pressure, and demands. We all know this kind of stress and have experienced its impact on our minds and bodies. In addition, we have all heard reports regarding the negative impact of emotional stress on our physical well-being. Many different diseases and disorders have been linked directly and indirectly to feelings of pressure and strain and anger. Emotional stress can lead to higher insulin levels and a strong increase in Profactor-H risk. Emotional (or psychological) stress is the first of two major kinds of stress that our bodies may be forced to endure.

There is, however, a second major type of stress that is rarely considered: physical stress, stress that comes from the body's coping with unexpected demands.

Extreme cold or heat, alcoholic beverages, smoking, strenuous physical exertion, strong medications, preservatives and additives, allergic reactions, illness, fever, surgery—all can stress the body beyond its normal limits.

When we are either emotionally or physically stressed, our bodies try to adjust by releasing *stress hormones*. Stress hormones are meant to help us handle increased demands, but they can also affect insulin levels and, in doing so, raise your Profactor-H risk.

In addition to releasing stress hormones, our bodies respond to emotional and physical demands by activating the sympathetic nervous system, which, in turn, can increase insulin levels and Profactor-H risk even more.

Stress-Reducing Options are designed to lower your insulin levels by "disconnecting" the impact of stress hormones on your nervous system and insulin release. Stress-Reducing Options carry values from 1 through 12. Stress-Reducing Options work with your Nutrition and Activity Options to help you reduce your Profactor-H risk and to keep it low in the face of unexpected or extreme demands.

There is little we can do to remove ourselves from the physical stress of fever, illness, or surgery, but reducing the physical stress that comes from drinking or smoking is quite a different matter. Studies on the impact of alcohol consumption report varying findings. Almost all research shows that heavy, frequent drinking results in a higher risk of poor health and disease, but in addition some studies show that drinking as little as one and a half drinks each day can increase your chances for breast cancer. Other scientists claim that a little wine or beer may be a key in keeping blood fat levels low, though more recent reviews cast some doubt on alcohol as the sole and essential factor.

In our research, the one consistent connection we have found is the impact of alcohol consumption on Profactor-H risk. Frequent alcohol intake raises Profactor-H levels two ways: by increasing your body's production and release of insulin (Cofactor-p) and by increasing your body's resistance to removing insulin from the bloodstream (Cofactor-r). As alcohol consumption raises insulin levels, it raises your Profactor-H risk.

If you enjoy alcoholic beverages, choosing a Stress-Reducing Option that confines alcohol to a specific time each day (at dinner, for instance) can greatly reduce your Profactor-H risk. Select this Option only if you currently consume alcoholic beverages at other times.

Smoking, a major stress on the body, has been repeatedly linked to heart disease, high blood pressure, stroke, some forms of cancer, and other illnesses. We strongly believe that smoking's health-diminishing impact is due, in part at least, to its ability to raise and maintain high Profactor-H levels. If you smoke, choosing a Stress-Reducing Option that reduces or eliminates your smoking may greatly reduce your Profactor-H risk. Select this Option only if you currently smoke.

Reducing the impact that emotional stress can have on your body can easily become a part of your Profactor-H Program. Removing yourself, in thought or body, from the source of the stress may help you to decrease your physical response to it and, in doing so, lower your Profactor-H risk. If you find yourself regularly in stressful situations, at home or at work, choosing a Stress-Reducing Option that "disconnects" you from that situation can help decrease your Profactor-H risk. Select this Option only if you find yourself under stress at home, at work, or both.

Stress-Reducing Options can be selected individually or in combination. Do not select more than one *new* Stress-Reducing Option in any one week. If you wish to choose more than one Stress-Reducing Option, select one and continue it for an entire week—then maintain it while you select a new Option.

Remember that it is more important to be consistent with the Options you have chosen than to add one Option after another. While you can add any new Option, Stress-Reducing or other, each week, add a *new* Option only when you feel comfortable with the Options you have already chosen.

Risk-Reducing Options may be far easier than you anticipate. Benefits from other Options may increase your comfort and ability to leave many of these past habits behind.

Glucose Tolerance Factor (GTF) Chromium, for instance, a Bonus Option that we will discuss in chapter 19, has been recommended as a reducer of smoking withdrawal symptoms. Adding the Bonus Option of GTF Chromium, then, may make the Stress-Reducing Options related to reducing smoking far easier than they have been in the past.

The Options in this Program have been designed to complement and build on other Options; you will probably find yourself happily surprised at how easy and enjoyable your Options can be.

If you are one of the rare and lucky individuals who neither smoke nor drink and have little or no stress in your work or at home, or if you do not wish to choose one of these Options, please select a Bonus Option in place of your Stress-Reducing Option at any or all Steps.

Bonus Options

Bonus Options give you extra flexibility on the Program. You may choose a Bonus Option in place of a Nutrition, Activity, or Stress-Reducing Option, or add it to your Options for additional risk-reducing benefit. Bonus Options include adding Glucose Tolerance Factor (GTF) Chromium as a supplement each day or removing monosodium glutamate (MSG), artificial sweeteners, caffeine, gum, or between-meal snacks from your diet.

Glucose Tolerance Factor (GTF) Chromium is so important to Profactor-H risk reduction that we have given it its own chapter, "Chromium: The Missing Link" (chapter 19). The Chromium Bonus Option is an exciting one; we would urge you to read chapter 19 and, with your physician's approval, add GTF Chromium to your program.

Diabetics and others taking insulin should be aware that the impact of GTF Chromium can be so great that it can reduce your need for medication. If you are taking insulin, then, be sure to have your physician regularly monitor your need for medication.

Bonus Options that ask you to remove substances—monosodium glutamate (MSG), artificial sweeteners, caffeine, gum, or between-meal snacks—from your diet have been designed to reduce your Profactor-H risk by reducing your production and release of insulin (Cofactor-p), reducing your body's resistance to insulin (Cofactor-r), and reducing the triggering of your sympathetic nervous system. Eliminating one or more of these Profactor-H agitators may combine with your other Options to help keep you healthy, happy, and fit.

Bonus Options can be selected individually or in combination, but, as always, choose one Option at a time and continue it for a week before selecting another. Each Bonus Option carries a Risk-Reducing Value of 6 points.

A Valuable Combination

Your Profactor-H Program is more than the sum total of its various Options. It has been carefully designed to work as a unit, so that each Option complements and increases the power of other Options.

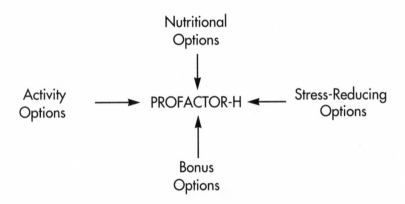

The Risk-Reducing Values that have been assigned to each Option are based on the assumption that, over time, you will select and continue Options in combination, one with others. Their values (in points) will help you compare the expected impact of an Option on your Profactor-H risk and, in addition, help you visualize the progress you are making as you may be literally changing your life. It is *not* necessary to keep track of your risk-reducing gains, but it can be fun and satisfying to see your progress.

No one Option and no one Value stands alone. They work in combination, as part of an entire Profactor-H risk-reduction program, a program that has been designed to be beneficial and enjoyed—for life.

CHAPTER 17

Step #2—The Intermediate Program: Reaping the Benefits

Step after step, the ladder is ascended.
—George Herbert

You have reached a very important milestone. You have shown, by your actions, that taking good care of yourself is important to you, important enough for you to make decisions and changes that can affect the rest of your life.

But we want to alert you; this is a critical point. The decisions you make in the next few weeks can be of utmost importance. So, while you have certainly taken the first steps toward reducing your Profactor-H risk, please do not relax and coast on your previous good work.

We encourage you to keep making new selections, adding a new Risk-Reducing Option each week. Imagine that you are climbing a stairway to good health and well-being. You are moving, one step at a time, climbing surely and steadily to the top. Keep your eyes fixed on your goal, do not look down, and don't stop moving.

In Step #2, the Intermediate Program, your Options will bring you greater relative risk reduction, and as you continue, you will more fully begin to reap the benefits of the Program.

Each of the Intermediate Risk-Reducing Options* that follow will take very little more of your time or effort than did the Beginner's

---

*Please select Options only if they do not conflict with your personal physician's recommendations.

Options. Each Intermediate Option has been designed to flow naturally and easily from your past choices, bringing you one step closer to your goal.

HOW TO BEGIN YOUR INTERMEDIATE PROGRAM

Intermediate Week #1: Nutrition

1. Look over Intermediate Nutrition Options A, B, and C, which follow.

2. Choose one Option as your first Intermediate Nutrition Option. For one week, add that Option to your regular routine *in place of* one of the Beginner's Nutrition Options that you have been following. At the same time, continue all other Options you have selected in the past.

   If you made no Nutrition selection in the past and want to choose one now, simply add your new Nutrition Option to your daily routine.

   If there is no Intermediate Nutrition Option that is appropriate or that you want to choose, see the "Special Circumstances" section on page 238.

Intermediate Nutrition Options

A. Include a large Risk-Reducing salad (at least 2 cups) and a Risk-Reducing vegetable with your usual dinner. **(3 points)**
   Continue eating any Essential Balance Foods and Risk-Reducing Foods you normally have at any meals, and at any snacks you usually have. Risk-Reducing and Essential Balance Foods are listed on pages 220 to 223.

B. Include an average portion (about 1 cup *each*) of *two* Risk-Reducing vegetables as part of your usual dinner. **(4 points)**
   Continue eating any Essential Balance Foods and Risk-Reducing Foods you normally have at any meals, and

---

at any snacks you usually have. You can find a full list of Risk-Reducing and Essential Balance Foods on pages 220 to 223.

SPECIAL NOTE: As an alternate to adding both Options A and B, add a *total* of two Risk-Reducing vegetables (1 cup each) and one large salad to your dinner, and credit yourself with a total of 5 points.

C. Eat *only* Risk-Reducing Foods, including protein, vegetables, and/or salad, at lunch *and* at any snacks. **(5 points)** If you choose to have snacks, make them about half the size of an "average-size" lunch. Continue eating any Essential Balance Foods and Risk-Reducing Foods you normally have at breakfast and dinner only. See pages 220 to 223 for a full list of Risk-Reducing and Essential Balance Foods and page 303 for Sample Meals and Snacks.

To chart your progress, use the Intermediate Progress Chart on page 242. For guidance, see the "Charting Your Progress" section on page 239.

3. When you are ready to select your new Intermediate Option for the week to come, read the "Intermediate Week #2: Activity" section, which follows.

Intermediate Week #2: Activity

1. Look over Intermediate Activity Options A, B, and C, which follow.

2. Choose one Option as your first Intermediate Activity Option. For one week, add that Option to your regular routine *in place of* one of the Beginner's Activity Options that you have been following. At the same time, continue all other Options you have selected in the past.

If you made no Activity selection in the past and want to choose one now, simply add your new Option to your daily routine.

If there is no Activity Option from this Step that is appropriate or that you are willing to select, see the "Special Circumstances" section on page 238.

Intermediate Activity Options

A.   Walk for ½ hour, three times each week, or 15 minutes every day.

Any Light Activity Option from the list on page 227 may be substituted.   **(3 points)**

B.   Swim, jog lightly, or bike (on a regular or stationary bike) for ½ hour, three times each week, or 15 minutes every day.   **(4 points)**

Any Moderate Activity Option from the list on pages 227 to 228 may be substituted.

C.   Play tennis or racquetball, jog briskly, or do step aerobics for ½ hour, three times each week, or 15 minutes every day.   **(5 points)**

Any Vigorous Activity Option from the list on page 228 may be substituted.

---

3.   When you are ready to select your new Intermediate Option for the week to come, read "Intermediate Week #3: Stress Reduction," which follows.

Intermediate Week #3: Stress Reduction

1.   Look over Intermediate Stress-Reducing Options A, B, and C, which follow.

2.   Choose one Option as your first Intermediate Stress-Reducing Option. For one week, add that Option to your regular routine *in place of* one of the Beginner's Stress-Reducing Options that you have been following. At the same time, continue all other Options you have selected in the past.

If you made no Stress-Reducing selection in the past and want to select one now, simply add your new Option to your daily routine.

If there is no Stress-Reducing Option from this Step that is appropriate or that you are willing to select, see the "Special Circumstances" section on page 238.

NOTE ON STRESS-REDUCING OPTIONS: As in the Beginner's Program, if you do not smoke or drink alcoholic beverages on a regular or semiregular basis, do not choose a Stress-Reducing Option that asks you to limit or eliminate these practices (Stress-Reducing Options B or C). If you do not regularly find yourself in a stressful situation either at home or at work, do not choose Stress-Reducing Option A.

Intermediate Stress-Reducing Options

A. At least three times each week, for at least ½ hour at a time, or for 15 minutes every day, remove yourself from an environment (home, work, or other) that you find stressful. **(3 points)**

You may want to physically remove yourself by leaving the premises or you can close the door (and your eyes) and listen to some soothing music or to one of the many relaxation audiotapes available commercially. You might want to meditate or simply take a nap. You may want to take a book or audiotape and sit alone for a while in your car. Or, if no other private place is available, remove yourself to a bathroom stall.

B. Confine all alcoholic beverages to dinner only. (Select this Option only if you have one or more alcoholic drinks at times other than dinner on a rather regular basis.) **(4 points)**

C. If you smoke (cigarette, cigar, or pipe), reduce your smoking by about one half. If you selected this Option in the Beginner's section as well, your smoking in total now will be cut to one fourth the amount prior to your starting the Program. **(5 points)**

---

3. After incorporating your Intermediate Stress-Reducing Option into your regular routine for one week, move to the "In the Weeks to Come" section on page 238.

Special Circumstances

If there is no Intermediate Nutrition, Activity, or Stress-Reducing Option that is appropriate or that you want to choose, select a new Bonus Option and continue following all previous Options.

Remember, in order to best reduce your Profactor-H risk, we urge you to choose from that week's Activity, Nutrition, or Stress-Reducing Option when appropriate. But choosing the usual selection is not always possible or advisable, so don't worry, you can choose a Bonus Option in its place.

Bonus Options

As you know, Bonus Options can always be used as a substitute for Nutrition, Activity, or Stress-Reducing Options. Bonus Options remain the same at the Beginner, Intermediate, or Advanced levels of the Program. A full list of Bonus Options can be found on page 209.

Bonus Options remain the same at the
Beginner, Intermediate, or Advanced levels of the Program.
A full list of Bonus Options can be found on page 209.

In the Weeks to Come

Once you have exchanged a Nutrition, Activity, and Stress-Reducing Option (or added Bonus Option alternatives instead) from this Step into your daily routine, all of the Options in this Step are open to you.

First, look over this Step's Nutrition Options and see if there is another Nutrition Option that you wish to add. If so, add any new Nutrition Option one week at a time. Each time you add a new Nutrition Option from this Step you can, at the same time, drop a Nutrition Option from your previous Step. If you have no more Nutrition Options from previous Steps to drop, or if you like, rather than exchanging a Nutrition Option you can simply add a new one to your previous choices. Do the same with Stress-Reducing Options. Again, add or exchange only one Option from that category during any one-week period.

When it comes to Activity Options, you may not want to add an Activity Option to your other previous Activity selections. Instead, you will probably prefer to exchange one Activity Option for another from this or previous Steps. If, however, you feel so inclined, you can add Activity Options rather than exchanging them for previous Activity choices.

For best Profactor-H risk reduction, over time try to add as many Options as possible given your needs, preferences, and physical limits.

When You Need a Change

If you find an Option overdemanding or underdemanding, or simply not to your liking, you can exchange it for another in the same category or for a Bonus Option instead.

At Your Own Pace

Weekly additions and exchanges of Options often bring satisfaction and success. They keep you motivated and can help to steadily decrease your Profactor-H risk. On the other hand, you should keep in mind that you are an individual with personal needs and preferences. If you want to adjust your pace and stay where you are for a while, do it; just keep to a regular schedule and try to maintain the wonderful risk-reducing choices you have already made.

Charting Your Progress

If you have charted your progress before, use the same method that you used in your Beginner's Program. Continue to use the same Risk-Reducing Percentage Chart you used before (see page 502); however, for this Step you will use the Intermediate Progress Chart

Guide on the next page. Your point total for each week will include points from continuation of your Beginner's Options as well as points for your new Intermediate Options.

Even if you have not charted your progress before, it is not too late to begin to keep track of your success. Remember, charting your progress on a weekly basis is completely optional, but it can be very motivating and quite enjoyable as well. See "Charting Your Progress" on pages 212 to 213 for details. For this level, remember to use Guide on the next page and the Intermediate Progress Chart at the end of this chapter.

The Next Step

After you have selected all of the Nutrition, Activity, and Stress-Reducing Options, and/or Bonus Options, that you want from this Step, and have made them a part of your regular routine, you can choose to move to Step #3, the Advanced Program: Reducing Your Risk—For Life.

You may choose to stay at any Step for good.

You may decide to stay at the Intermediate level for a while, or you may choose to stay for good. Remember that it is better to remain indefinitely at any Step that is comfortable and fits into your normal routine than to move to the next Step, which may be less appropriate or too challenging.

If you find the Intermediate Step to be "right" for you, comfortable and do-able, stay here. In the future you may find that you are ready for a new Step, but for now you have found a livable way to reduce your Profactor-H risk. Stay with this Step and enjoy the benefits you find here.

Whether you stay here or move on, chapters 20 and 21 provide important information that will help you tailor the Program to fit your needs and preferences and help you with strategies for success. Take time to read them; they will help you stay motivated and successful in your new, exciting, and commendable way of life.

STEP #2: INTERMEDIATE PROGRESS CHART GUIDE

Use this guide to count up your total Option points each week. Keep track of your progress on the chart that follows on the next page.

**Intermediate
Nutrition Options**   **Risk-Reducing Values
for Each Week**

A. Include mixed green salad *and* a Risk-Reducing
   vegetable with your usual dinner .... 3 points
B. Include two Risk-Reducing vegetables as part of
   your usual dinner.. 4 points
   SPECIAL NOTE: If Options A and B are chosen in
   combination, only two Risk-Reducing vegetables
   and one salad need be included as part of dinner .... 5 points
C. Eat *only* Risk-Reducing Foods at lunch as well as for
   any snacks... 5 points

Activity Options

A. Light activity: ½ hour, three times each week, or
   15 minutes every day .... 3 points
B. Moderate activity: ½ hour, three times each week, or
   15 minutes every day .... 4 points
C. Vigorous activity: ½ hour, three times each week, or
   15 minutes every day .... 5 points

Stress-Reducing Options

A. Leave stressful environment, ½ hour, three times each
   week, or for 15 minutes every day .... 3 points
B. Confine all alcoholic beverages to dinner .... 4 points
C. Reduce smoking by about half again
   (equal to a quarter from start of program)...................... 5 points

Bonus Options

Take 200 micrograms of GTF-Chromium with dinner
   every night... 6 points
Refrain from gum chewing/mint eating (regular or
   artificially sweetened)... 6 points
Avoid all MSG (monosodium glutamate) .... 6 points
Avoid all caffeine .... 6 points
Avoid all artificial sweeteners.. 6 points
Avoid all between-meal snacks .... 6 points

STEP #2: INTERMEDIATE PROGRESS CHART

Week Beginning (Date)	Total Points for Week (Nutritional, Activity, Stress-Reducing, and Bonus)	Profactor-H Risk-Reduction Percentage*

*See Risk-Reducing Percentage Chart on page 502. Risk-Reduction Percentages are relative and are based on the continuation and combination of Risk-Reducing Options. Calculations have been based on the scientific data we have found available.

Too Young to Be Getting Old: Sheila's Story

Sheila had everything a woman could hope for. Her husband, Steve, was a fine and successful physician, handsome, intelligent, and well-respected. He was attentive to her needs and concerns, and when he called us, his voice was filled with distress. He had consulted us, in the past, regarding several of his patients and said that he had been pleased with the "turnaround" he saw in them. Now, he said, he wanted our help with his wife.

He described his wife in loving but professional terms. She was forty-four years old, about thirty pounds overweight—most of which she gained during her two pregnancies, though he admitted she might have put on "a little extra recently." Though she was not actually ill, Sheila was showing signs of less than ideal health.

We asked Steve to answer a few focused questions about his wife's family and personal medical history and learned that her parents were both quite ill—her mother with breast cancer and her father with recently diagnosed heart problems. Her father was being scheduled for surgery even as we spoke.

Steve said that he was concerned that his wife might be feeling depressed. She had lost interest in many of the things that used to please her. A fine cook, specializing in Oriental cuisine, she had not had any guests over for quite a while and had started, on a regular basis, buying take-out food for the family or going out to eat. Though he was quick to tell us that he was not asking to have Sheila "tied to the kitchen," Steve told us that he knew that cooking for the family and entertaining was something his wife truly enjoyed and he was concerned at her change and loss of interest. At first he thought her lack of energy was simply due to her parents' ill health, but a recent physical exam showed some new and distressing signs.

In the year and a half since her last examination, Sheila's blood pressure had jumped. The fat levels in her blood had gone from normal to high-risk levels, and she had put on over twelve pounds. She told the doctor that she had been having headaches and feeling weak and shaky at times. She said that she had little desire to do anything. Many days, she would spend hours in front of the television or napping and rouse herself only when she knew her husband or her daughters would be coming home.

Though her physician could find nothing physically wrong with her, other than the rising risk indicators shown by her blood pressure, her weight, and the levels of fat in her blood, he too was concerned.

We agreed to see Sheila the following week, and she entered our offices looking far older than her forty-four years. The feeling of advancing age came not from Sheila's looks but from her attitude and movement. She seemed tired. She had no energy and, with great effort, sat down across from us.

We spoke a while and then gave Sheila our Profactor-H Evaluation. Her overall score placed her at High Risk. Her highest concentration of risk seemed to come from her Family History subscore. While this would certainly place her at High Risk for Profactor-H, this fact alone was not enough to explain the sudden and dramatic changes in her health and well-being. She said that she had not changed her eating or diet, although she had been sleeping a great deal more lately.

> "I feel so tired," she said, "and I can't seem to shake myself out of it."

When we talked of other recent changes, including her parents' illnesses, Sheila's pain and worry broke through. With honest emotion she told us of her fear of breast cancer and that watching her mother's pain was almost more than she could bear. Her anger with her father for smoking and eating "his way to the grave" was matched by her guilt at being unable to stop him. She wanted to help them, she told us, but she felt as if she were being pulled in twenty directions all at once—to the point where, she told us, "sometimes I feel almost paralyzed."

Sheila could barely summon the energy to keep her own life together, she admitted, much less start a new program. "I feel so tired, so old," she said, "and I can't seem to shake myself out of it." Then she added, "This couldn't all be coming from my parents . . . could it?"

Oh, yes, it could, we told her. But not in the way she thought. Many of Sheila's difficulties could easily be coming, not from her parents directly, but rather from the way her body handled—or was unable to handle—stress. Before her parents became ill, Sheila had shown many signs of Profactor-H. Her carbohydrate cravings, weight gain, and occasional signs of low blood sugar were something she had tried to learn to live with. She had wondered as to the cause of it all but had blamed it on what she called her own "bad eating habits."

When both of her parents' illnesses were diagnosed within two weeks of each other, however, Sheila felt "like the carpet had been pulled out" from under her. The stress had been un-expected and great.

In trying to cope, we told Sheila, she was almost certainly producing stress hormones, called *glucocorticoids*. Now her blood pressure, weight, and blood fat levels were reflecting a far more advanced stage of Profactor-H than before, and she might, indeed, feel the difference.

> In trying desperately to cope, Sheila could be expected to produce excess levels of "stress hormones." The rises in her weight, blood pressure, and blood fat levels were reflecting typical effects of stress and the Profactor-H levels it produced.

We helped Sheila understand that while no one could take away the problems with which she was dealing, we could help her body better handle the stress. Our Program was designed to correct her body's *response* to the stress, we told her, and should be able to help her reduce her blood pressure, blood fat levels, weight, and lack of energy—all at the same time.

"You hear about what stress can do," she told us, "but you think you're invulnerable. You know, you get tired, but you don't really expect to get *sick*. It's hard to believe this is all coming from the stress of dealing with my parents' problems," she said, "but I'm willing to give it a try."

Sheila was as good as her word. She moved through the Program quickly and easily, enjoying her progress and feeling better than she had "in years." As we suggested, given the stress in her life, Sheila concentrated on her Stress-Reducing Options in addition to her Nutrition and Activity Options, and most important, with our encouragement, she stayed centered on *her* needs and *her* health.

At each visit to her physician, her health indicators improved, and after she completed the Intermediate Program, her physician confirmed that she was on "a sure path" to better health. Sheila was relieved, and her husband was delighted.

They both dropped in to see us about a year or so after that first visit. Sheila looked wonderful and well. She had weathered her mother's illness and helped her through her father's passing. She had stayed with the Intermediate Program, she told us, because she found it "easy to maintain." "Besides," she added, "it seems to be doing the trick." Sheila told us that her blood pressure and laboratory results had remained well within normal limits, and we could see a change in her appearance that was truly startling.

As Sheila was leaving the office, one of our research assistants commented on how well Sheila looked. She smiled and said, "I never felt better. I've lost fifty pounds . . . and I feel twenty years younger."

"Well, you certainly look it," our assistant said, and Sheila smiled and waved good-bye.

Stress does amazing things to our bodies—especially if we are Profactor-H Positive. It can move us from Low Risk to Moderate Risk—or, in some cases, to High Risk. It can add a second cofactor and increase the effect of Profactor-H manyfold. It can lower our resistance to illness or, in some cases, directly cause damage to our bodies. It can make us feel and look old, long before our time.

In this country, we have come to accept stress as part of our lives. We have started to tell ourselves that stress has no effect, or should have no effect, on us. In truth, the effects of stress can be devastating. Reducing or eliminating stress must involve more than meditation or deep breathing—it means a complete and simple program that can, without deprivation or sacrifice, reduce both the physical and the psychological demands on your body. Reducing stress means changing the way stress affects *your particular body* so that you too can enjoy your life, your health, and your peace of mind.

CHAPTER 18

Step #3—The Advanced Program: Reducing Your Risks—For Life

When seeking to reach the top of a staircase, look forward only and mount one small step at a time.
—Dr. Richard F. Heller

You've done it. Your good work and commitment have brought you to the homestretch of a program that you will be able to follow—for life. You have shown the ability to do what almost every health recommendation says is essential to all health-promoting programs: You have changed your lifestyle.

Step by Step, Option by Option, you have made positive choices, and this final group of Options will now come easily and naturally to you.

You are almost where you always wanted to be. You are making real change and we congratulate you. But a word of caution: Don't feel too sure of yourself. It is far too easy to take for granted your own conscientious efforts. Do not be fooled into "taking some time off" or "taking it easy for a while" just because you are pleased with yourself. You have done too well for that kind of temptation.

Listen to yourself. Remember how good you feel in making change, and for some extra reinforcement, from time to time read over chapters 1 and 21: "New Bodies, New Hopes, New Lives" and "Strategies for Success." Each of these chapters contains the personal experiences of ourselves and others and has been included for your repeated use—when you need it, and even when you think you don't. These chapters are our way of saying, "We know; we've been there. It's great on this side and we'll help you keep it up!"

In Step #3, the Advanced Program, your Options will bring you even greater Profactor-H relative risk reduction.

Each of the Advanced Options* that follow will be an easy extension of your Intermediate Options, and in the weeks to come, you will enjoy, even more, watching yourself continuing to reduce your Profactor-H risk.

How to Begin Your Advanced Program

Advanced Week #1: Nutrition

1. Look over Advanced Nutrition Options A, B, and C, which follow.

2. Choose one Option as your first Advanced Nutrition Option. For one week, add that Option to your regular routine *in place of* one of the Intermediate Nutrition Options that you have been following. At the same time, continue all other Options you have selected in the past.

    If you made no Nutrition selection in the past and want to choose one now, simply add your new Option to your daily routine.

    If there is no Advanced Nutrition Option that is appropriate or that you want to choose, see the "Special Circumstances" section on page 253.

Advanced Nutrition Options

A. Include a large Risk-Reducing salad (at least 2 cups) and two Risk-Reducing vegetables (at least 1 cup each) with your usual dinner. **(5 points)**

   Continue eating any Essential Balance Foods and Risk-Reducing Foods you normally have at any meals, and for any snacks you usually have. Risk-Reducing and Essential Balance Foods are listed on pages 220 to 223.

---

*Please select Options only if they do not conflict with your personal physician's recommendations.

B. Eat a Risk-Reducing salad (at least 2 cups) *before* dinner
and include two Risk-Reducing vegetables (at least 1 cup
each) as part of your usual dinner. **(6 points)**

Continue eating any Essential Balance Foods and Risk-
Reducing Foods you normally have at any meals, and
for any snacks you usually have. You can find a full
list of Risk-Reducing and Essential Balance Foods on
pages 220 to 223.

C. Eat *only* Risk-Reducing Foods, including protein, vegetables, and salad, at all breakfasts, lunches, *and* for any
snacks. If you choose to have snacks, make them about
half the size of an "average-size" lunch. **(12 points)**

Include a balance of both Essential Balance Foods and
Risk-Reducing Foods at dinner. See pages 220 to 223
for a full list of Risk-Reducing and Essential Balance
foods; see pages 294 to 296 for a guide to balancing
your dinner; Sample Meals begin on page 298.

To chart your progress, use the Advanced Progress Chart at
the end of this chapter.

3. When you are ready to select your new Advanced Option for
the week to come, read "Advanced Week #2: Activity," which
follows.

Advanced Week #2: Activity

1. Look over Advanced Activity Options A, B, and C, which follow.
2. Choose one Option as your first Advanced Activity Option.
For one week, add that Option to your regular routine *in
place of* one of the Intermediate Activity Options that you
have been following. At the same time, continue all other Options you have selected in the past.

If you made no Activity selection in the past and want to
choose one now, add your new Option to your daily routine.

If there is no Advanced Nutrition Option that is appropriate or that you want to choose, see the "Special Circumstances" section on page 253.

Advanced Activity Options

A. Walk for 1 hour, three times each week, or ½ hour every day. **(5 points)**

Any Light Activity Option from the list on page 227 may be substituted.

B. Swim, jog lightly, or bike (on a regular or stationary bike) for 1 hour, three times each week, or ½ hour every day. **(6 points)**

Any Moderate Activity Option from the list on pages 227 to 228 may be substituted.

C. Play tennis or racquetball, jog briskly, or do step aerobics for 1 hour, three times each week, or ½ hour every day. **(7 points)**

Any Vigorous Activity Option from the list on page 228 may be substituted.

3. When you are ready to select your new Advanced Stress-Reducing Option for the week to come, read "Advanced Week #3: Stress Reduction," which follows.

Advanced Week #3: Stress Reduction

1. Look over Advanced Stress-Reducing Options A, B, and C, which follow.

2. Choose one Option as your first Advanced Stress-Reducing Option. For one week, add that Option to your regular routine *in place of* one of the Stress-Reducing Options that you have been following. At the same time, continue all other Options you have selected in the past.

If you want to choose a new Stress-Reducing Option but chose none in the past, simply add your new Option to your daily routine.

If there is no Stress-Reducing Option from this Step that is appropriate or that you are willing to select, see the "Special Circumstances" section on page 253.

NOTE ON STRESS-REDUCING OPTIONS: As in the Intermediate Program, if you do not smoke or drink alcoholic beverages on a regular or semiregular basis, do not choose a Stress-Reducing Option that asks you to limit or eliminate these practices (Stress-Reducing Options B or C). If you do not regularly find yourself in a stressful situation at either home or at work, do not choose Stress-Reducing Option A.

Advanced Stress-Reducing Options

A.   At least three times each week, for at least 1 hour at a time, or for ½ hour every day, remove yourself from an environment (home, work, or other) that you find stressful. **(5 points)**

   You may want to physically remove yourself by leaving the premises or you can close the door (and your eyes) and listen to some soothing music or one of the many relaxation audiotapes available commercially. You might want to meditate or simply take a nap. You may want to take a book or audiotape and sit alone for a while in your car. Or, if no other private place is available, remove yourself to a bathroom stall.

B.   Confine all alcoholic beverages to dinner only *and* cut your normal intake by one half. You need not reduce your intake below one drink.   **(6 points)**

   (Select this Option only if you have one or more alcoholic drinks at times other than dinner on a rather regular basis.)

C.   If you are still smoking (pipe, cigar, or cigarettes), stop smoking altogether.   **(12 points)**

---

3.   After adding your Advanced Stress-Reducing Option to your previous Options and incorporating your new Option into your regular routine for one week, move to the "In the Weeks to Come" section on page 253.

Special Circumstances

If there is no Advanced Nutrition, Activity, or Stress-Reducing Option that is appropriate for you or that you want to select, choose a new Bonus Option in its stead and continue following all previous Options.

You know that we would like you to choose Activity, Nutrition, or Stress-Reducing Options whenever possible, but we also know that that is not always possible or desirable. You can always choose a Bonus Option in place of your usual selection and add it to your routine and continue as described above.

Bonus Options

Bonus Options are your "wild cards"; they can always be used as substitutes for Nutrition, Activity, or Stress-Reducing Options when you cannot or do not want to select one of the usual Options for that week. Bonus Options remain the same at the Beginner, Intermediate, or Advanced levels of the Program. You can find a full list of Bonus Options on page 209.

Remember: Bonus Options remain the same at the Beginner, Intermediate, or Advanced levels of the Program. You can find a full list of Bonus Options on page 209.

In the Weeks to Come

Once you have exchanged a Nutrition, Activity, or Stress-Reducing Option (or added Bonus Option alternatives instead) into your daily routine, by adding them one week at a time, all of the Options in this Step are open to you.

First, look over this Step's Nutrition Options and see if there is another Nutrition Option that you wish to add. If so, add any new Nutrition Option, still at a rate of one per week at a time. Remember, each time you add a new Nutrition Option from this Step you can, at the same time, drop a Nutrition Option from your previous Step.

If you have no more Nutrition Options from previous Steps to drop or, if you like, rather than exchanging a Nutrition Option, you can simply add a new one to your previous choices. Do the same with Stress-Reducing Options. Again, add or exchange only one Option from that category during any one-week period.

As you know, when it comes to Activity Options, you may not want to add an Activity Option to your previous Activity selections; instead, you will probably prefer to exchange one Activity Option for another. If, however, you feel so inclined, you should feel free to add Activity Options rather than exchanging them for previous Activity choices.

Remember, the more Options you select, one at a time, the greater your relative Profactor-H risk reduction.

When You Need a Change

There may come a time when you want to exchange one Advanced Option for another Advanced Option. Look over the Options in the *same category* as the one you wish to exchange—Nutrition, for instance. Choose your new Option and exchange it for your previous same-category selection by adding it to your regular routine. Be sure to continue your new Option for an entire week, in combination with the other Options you had been following (other than the one you exchanged) before moving on to your next Option choice.

If no same-category Option can be satisfactorily exchanged, a Bonus Option can be substituted in its stead.

At Your Own Pace

By now you know that, although we recommend adding or exchanging one Option each week, you are free to move more slowly. If you do not add any new Options in any given week, be sure to continue all previously selected Options. Given your progress, we have confidence in your motivation and commitment, but be careful to be on the watch for any backsliding. You've done so well!

Charting Your Progress

It is never too late to begin charting your progress—though, as always, it is your choice. See "Charting Your Progress" on page 212 for details. For this level, however, you will use the Advanced Progress Chart Guide on the following page and your Advanced Progress Chart at the end of this chapter for recording your score.

Moving On

After you have selected all of the Advanced Options that you wish and have made them a part of your regular routine, you will have mastered all of the basic guidelines of the Profactor-H Program.

The four chapters that follow will help you tailor the Program to fit your needs and preferences and help you with strategies for success.

Sharing Your Success

Now, or at some time to come, you may be tempted to try to change some of the people around you—spouses, friends, family, co-workers. Chances are you will meet with opposition. This is not unusual. People change only when they are ready to; sometimes that's never. Let them come to you and ask you for your advice; then you can share your experiences with them. Until that time, most folks will simply be unable to hear what you have to say.

In time, as people notice the changes in you, many will come, but the sad truth is, some will not. And that is how it must be. Keep your focus on yourself and your own life. Don't get pulled into helping others who do not really want your help. The best thing you can do, for everyone concerned, is to put your time and energy into taking good care of yourself.

It has been said that "living well is the best revenge." We agree, but we would add that "living well is also the best example."

STEP #3: ADVANCED PROGRESS CHART GUIDE

Use this guide to count up your total Option points each week. Keep track of your progress on the chart that follows on the next page.

Advanced Nutrition Options	Risk-Reducing Values for Each Week

A. Include mixed green salad *and* two Risk-Reducing vegetables with your usual dinner .... 5 points

B. Include mixed green salad *before* dinner and two Risk-Reducing vegetables with dinner .... 6 points

C. Eat only Risk-Reducing Foods at breakfast, lunch, and for any snacks. Eat a balanced dinner that includes Risk-Reducing and Essential Balance Foods .... 12 points

Activity Options

A. Light activity: 1 hour, three times each week, or ½ hour every day .... 5 points

B. Moderate activity: 1 hour, three times each week, or ½ hour every day .... 6 points

C. Vigorous activity: 1 hour, three times each week, or ½ hour every day .... 7 points

Stress-Reducing Options

A. Leave stressful environment, 1 hour, three times each week, or ½ hour every day .... 5 points

B. Confine alcoholic beverages to dinner and cut normal intake by one half .... 6 points

C. Stop smoking altogether .... 12 points

Bonus Options

Take 200 micrograms of GTF Chromium with dinner every night .... 6 points

Refrain from gum chewing/mint eating (regular or artificially sweetened) .... 6 points

Avoid all MSG (monosodium glutamate) .... 6 points

Avoid all caffeine .... 6 points

Avoid all artificial sweeteners .... 6 points

Avoid all between-meal snacks .... 6 points

STEP #3: ADVANCED PROGRESS CHART

Week Beginning (Date)	Total Points for Week (Nutritional, Activity, Stress-Reducing, and Bonus)	Profactor-H Risk-Reduction Percentage*

*See Risk-Reducing Percentage Chart on page 502. Risk-Reduction Percentages are relative and are based on the continuation and combination of Risk-Reducing Options. Calculations have been based on the scientific data we have found available.

CHAPTER 19

Chromium:
The Missing Link

The balance of the human body is more beautiful and wondrous than the finest flower.   —Lao-tzu

Suppose you were to learn that scientists had discovered a natural Profactor-H "fighter" that, when combined with this Program, could boost the impact of every single Option you selected: a simple nutrient that could even further help reduce your risk for Profactor-H and the many diseases and health risk factors related to it.

Then imagine how you would feel if you learned that this nutrient was not only inexpensive but also easy to get—sold over the counter at many health food stores.

Consider this. A special form of the nutrient chromium, called *Glucose Tolerance Factor (GTF) Chromium,* is being reported to have so many health-promoting benefits that scientists have begun to hail its importance in reports and studies in medical and scientific journals—reports that multiply and increase by the day.

Though chromium* occurs naturally in our foods, so few of us are getting adequate amounts of this nutrient that studies are now revealing that as many as nine out of ten of us have diets that are deficient in chromium.

---

*Throughout this book, unless otherwise indicated, the term *chromium* can be assumed to mean the trivalent, nutritional form of chromium.

> Researchers from the U.S. Department of Agriculture
> are reporting as many as nine out of ten of us
> have diets that do not supply enough chromium.

Being deficient in chromium is no small matter. The impact of not having enough chromium—in particular, the effect of not having enough GTF Chromium—can *greatly* increase your likelihood of getting Profactor-H and increase your risk for heart disease, high blood pressure, diabetes, hypoglycemia, and more.

The information on GTF Chromium that you find in this chapter is essential to your continued good health and to reversing your Profactor-H risk. We will show you:

Which foods are high in chromium
Which foods literally deplete your body of this important nutrient
Why your multivitamin pill may contain a form of chromium that is *unusable* for Profactor-H risk reduction
What you can easily do to get the right kind of chromium that your body needs

A Special Kind of Chromium

GTF Chromium is a nutrient that contains the naturally occurring element chromium in a very special form. This special form of chromium is called *trivalent* or *nutritional chromium* and it is "biologically active"—usable by the body. In addition, in the GTF form of chromium, it is combined with niacin and the antioxidant glutathione.

While chromium is essential to your health and well-being, very little is needed in order to maintain good health. That is why chromium is called a *trace element*. The National Research Council says that 50 to 200 micrograms of trivalent chromium each day is the "safe and adequate" intake for adults, but researchers have shown that most

Americans take in far less than this amount and they are, in most probability, chromium deficient.*

In 1985, Dr. Richard Anderson of the Vitamin and Mineral Nutrition Laboratory of the U.S. Department of Agriculture studied the diets of both men and women and found that "approximately 90% of the diets analyzed were below the minimum suggested safe and adequate daily intake for chromium of 50 micrograms." Two years later, in a new study, he added that impaired chromium nutrition or the ability to metabolize it well may be a factor in the cause of reactive hypoglycemia. The following year, in the medical textbook *Modern Nutrition in Health and Disease,* Dr. Anderson repeated his concerns, warning researchers and physicians that chromium intake in the United States may be less than that which is suggested as safe and adequate.

Even a good working knowledge of general nutrition may not make much of a difference in awareness of chromium's importance. Dr. Anderson found that one third of the diets designed by a nutritionist contained less than the minimum safe and adequate intake of 50 micrograms of chromium.

Dr. Anderson's repeated concerns went unheeded, and in 1989 he wrote: "Dietary chromium intake in the U.S. and other developed countries is roughly half of the minimum suggested intake of 50 micrograms." Then he added an important warning: ". . . marginal dietary chromium intake is widespread in the general population and may lead to serious health problems." Such problems include low blood sugar levels, undesirable blood fat levels, adult-onset diabetes, and cardiovascular diseases.

In the area of medical research and practice it is often said that unless the public learns of a medical breakthrough, a discovery can remain indefinitely within the medical school libraries, unrecognized and unused. The grave consequences that may be related to chromium deficiency are just starting to make their way into public awareness, and at this time most health professionals still remain unaware of its importance.

---

*Individual health needs and concerns should be considered; therefore check with your physician before adding GTF Chromium supplementation to your diet. GTF Chromium may reduce the need for insulin; if GTF Chromium is taken, diabetics should be closely monitored by their physicians.

To this day, most health professionals remain unaware of the importance of GTF Chromium.

Insulin's Valuable Assistant

Chromium, in particular GTF Chromium, acts like an insulin "helper," assisting insulin in doing its job. Without chromium, insulin cannot move adequate amounts of blood sugar from your bloodstream to the cells that need it. Your body is resourceful, however, and if it does not get enough chromium, in many cases it will try to find ways to compensate.

One way your body may try to make up for not having enough chromium is to overproduce and overrelease insulin—releasing more and more insulin (Cofactor-p) in the hope of getting the job done. In addition, deprived of adequate amounts of chromium, your body may not be able to allow appropriate amounts of insulin to leave your bloodstream; the result—Cofactor-r. In both cases, you greatly increase your risk for Profactor-H and the diseases that so often come along with it.

"Insulin is required to remove glucose from the blood," explains Dr. Anderson. "When sugar levels in the blood are high, the pancreas dispatches insulin, which stimulates the cells to take up the glucose and burn it for energy. Chromium makes insulin more efficient at this task, so you need less to accomplish the job," he goes on. "And that's beneficial, because high insulin levels in the blood are thought to be associated with hardening of the arteries."

Chromium, in particular GTF Chromium, is an essential part of the process we call *metabolism*. Without enough chromium, our body tries to "make do," but the imbalances that result can be devastating and, in the end, may be life-threatening as well.

Chromium Sources

Although it is so vital to our health, and though our bodies need very small amounts of chromium, still, most people do not seem able to take in the chromium they need.

Many foods contain chromium. Brewer's yeast has the highest chromium content, followed by many other chromium-rich foods such as beef, beer and wine, black pepper, calves' liver, fish and shellfish, cheese, and many vegetables, including mushrooms and potatoes (with skins) and whole grains. Fresh fruits contain chromium as well, but as you will soon see, if fruit is eaten often it can actually rob your body of its chromium reserves.

CHROMIUM SOURCES

Though nutritional science has yet to quantify the exact amount of chromium in food, these foods have been shown to be rich in chromium:

Beef
Beer and wine (red and white)
Black pepper
Brewer's yeast (highest)
Calves' liver
Cheese
Fish
Fresh fruit

Shellfish (clams, lobster, scallops, etc.)
Thyme
Vegetables (in particular, mushrooms and potatoes with skin)
Whole grains

With Chromium, Good Nutrition May Not Be Good Enough

Eating good, chromium-rich food may not protect you from chromium deficiency. If naturally chromium-rich foods are grown in soil that is enriched with chemical fertilizers, the food may not contain the chromium levels you thought you could count on.

Even if you are eating adequate, or more-than-adequate, amounts of chromium, other foods and factors may *remove* the chromium from your body and leave you chromium deficient.

Eating adequate amounts of chromium-rich foods is not enough.

There are two major ways in which we strip our bodies of chromium. First, we lower our chromium levels by eating refined carbohydrate-rich foods *frequently;* and second, our bodies are depleted of chromium by the emotional and physical stress with which we so often are forced to cope.

Eating certain carbohydrate-rich foods, and eating them frequently, depletes our bodies of their precious chromium stores by raising our insulin levels. In particular, simple sugars, refined and processed foods, and milk are the worst chromium thieves.

Most people do not realize that fresh fruit is a simple sugar and that the apple you grab for a snack, as well as that cookie—even the yogurt that you eat while thinking you are being so "good"—may all flush essential chromium stores from your body out into your urine.

So, although fruit is chromium-rich, when it is eaten frequently the insulin rise it produces may strip your body of more chromium than the fruit contributes and you may end up with less chromium than when you started.

**Fruit, eaten often during the day,
can take away far more chromium than it provides.**

Frequently eating refined and processed foods, simple sugars (including fruit, sweets, and desserts), and drinking milk can strip your chromium reserves. By following the Profactor-H Program, you can greatly reduce the number of insulin insults that your body endures and that can rob your body of its precious chromium stores. Still, it is important to understand that even though the Profactor-H Program reduces the likelihood of repeated insulin insult, other factors may deplete your chromium reserves. Supplementing your chromium intake can be very important.

Not only can inadequate amounts of chromium in your diet leave you vulnerable, but physical and emotional demands can lower your chromium levels even further. Emotional stress or physical stresses such as strenuous exercise, trauma, surgery, fever, pregnancy, lactation, or even the simple act of aging, can all, in their own ways, reduce your body's precious chromium reserves.

Adriane Kozlovsky and her research team, working at the United States Department of Agriculture, warned scientists and physicians that since most diets may contain less than suggested safe and adequate levels of chromium, and since these diets also contain high levels of refined sugars that have been shown to lower chromium levels, "chromium depletion seems almost inevitable." Low levels of chromium, she added, are associated with problems in blood sugar levels and undesirable blood fat levels as well.

Dr. Jeffrey A. Fisher, studying the work of many scientists, concluded that "chromium, as a partner of insulin, is an essential cofactor," adding that "stress can deplete chromium." Dr. Richard Anderson agreed, noting that stresses deplete chromium stores: "Strenuous exercise, physical trauma as experienced in an accident, infections of various types and certain disease states are all known to reduce chromium in the body."

In the medical research journal *Sports Medicine,* Dr. W. W. Campbell reported that exercise led to great losses of chromium in the urine. This researcher found that during exercise days, the people he studied showed increased chromium loss as compared with rest days. When you combine low levels of chromium intake, which are common in the general population, with the losses that can come from exercise, the "nutritional status and overall health of exercising individuals may be suboptimal."

> ### Stress can greatly deplete your body's chromium stores.

In addition to emotional stress and the demands of exercise on the body, the physical stress of eating foods high in sugar content, an infection or injury, and pregnancy and breast-feeding have all been shown, as well, to decrease the body's chromium levels.

Supplementing your chromium intake could easily mean the difference between good health and poor health.

Vital Signs and Signals

There are several signs and symptoms of chromium deficiency that many people may not recognize or may simply ignore. Though many people can be chromium deficient and show no outward signs (for the time being), low levels of chromium in the body can lead to undesirable blood fat levels or abnormal blood sugar levels or both.

There are signs of chromium deficiency that people do not recognize or, even worse, may simply ignore.

Abnormal blood sugar levels are one of the first signs of chromium deficiency and are often followed by problems in blood fat levels. Low levels of chromium can lead to signs and symptoms similar to those associated with diabetes and cardiovascular disease—or to these diseases themselves.

As far back as 1977, Dr. K. N. Jeejeebhoy and his colleagues reported in the *American Journal of Clinical Nutrition* that chromium deficiency resulted in abnormal blood sugar levels, high blood fat levels, and slower metabolic rates. Five years later, in 1982, Dr. Richard A. Passwater, researcher and author, reported: "Chromium deficiency is common to heart disease and diabetes." He added that, in particular, Glucose Tolerance Factor (GTF) Chromium deficiency "results in arterial plaque formation, which in turn can induce blood clotting, which causes a heart attack."

Though it will take some time for this information to make its way into physicians' and nutritionists' practices, most research scientists in the area of nutrition are well aware that chromium deficiency may show itself as the beginning or progressing of atherosclerosis, heart disease, diabetes, or high blood pressure.

Though lack of chromium can lead to medical problems in all of us, particularly those of us who are Profactor-H Positive, it has been found that in diabetics an unknown chromium deficiency may play a particularly crucial role. In Dr. S. Fujimoto's 1987 study of diabetics, blood chromium levels were found to be the lowest in those with the most severe complications. "Therefore, it appears," concluded Dr. Fujimoto, "that [lack of] chromium plays an important role in advancing diabetes mellitus." In 1986, Dr. A. S. Kozlovsky's study in the journal *Metabolism* confirmed the now well-established chromium-diabetes connection. The long-term effects of inadequate chromium intake, combined with an excess intake of refined sugars, she reported, may lead to a chromium deficiency that is linked to adult-onset diabetes and cardiovascular disease.

Scientists have found that the effects of chromium deficiency include a wide variety of diseases and risk factors, all connecting chromium deficiency to blood sugar imbalances, metabolism, and Profactor-H:

1. High insulin levels in the blood that, over time, become Profactor-H
2. High levels of blood sugar after eating that in time may lead to adult-onset diabetes
3. Abnormally high levels of sugar in the urine
4. Undesirable fat levels in the blood
5. Narrowing of blood vessels (atherosclerosis)
6. Low blood sugar an hour or two after eating (reactive hypoglycemia)
7. A weakness or numbness in the arms or legs (peripheral neuropathy)
8. Mental confusion
9. Shortening of the life span

When you are chromium deficient,
your body can no longer function normally.

When you are chromium deficient, your body can no longer function normally. As time goes on, results from physical examinations or blood tests may begin to show evidence of problems: High blood fat levels may appear and high or low blood sugar levels, signs of atherosclerosis, and high blood pressure may begin to emerge.

You may blame yourself, your diet, your lack of exercise, your genetics. You may try to lose weight through traditional diets, eat "more healthfully," and rigorously increase your exercise regime—and in doing so, you may eat the very foods and do the very things that will make you even more chromium starved.

The Chromium Correction

As far back as twenty-five years ago, researchers were beginning to see the importance of chromium, especially in its ability to reduce blood fat levels. In 1969 in the well-respected journal *Science,* Drs. H. W. Staub, G. Reussner, and R. Thiessen confirmed earlier reports of chromium's health-bettering effects and added that the results of their experiment "confirm and extend Schroeder's finding that chromium can lower serum cholesterol."

Unfortunately, at the time scientists did not understand the significance of blood fat levels and so the magnitude of this discovery was lost. Now, when we understand the relevance of blood fat levels to heart disease, high blood pressure, and the like, this research has far more exciting implications.

Today's research is verifying these past scientists' reports and, most important, is revealing even more essential information. Dr. Richard Anderson found that adding supplemental chromium to diets was associated with "improvements of risk factors associated with maturity-onset diabetes and cardiovascular diseases." In 1989, he reported that many studies demonstrated beneficial effects of supplemental chromium on blood sugar levels, blood fat levels, reducing Profactor-H risk, and low blood sugar levels and symptoms. In his paper presented at the meeting of the American Institute of Nutrition, Dr. J. S. Striffler reported that his research showed that dietary chromium improves the body's ability to handle sugars and decreases the risk for Profactor-H.

Dr. J. A. Fisher found that when chromium was administered to diabetics with Profactor-H, blood sugar improved, cholesterol and triglycerides dropped to normal levels, and Profactor-H levels normalized.

Not All Chromium Is Created Equal

There are several kinds of chromium that you may have read about recently: chromium picolinate, inorganic chromium, and GTF (Glucose Tolerance Factor) Chromium. It is essential that you choose the right chromium for Profactor-H risk reduction.

First, it is important to choose only certified, biologically active, Glucose Tolerance Factor (GTF) Chromium. Inorganic chromium, the kind most often found in multivitamin pills, has *not* been shown to be as effective in lowering blood fat levels as GTF. GTF Chromium has been shown to be much more absorbable and better at stabilizing blood sugar than the inorganic chromium you typically get in your vitamin pill. So, for Profactor-H risk reduction, choose biologically active, rather than inorganic, chromium.

There is some debate as to whether or not chromium picolinate is as good as GTF Chromium in the benefits described here. Certainly, some research has been published on picolinate's positive impact on muscle building, but these reports are relatively recent, and studies on picolinate's effect on blood fat and blood sugar levels do not nearly equal the amount of research we have seen on GTF.

The chromium supplement that we would suggest, with your physician's approval,* is GTF (Glucose Tolerance Factor) Chromium. The label should say that it is "certified biologically active" and that it contains molecules of niacin and glutathione (an antioxidant) and an atom of trivalent chromium.

---

*Individual health needs and concerns should be considered; therefore check with your physician before adding GTF Chromium supplementation to your diet. GTF Chromium may reduce the need for insulin; if GTF Chromium is taken, diabetics should be closely monitored by their physician.

> There are several brands on the market
> that meet these guidelines. We use
> Solgar's GTF Chromium (Trivalent).

There are several brands that meet these guidelines and that will help you be sure that you are, indeed, getting the correct form of chromium. We use Solgar's GTF Chromium (Trivalent). But be careful. Even Solgar distributes several different chromium products. Look carefully to see what *kind* of chromium you are purchasing. Choose GTF only.

Sadly, there are some manufacturers that may try to fool you. They combine chromium with high doses of niacin and leave out the glutathione. This is not GTF Chromium as we know it. These companies may be trying to produce new patents for themselves by contriving new combinations and using similar names. We know of no research that supports any claims they may make regarding Profactor-H risk reduction related to their formulations. Again, choose only GTF.

Read the label carefully and take your time. If you are in doubt, you might want to compare any other brand with Solgar's GTF Chromium.

If your health food store does not have the correct kind of chromium or the brand that you prefer, do not let them talk you into purchasing the kind they have in stock. Strongly request that they order, for you, the GTF Chromium you want; it is well worth the wait.

The National Research Council says that 50 to 200 micrograms of trivalent chromium each day is the "safe and adequate" intake for adults. Each Solgar pill contains 200 micrograms, so one pill each day fulfills the "safe and adequate" daily intake recommendation. Not all brands contain 200 micrograms, so it is important to read the label.

Your GTF Chromium is best taken with your dinner. Remember to take it every day. Chromium's effects take at least a month, sometimes as long as several months, to become evident, but this inexpensive and easy way to increase the power of this Program is an exciting and easy bonus.

A Word of Caution

Do *not* rely on GTF Chromium alone to help reduce your Profactor-H risk. GTF Chromium intake should be *combined* with the Profactor-H Program in order to best help you restore your chromium balance. It is the combination of the Program and GTF supplementation that best brings it all together.

Do *not* rely on GTF Chromium alone.

A World of Difference

We believe that it is no coincidence that in other countries where dietary fat intake is high (France, for instance) but where snacking is less frequent and where increased intake of chromium-rich foods such as wine, mushrooms, cheese, black pepper, and thyme are part of the typical fare, you also find far less heart disease. To us, the reasons are obvious.

Here, in the United States too, chromium could make all the difference "in the world."

CHAPTER 20

Personalizing Your Program

I am what I am. —Popeye

This is not a one-size-fits-all plan; we will never tell you that you *must* eat two ounces of this or four ounces of that, and unless your physician says otherwise, there are no foods that you cannot have. The Profactor-H Program merely provides you with simple guidelines and Options based on what we, and other scientists, have found best reduces your Profactor-H risk. Within the Program, you are free to follow your own preferences or needs, and *within* each Option, to shape the Program to fit *your* likes and dislikes.

Choosing an Option that asks you to eat only Risk-Reducing Foods at lunch, for instance, is only the beginning. Within this Option—as a vegetarian, for example—you may make nonmeat selections from the Risk-Reducing Foods list. Or, depending on your preference, you may select low-fat choices, or low-salt, or both. If meat is your delight, you may choose that as well. In the same way, an Option that asks you to eat a well-rounded dinner that includes lots of Essential Balance Foods still leaves it up to you to decide if you want to include bread, pasta, rice, or potatoes and fruit or sweet desserts in that meal.

This chapter is about making choices within each of your Options. Choices should be based on what your goals are, what you prefer, and what you will enjoy. After all, to incorporate any program into your life, to make lifestyle changes, a program must be suited to the way you really live and what you really want—not someone else's idea of how you *should* live and what you *should* want.

If you think that you are going to hear the same old
advice that you have heard all your life,
you are in for a surprise.

Fruit and Table Sugar:
The Simple and Surprising Facts

We have all been told that table sugar is bad for us and that fruit is good. "Grab a piece of fruit, rather than that candy bar," we've been told. "Fruit is good for you." "An apple a day keeps the doctor away," they add. "What could be better for you than a glass of orange juice?" The answer is, plenty!

First of all, fruit and fruit juices are high in carbohydrates and are basically made up of water, fiber, and fruit sugar (called *fructose*). Fructose is *not* a complex carbohydrate; it is a simple sugar. Fructose is easily and quickly digested, and in many people, it has been shown to bring about a Profactor-H response.

Despite the great reputation that they have, fruit and fruit juices, especially when they are consumed more than once a day, can greatly increase your Profactor-H risk. The idea that fruit and fruit juice can increase your risk for illness may be difficult to believe at first; after all, we have been told exactly the opposite all of our lives. But fruit's potentially negative impact on our health is true and the scientific evidence is more than convincing.

In her excellent report, "Metabolic Effects of Dietary Fructose," Dr. Judith Hallfrisch of the National Institute on Aging found that there is "overwhelming evidence" that fruit sugar increases triglycerides in the blood. In addition, she reported, fruit sugar is more fat-producing than starches and usually causes greater elevations in triglycerides and sometimes in cholesterol than other carbohydrates. Reviewing the research of many other fine scientists, Dr. Hallfrisch concluded that dietary fruit sugar results in increases in uric acid (which can lead to gout) as well as increases in blood pressure.

Dr. Hallfrisch's recommendations are clear. In patients with hypertension, excess weight, undesirable blood fat levels, or gout, it may be more harmful than helpful to substitute fruit sugar for other sugars. In particular, she points out, people who are Profactor-H Positive, have high blood pressure, high triglycerides, adult-onset diabetes, or are postmenopausal are most susceptible to the effects of fruit sugar.

The Surgeon General of the United States has reported similar findings, explaining that some of us (those we call Profactor-H Positive and to whom he refers as "carbohydrate sensitive") respond to sugars in our foods with different physical reactions than the average person. In these people, he reports, table sugar *and* fruit sugar have been shown to promote high triglyceride levels. He adds that "men appear to be more susceptible than premenopausal women, older persons more than younger persons, and those with high triglyceride levels more than those with normal levels of triglycerides."

Other renowned scientists have independently reported the same compelling discovery. Stanford School of Medicine's Dr. Gerald Reaven learned that high blood pressure could be produced by a diet high in fruit sugar—the same diet that he found leads to Cofactor-r and Profactor-H. Researchers from the Carbohydrate Nutrition Laboratory of the Beltsville Human Nutrition Research Center found that a diet high in fruit sugar in combination with saturated fat and cholesterol increased the risk for heart disease, especially in Profactor-H Positive men.

The impact of frequent intake of fruit extends to the area of cancer as well. A 1991 report in *The British Journal of Cancer* advised physicians and scientists that fruit sugar, through the actions of Profactor-H, appeared to enhance the growth of tumors.

With so many scientists saying that fruit sugar may be so harmful, where did we get the idea that fruit and fruit juices are healthful, that these are foods that could never do us any harm? It is hard to know for sure where unfounded beliefs spring from, but in the area of nutrition, as in other areas of life, once a rumor gets started, it is hard to stop it.

We believe that the "good fruit image" comes from a time when diseases due to lack of available fruit were rampant. At those times, people would suffer the ravages of scurvy and the like simply for the lack of fresh fruit. Sailors, away from land for months or more at a time, would endure swollen, bleeding gums, open wounds in the skin, even death, all for want of the vitamin C found in a single orange. Fruit, so precious and rare then, would be given as a Christmas present, hidden in a fortunate child's stocking.

Today, when our vitamin C comes to us in a myriad of readily available foods and drinks as well as in multivitamin tablets, the healthful, though unwarranted, reputation of fruit lingers on.

Certainly, the effects of fiber are beneficial, as are the many vitamins that fruit may provide, but these advantages can often be achieved by eating other, less-insulin-releasing foods (such as those you can find in the Risk-Reducing Foods list on pages 220 to 221). If Profactor-H risk reduction is your goal, you may want to confine your fruit intake to one meal each day; dinner, for instance.

The sugar* that you find on your table, technically known as *sucrose,* is a relatively simple sugar. Although most people do not know it, sucrose is made of two simpler sugars, fructose (fruit sugar) and glucose. Table sugar has been shown to increase tumor growth (see chapter 9, "The Cancer Tie-in"), and recently its impact on high blood pressure, high blood fat levels, and heart disease, along with its connection to Profactor-H, has become even more evident.

In their 1991 report to the *Journal of Human Hypertension,* Drs. M. J. O'Donnell and P. M. Dodson reported that, in people with normal blood pressure, simple sugars bring on abnormal salt retention and a significant rise in blood pressure. Reporting in the *Journal of Nutrition,* Dr. Sheldon Reiser and his research team concluded that the sugar intake common in the American diet could, in Profactor-H Positive men, lead to the undesirable blood fat levels associated with coronary risk.

Over ten years ago, Stanford School of Medicine's Dr. A. M. Coulston concluded that the commonly accepted diabetic diet, one that is low in fat and high in carbohydrates with only moderate amounts of added sugar, when consumed by adult-onset diabetics for only two

---

*Unless otherwise indicated, the term *sugar* refers to table sugar (sucrose).

weeks, resulted in significant increases in Profactor-H, blood sugar levels, triglycerides, and a decrease in "good" cholesterol (HDL) concentrations.

Dr. Coulston pointed out that similarly negative health indicators had been shown in nondiabetic subjects as well, and in patients with high triglyceride levels. She concluded that these unhealthful physical changes could be assumed to be the result of the diet, a diet that is often recommended to the patient as supposedly healthful.

Four years later, in her report in the *American Journal of Medicine,* Dr. Coulston and her research team concluded that these same diets, in keeping with the recommendations of the American Diabetes Association, have harmful effects when consumed by diabetic patients for only fifteen days. Dr. C. Hollenbeck, reporting in *Diabetes Care,* gave even further evidence and explained that the recent addition of sugar to their diet appears to lead to Profactor-H and to high blood sugar, triglyceride, and cholesterol levels, along with a reduction in good cholesterol levels in diabetics.

Sugar is known to reduce the body's chromium supplies by raising and maintaining Profactor-H levels, and as the research continues, scientists uncover additional evidence that supports their colleagues' findings regarding sugar's connection to Profactor-H. As Dr. L. H. Storlein concluded in his report in the *American Journal of Clinical Nutrition,* sugar produces major difficulties leading to Profactor-H–related problems.

It is important to understand that, in most cases, laboratory experiments involving the impact of sugar on Profactor-H risk, and health in general, have examined the effects of frequent and repeated sugar intake.

If you want to eat table sugar, in order to decrease your probability of Profactor-H impact and the risks you have seen to be associated with high insulin levels, it may be best to confine your sugary and sweet foods (including honey), desserts, cakes, cookies, ice cream, and the like to one meal each day—a meal, like dinner, that already includes Essential Balance Foods.

Fat Facts

Though you may have heard otherwise, there is a great debate among scientists as to whether or not fats are bad for you, if some fats are good, and which fats fall into which category. While the debate continues, we all have to try to make the best decisions we can.

The one fact that does seem clear is that fat, in combination with the *frequent* intake of carbohydrate-rich foods (including starches, snack foods, sweets, and fruit), can greatly increase your Profactor-H risk. So, by following the Profactor-H Program, you are helping reduce your risk for many of the ill effects related to fat consumption.

This is not to say, by any means, that you are free to eat all the fat you desire, but is simply meant to inform you that you are, already, taking positive action.

For more information about the impact of dietary fat on your Profactor-H risk, read chapter 7, "Fats and Fiber: Fears, Facts, and Fallacies." If, in addition, you wish to lower your intake of fats on the Profactor-H Program or change the kinds of fats you eat, we have provided information in the section that follows, "Big Fat Lowdown." Guidelines in keeping with recommendations of health agencies, such as the American Heart Association, the United States Department of Agriculture, and the Department of Health and Human Services, are detailed on page 345.

Big Fat Lowdown

Among other things, fats and oils are made up of fatty acids. These fatty acids vary in how *hydrogenated* they are, which means how much hydrogen each fatty acid contains. The more hydrogen a fatty acid contains, the more *saturated* it is said to be. You could say the fat is saturated with hydrogen.

An easy general guide to knowing the difference between saturated and unsaturated fats is this: At room temperature, unsaturated fats are usually liquid, while saturated fats are usually solid or semisolid.

The oils and fats you eat are made up of combinations of fatty acids. When you hear someone refer to a "saturated fat," what they are really saying is that the fat contains a greater proportion of saturated fatty acids than unsaturated (monounsaturated or polyunsaturated) fatty acids. That is not to say that it is totally made up of saturated fatty acids. The difference is important because, in fat nutrition, as in many things, there are no easy and distinct lines.

A saturated fat, then, can contain high levels of unsaturated fatty acids, but if the balance is only slightly in the direction of saturated fatty acids, it is called a saturated fat. Peanut oil is considered a monounsaturate, like olive oil, although peanut oil has almost one third less monounsaturated fatty acid than olive oil. The quantity of fatty acids that each contains does not matter. Since both peanut oil and olive oil have more monounsaturated fatty acids than other fatty acids, both are considered monounsaturates.

The difference is important because, in the years ahead, as you read and hear many of the scientific reports that are sure to pass your way, you will now be aware that the grouping "saturated" versus "unsaturated" is not as clear-cut as a reporter or an article may imply. The terms *saturated* and *unsaturated* do not refer to absolutes; they simply refer to the highest proportion of one or the other type of fatty acids within a combination. By looking at the chart on pages 278 and 279, you will see that you could eat mostly "unsaturated" fats (in the form of monounsaturates and polyunsaturates) and still take in a great deal of saturated fatty acids.

While the facts on the "best" kinds of fat to eat are still under investigation, the general agreement, for the time being, seems to be the following:

Saturated fatty acids, in general, tend to raise cholesterol levels in the body (though research is pointing to important exceptions such as stearic acid).

The higher the ratio of polyunsaturated fat to saturated fat, the greater the cholesterol-lowering effect, and likewise, the more saturated fat you eat as compared to polyunsaturated fat, the more you can expect to raise your blood cholesterol levels.

When possible, replace saturated fats with monounsaturates (like olive oil).

Limit overall fat intake to between 10 and 20 percent of your daily in-take of calories. (Some recommendations still allow 30 percent.)

In addition, some researchers have reported saturated fats to be the main problem in cholesterol control and have shown that by simply replacing saturated fats with monounsaturates (like olive oil) and some polyunsaturates (like vegetable oil), though not changing total intake of fat whatsoever, you can significantly reduce your blood fat levels.

In the end, the fat decision must be up to you and your physician. There are as many different fat recommendations as there are re-searchers, which leads us to believe that no one recommendation works for everyone. If it did, it would have been proven repeatedly. And that has not been done to date.

So, for now, check with your doctor and rest assured that with the guidelines on page 345, you may choose to incorporate into your Pro-factor-H Program any dietary fat recommendation that is appropriate.

COMPARISON OF DIETARY FATS*

Type of Dietary Fat	Saturated Fatty Acids (% of fat)	Monounsaturated Fatty Acids (% of fat)	Polyunsaturated Fatty Acids (% of fat)
Animal fats (including dairy)			
Beef fat	48	42	5
Butter	51	24	3
Chicken fat	31	42	11
Lamb fat	47	39	8
Lard	39	45	11
Tuna fat	29	29	20

*Percentages based on United States Department of Agriculture and data base source information. Data based on average percentage of total weight, and therefore may not equal 100%.

Type of Dietary Fat	Saturated Fatty Acids (% of fat)	Monounsaturated Fatty Acids (% of fat)	Polyunsaturated Fatty Acids (% of fat)
Vegetable oils and shortenings			
Canola oil	6	60	30
Coconut oil	86	6	1
Corn oil	13	24	59
Cottonseed oil	26	20	52
Margarine			
Imitation	8	16	14
Regular			
Hard, stick	16	36	26
Soft, tub	14	29	34
Spread			
Hard, stick	14	26	18
Soft, tub	13	31	14
Olive oil	14	74	9
Palm oil	47	41	8
Palm kernel oil	84	12	2
Peanut oil	17	46	32
Safflower oil	9	12	74
Soybean oil (partially hydrogenated)	15	43	38
Soybean and cottonseed blend (hydrogenated)	15	43	38
Sunflower oil	10	19	66
Vegetable shortening (can)	25	44	26
Walnut oil	8	24	66

Salt Concerns

Incorporating a low-salt diet into the Profactor-H Program is easy. The guidelines we have provided on page 345 will help you and, as you know, you should be guided by your physician.

The good news is, however, as you continue on the Program, you may be in for a pleasant surprise. The high insulin levels that are the hallmark of Profactor-H have been shown to influence salt and water retention and may be causing you to hold far more water than is desirable. As you continue on the Program, and as your Profactor-H levels naturally decline, you may find that water retention is far less of a concern or no longer a problem at all.

Vegetarian Choices

Within the guidelines of the Program, you are free, if you like, to refrain from eating red meat, all meat, or any animal products whatsoever. This choice is *not* a suggested part of the Program, but you are free to make vegetarian choices if you like. Being a vegetarian may limit some of your Option selections, but there are so many Options available that you should have no difficulty in personalizing the Program to fit your preferences.

If, for instance, you eat no animal products whatsoever, you would *not* want to choose the Advanced Nutrition Option that asks you to eat only Risk-Reducing Foods at all meals except dinner. Without any animal products at all, you would find your breakfast and lunch choices limited to eating tofu as your main source of protein, and after a time, as a vegetarian you might find this Option too limiting. If, on the other hand, instead you choose the Advanced Nutrition Option that asks you to add salad and vegetables to your dinner, chances are you would have no difficulty at all.

While you should be monitored by a physician to insure proper nutrition, for the vegetarian, then, the Profactor-H Program will allow you to select Options in keeping with your preferences and goals. Look over your choices carefully and make your selections while keeping your personal food preferences in mind. This Program has been designed to fit you and your needs; the wide variety of choices will make it easy for you to make this Program yours.

Weighty Decisions

As you move through the Program, you may find an unexpected, and welcome, loss in weight. In general, this loss will slow down and stop as you approach your ideal weight level.

If you do not want to lose weight, or if the weight loss continues beyond your goal weight, make sure that you are eating enough Essential Balance Foods at dinner. Essential Balance Foods should make up about one quarter of the total proportion of food you take in at your evening meal. If you are taking in enough Essential Balance Foods with dinner, and still want to slow down your weight loss, simply add a snack or two made up of Risk-Reducing Foods during the day.

Ideal snack times are mid-afternoon and evening. While keeping track of your weight, add only one snack of Risk-Reducing Foods a day for a week or two. If your weight continues to drop, add a second snack of the same types of food and adjust according to your weight level.

If, for some reason, you have started to gain weight on the Program, make sure that you are including Essential Balance Foods in the correct proportions, as described in chapter 21.

**In the chapter that follows,
we will share our personal secrets to success.**

More to Come

In chapter 21, which follows, we will give you our best strategies for success. You will learn how to take your program through the holidays and on vacation. You will learn which triggers may tempt you to break your program, how to balance your meals for optimal

Profactor-H risk reduction, and how to swap meal times to give you even greater freedom and flexibility. Best of all, you will learn the secrets to success that come from over ten years of healthy victories.

Toni in Wonderland: A Vegetarian's Story

Antoinette (Toni) M. entered our offices wrapped in a full man-styled coat with padded shoulders. Her less than five-foot frame seemed dwarfed by the huge coat. When she slipped it off, we could see that she dressed in overly large clothes beneath her outer coverings. She was wearing a huge loosely knit sweater that came below her hips and a loose-fitting skirt that came almost to her ankles. The little bit of ankle that was visible was covered in heavy black stockings. She clearly seemed to be hiding her body. Although we are quite familiar with estimating the weight of the people with whom we work, we had no idea whether Toni had ten, twenty, thirty, or more pounds to lose. She looked large and tiny at the same time.

Toni came from a traditional Italian family where food was both pleasurable and plentiful: "Almost every woman over thirty in my family is fat." Toni estimated that two of her aunts and her mother were each well over a hundred pounds overweight. Toni, now twenty-two, was "seriously dating" a young man who, although also of Italian descent, did not appreciate her recent weight gain. He did not tease her, nor did he hint about her weight. He clearly told her that he cared a great deal for her but that he was concerned about the fact that she was "putting on pounds."

In reality, Toni had been about fifteen pounds overweight when she met Vincent and had gained about ten pounds more during the time they were together. Toni tried to shrug it off to "being happy," but her doctor noted that her blood pressure was far too high, especially considering her young age. Vincent was distressed by the change in her blood pressure and begged Toni to "do something." Still Toni put off taking any real action.

The turning point came for Toni after her cousin's wedding, when, after struggling to dance, her mother had her second heart attack. Vincent admitted that he was afraid to get more serious with Toni because he was concerned that she would "end up like her mother"—a woman carrying nearly twice her normal weight and suffering from high blood pressure, heart disease, and diabetes. "I really don't want that kind of life for myself," he said. "And I don't think that you do either," he added.

Toni admitted that she was terribly hurt, but in a way, she could see his point. Instead of blaming him, she became determined to do something about her weight and her health.

"My mother and my aunts constantly cook and talk about food. That's all they live for. They spend their whole day planning, shopping, and cooking dinner. That's all they think of. They cook and taste all day long. And they used to constantly involve me in their obsession with food. Sometimes I'd go along and taste things. Sometimes I'd go to the school library just to get out of the house. Whenever I would try to lose weight, they'd nag me and prod me and make me feel guilty. If I was able to even approach normal weight, they would tell me I looked terrible. I know it sounds like a movie, but it's true. Most of all, they'd make fun of me. They'd tell me it was in my 'genes' and there was nothing I could do about it. I got to the point where I couldn't lose more than a few pounds or go for more than a few days without giving in.

"Finally, after my cousin's wedding, I decided to do what I always wanted to do—become a vegetarian. My family thought I was nuts. They teased me and made me feel like I was weird, but I stuck with it. I was determined to lose weight and to get healthy. But the joke was on me.

"Not only didn't I lose weight but I gained over twenty pounds in a few months. Add that extra weight to the twenty-five pounds that I was already carrying and you have me well on the way to becoming my mother.

"It was crazy. The harder I tried, the more weight I gained. It was like everything was working in the opposite way that it should. I felt like Alice in Wonderland—where everything works backwards. Then my doctor said my blood pressure was becoming 'a serious concern.' He was talking about putting me on blood pressure medication—at twenty-two! I'm not eating meat, I eat nothing with any fat, I'm hungry all the time, I'm doing everything that should have worked, and as my reward, I'm getting sick and fat. The whole thing doesn't make sense, so if you can explain it, I'm listening."

Toni's story was not new to us. Vegetarians are not a singular group; they are different people with different needs and, if they are Profactor-H Positive, vegetarians can choose a pattern of eating that can quickly and intensely worsen their Profactor-H levels. Though vegetarians can find easy and enjoyable ways to follow the Profactor-H Program, first they must understand what they might have been doing wrong in the past and how they might have been increasing their Profactor-H levels by what they were told were health-promoting actions.

Toni had been eating three foods in place of meat: low-fat yogurt, whole-grain bread, and fruit. She was reaching for these three high-carbohydrate foods often during the day, and her Profactor-H Positive body was responding as we would have predicted. She was more hungry and tired, heavier, and less healthy than she was before her vegetarian change.

But we had unexpected good news for Toni. We could help her design an eating program that would allow her to be a vegetarian and reduce her Profactor-H risk at the same time. It was not the food that she was eating that was her problem, we explained, but rather how frequently she was eating it.

Fruit, in particular, was her downfall. She was "reaching for a piece of fruit or a glass of juice" several times a day—each time driving her Profactor-H levels higher and higher. Yogurt, a midday snack, and whole-grain bread or cereal at each meal were adding to her problem.

Toni began the Profactor-H Program with an open mind. "It makes sense," she explained. "It's the first time anybody could explain how I could be gaining weight on a vegetarian and *low-fat* program."

Toni's response to the Program was perfect. Though she stayed at the Intermediate level, her weight loss was steady. She lost about a pound a week virtually without hitting any plateaus. She wanted to lose at least forty pounds, but her weight naturally slowed to a stop at about the forty-five-pound weight loss mark. Toni was thrilled and so was her physician. Her blood pressure normalized and remained ideal. Her blood fat levels, though not yet a problem, became even better. She felt good and looked great. And she had no trouble staying with a program that was "ridiculously easy." Best, she had a way that would help her fight the illness and obesity that ran rampant in the women in her family. "Finally, things make sense. I follow the Program, I lose weight, and get healthier. That's all I was asking."

By the way, Vincent and Toni never married. She met someone new whom she "fell madly in love with" and married after only a few months. Two years later she "swears that it was the best thing that ever happened to me, except," she adds "for coming to see you." We agree on both counts. Toni is slim, now able to wear figure-revealing clothes, and happily maintaining her weight, her health, and her vegetarian lifestyle for the third consecutive year.

No longer Toni in Wonderland, she is finally able to keep control of her weight, her health, and her life.

DIET AND HEALTH RECOMMENDATIONS AND THE PROFACTOR-H PROGRAM

Several well-respected agencies, including the U.S. Department of Agriculture and the Department of Health and Human Services, the American Heart Association, and the Surgeon General of the United States, have issued dietary and health recommendations.*

These reports offer guidelines to aid Americans in the prevention of: adult-onset diabetes, cardiovascular diseases, cancer, chronic liver or kidney disease, obesity, high blood pressure, osteoporosis, and stroke.

These recommendations are completely compatable with, and easily included in, the Profactor-H Program. Suggestions for incorporating these dietary guidelines into your program can be found in "Health Agency Recommendations" on page 345.

*The Surgeon General's Report on Nutrition and Health; the U.S. Department of Agriculture and the Department of Health and Human Services' Report on Dietary Guidelines for Americans; the American Heart Association's diet, Eating Plan for Healthy Americans; and the American Cancer Society's Eat to Live.

CHAPTER 21

Strategies for Success

Forewarned is forearmed. —Benjamin Franklin

Forewarned is forearmed; to be prepared is half the victory. —Cervantes' *Don Quixote*

Don Quixote said it, Benjamin Franklin said it, and most important, you probably know it too. Forewarned is forearmed; to be prepared is half the victory. When you know what to expect, your chances of success are great, and when you have planned for all contingencies, your success is even more assured.

This chapter will help you anticipate the challenges that may come and will show you how you can be best assured of success.

Knowing Your Challengers

As you continue on your program, selecting and exchanging Options and personalizing them to fit your lifestyle, you can count on one thing: Challengers to your success will emerge at every Step of the Program.

Challengers to your success
will emerge at every Step of the Program.

Challengers to your success are the persons, feelings, and changes in your life that cause you concern, conflict, or additional stress and that tempt you to temporarily, or permanently, break your commitment to your program.

Challengers in the form of persons may include loved, or not-so-loved, ones who challenge your right to take care of yourself and put your own health needs before their desires, who continue to question and deny your belief in the precepts of the Program, or who subtly tempt you to do things that will sabotage your good intentions.

As spouses and other family members, co-workers, and friends see you begin to truly take your life and health into your own hands, their personal fears and concerns and issues of control, their hidden agendas, may all emerge and provoke surprisingly negative behaviors.

A husband who has been after his wife for years to "eat better" will suddenly start complaining that she is not serving his favorite (artery-clogging) meal. An otherwise wonderfully supportive wife may find herself teasing her husband about his new activity schedule or resenting the "time-out" he takes as part of his new Stress-Reducing Option. Family members suddenly emerge with junk food demands or always seem to leave their half-eaten snacks around the house.

The ways and means of "people sabotage" are infinite.
We have for you a surprisingly simple and success-filled
strategy. One that will linger in your mind for years to come.

The various methods of "people sabotage" are infinite and we can never avoid them all. We can, however, deal with them cleanly and effectively with a single surprisingly simple strategy, a strategy that has been repeatedly successful for years: JSC (Just Stay Centered).

People will challenge your commitment to your program, to yourself, and to your future. Stop yourself from reacting. Remember—JSC.

Do not get pulled from *your* intentions, *your* needs, *your* plans. Don't try to figure out *why* they are challenging you. Do not leave your place of strength to explain yourself or excuse yourself. Be the person you always wanted to be. Don't let them wear you down.

Take this book to a place where you can be alone. Reread it, over and over again. Open again to its words and ideas. Read and reread the chapters that are important to you. Write on it; underline in it.

It is important to stay focused on what *you* want and on the fact that you have a right to choose for yourself. Trust yourself. Friends and family do not know what is better for you than you do. This is your life; you have a right to live it as you think best. Don't defend or explain yourself. Just stay centered on yourself, on what you want. When in doubt, JSC.

Challengers in the form of feelings and change are, in many ways, easier for most of us to handle than people. We call these challengers "triggers" because they can trigger physical and psychological responses that pull us from our program.

Emotional triggers include feelings (especially those feelings you are not free to express) that usually reflect a discomfort with change, where you are prevented or think you are being prevented from doing what would make you feel better or would right the situation.

Anger, fury, rage, anxiety or anticipation, self-blame or blame of others, helplessness or powerlessness, worry, frustration, loss, sadness, stress, and pressure can all trigger higher Profactor-H levels and, at the same time, pull you away from the very Program that is designed to help you lower your risk. Even excitement, a happy feeling of anticipation, can cause similar kinds of physical and emotional changes.

To know these feelings and to expect them is half the battle; they are part of life—they will come and tempt you from your goals. It is essential to remember that each of these feelings is just that, a feeling, a passing emotion that will be replaced by another. No matter how intense a feeling may be, in itself it cannot hurt you. Just stay centered.

We know that it can be difficult to remain centered at times, and that is the battle we all face; be aware that you are not alone and, most important, that you can face these feelings squarely, without sacrificing your health, or your life, in the process.

You have met these saboteurs in the past; and in the future, together, we will be prepared, ready, and waiting for them. Remember, JSC. This is your life; you have a right to make it what you want.

> This is your life; you have a right to make it what you want.

EMOTIONAL TRIGGERS

The powerful effect that your feelings have on your body should not be taken lightly. The impact of emotions can directly influence your Profactor-H levels and can, in addition, pull you from your commitment to your program. Whether they influence you directly or indirectly, emotions can bring about the same result: an almost inevitable increase in Profactor-H risk.

Each of these emotions can trigger, directly and indirectly, an increase in your Profactor-H levels and risk:

Anger, fury, rage (especially feelings you are not free to express)
Anxiety or anticipation
Blame of self or others
Helplessness or powerlessness
Excitement
Fear
Frustration
Loss
Sadness
Stress and pressure

The Challenge of Change

Just when you think you have your life pretty much under control, just when it seems you might be getting a handle on things, just when life seems manageable—wham, it happens. Something changes. Sometimes the changes seem small—to other people. Sometimes the changes are clearly important and influence a great part of your life. In any case, they can throw you off balance and cause physical stress that translates into raised Profactor-H levels.

Though physical changes may be temporary, the most important impact of change lies in its ability to pull you away from your focus, your commitment to your program. Tempting you to attend to the immediate, rather than to your long-term goals, can undo your good and important work.

Change is inevitable. But as we love to say, the good thing about change is that it comes and goes. You must remain stalwart, strong and unbending, hold on to your resolve and your goals, and of course, just stay centered.

In the midst of change, make a safe place for yourself. Write down your feelings, put them into a diary or into letters you may never send. Put them into thoughts that you may someday pass on to your children. Your insights are important. Help yourself stay centered. In a little while, when this change passes, you will be happy to find that you still have your program—and yourself.

THE CHALLENGES OF CHANGE

Changes in your body and your environment can have great impact on your Profactor-H risk and can tempt you to compromise your commitment to your program. Be on the lookout for these Challenges of Change and just stay centered.

Allergic reactions	Medications, new or changed
Changes in homelife	Menopause
Changes in working conditions	Moving
Divorce	Pregnancy and breast-feeding*
Fever	Premenstrual changes
Jet lag	Quitting smoking
Lack of sleep	Seasonal changes
Loss or illness of friend or family member	Surgery

*Pregnancy and breast-feeding bring with them special needs and concerns. This Program is not meant to be used during pregnancy, nor during times when you are breast-feeding. See your physician for individual guidance regarding an appropriate program.

Stress with a Special Flavor

There is a special challenge that is important enough for us to give it its own section, a physical stress that often comes from eating restaurant-prepared Chinese food. In some cases, this stress response has been reported after eating Indian or other highly spiced foods as well.

You are probably familiar with jokes about being hungry an hour after eating Chinese food, or the less humorous reports of headaches and other reactions to MSG (monosodium glutamate). We have seen evidence that these responses, and those that may not even be perceived by the victim, indicate a stress reaction strong enough to raise Profactor-H levels significantly. In addition, the hunger, cravings, and disorientation that can result can throw you off your center and put a critical damper on your program resolve.

If you find that you have strong cravings for Chinese (or Indian or other spicy) food, if you do not feel really "good" after eating it—bloated perhaps, or just out of sorts—we recommend that you avoid it entirely or eat it only on rare occasions.

By the way, if you think that you can get Chinese food without any monosodium glutamate, keep this in mind: Soy sauce and Teriyaki, key ingredients in Chinese cooking, naturally contain MSG, so while your restauranteur may not be sprinkling it on, it may be in the food anyway.

Getting Away from It All

Vacations, holidays, and celebrations are meant to be enjoyed. Your Options have been designed to offer you the flexibility to take your program with you, on vacation or holiday or to special celebrations, all without sacrificing your fun or your good health. With a little planning, you can have it all.

Special times do *not* require sacrifice, but they do require some planning. You cannot expect to go on vacation and be assured of finding the salads and vegetables you need, for instance. If you do not plan ahead to have these available, you might come face-to-face with finding yourself unable to stay on your program.

Be honest with yourself. When you really want to do something, you know what needs to be done. Call first; make sure your hotel has the food you need as well as any other accommodations you require. Bring your own salad to a party. Don't be shy; this is your program and your choice. Perhaps you can offer to bring salad for everyone. In any case, don't explain. Take care of yourself. Be strong and be prepared.

Time Swapping

On vacation or during holidays, for certain social occasions or just for a change of pace, you might enjoy exchanging your meal times. On the Profactor-H Program you are free to change the time of any meal, or your meals in general.

If you have chosen the Advanced Nutrition Option that asks you to confine all carbohydrate-rich Essential Balance Foods to dinner, for instance, rather than having these foods with your evening meal, you might decide that a carbohydrate-rich breakfast would be a nice change of pace. Or you might want to take advantage of a wedding brunch with all its taste-tempting splendor. For that day, or any other day, you are free to swap dinner for breakfast.

In this case, you would have your Essential Balance Foods with your morning meal and have only Risk-Reducing Foods with dinner. (You would in that case, however, not have Essential Balance Foods at *both* of these meals.)

You are free to change back to your original plan the following day or to continue to swap for a while. As long as, in keeping with that Option, you confine your Essential Balance Foods to one meal each day, it does not matter whether it is breakfast, lunch, or dinner. You are free to make the trade.

You are also free, if you like, to change your meal times. Not all of us prefer a breakfast, lunch, and dinner schedule at standard hours.

The Late Show: Matt's Story

Matt K. is a wonderful example of a man who, like some of us, needed the freedom to fashion his own eating times. During his first two years of retirement, Matt had put on nearly twenty pounds and watched as his blood pressure and blood fat levels rose steadily. He tried to "eat sensibly" and watch his fat intake, but things only got worse. When we first saw him, he confessed he was worried.

"If I keep this up," Matt admitted, "I won't have very long to enjoy my retirement." His big stumbling block, we discovered, was trying to eat according to his old time schedule. In addition, he loved to snack in the evenings, but less activity meant easier weight gain. One change solved all of his problems. It was simple and obvious and the Program gave him the flexibility he needed.

Matt preferred to eat a late breakfast, around 11:00 A.M., and to skip lunch. The late breakfast satisfied him and he was more than willing to wait to eat dinner until 6:00 P.M.

Most important to Matt, by substituting a late brunch for both his breakfast and lunch he eliminated one meal during the day and was able, without adding extra food to his diet, to enjoy a very welcome evening snack every night. His weight came off easily, without struggle, and his blood levels quickly returned to normal.

Like Matt, you should feel free to change your times around. You may eat differently on weekends than during the week; you may have different preferences depending on the season or on what your work or home life demands.

You are free to make the Program fit your needs. One word of caution: If at all possible, follow each Option for a while, until you are comfortable and familiar with it. Then plan your changes beforehand and enjoy your freedom.

A Question of Balance

Essential Balance Foods are delicious and exciting, and these carbohydrate-rich choices may tempt you to include far more pasta, bread, and dessert in your dinners than Risk-Reducing vegetables and salad. When meals are out of balance you can raise your Pro-factor-H risk and reduce some of the benefits of the Options you have chosen.

In all of your meals, do not be as concerned with absolute amounts as with the choice of foods and balance. It does not matter, for instance, if at your Risk-Reducing lunch you have two, three, or four ounces of turkey. What is important is that you include vegetables or salad along with your protein.

In the same way, balancing meals that contain Essential Balance Foods is very important. You do not have to be concerned about amounts if you keep the meal balanced. Balance the starches, snack foods, sweets, and fruit with protein, salad, and Risk-Reducing vegetables.

With your physician's consent, we generally recommend that meals that contain Essential Balance Foods should be divided into four quarters:

¼   salad
¼   any protein (meat, fish, fowl, dairy or tofu substitute)
¼   Risk-Reducing vegetables
¼   Essential Balance Foods, including starches (bread, potatoes, rice, pasta), fruit and juice, snack foods and dessert

If Essential Balance Foods are included in your breakfast, you would probably not choose salad or vegetable, but again balance your carbohydrate-rich foods with protein-rich foods at that meal.

Meals that contain only Risk-Reducing Foods should be balanced between Risk-Reducing protein and Risk-Reducing vegetables and salad in equal portions.

Do *not* bother measuring or weighing; you cannot live like that.

Do *not* bother measuring or weighing; you cannot live like that. Just look at your plate and use your own judgment—approximate.

We have included examples of balanced meals in our Meal Plans chapter, beginning on page 298. A good guide is to think of a dinner that includes Essential Balance Foods as a mini-Thanksgiving meal: a well-rounded, moderate feast, a wonderful array of food of all kinds. Just make sure to keep it balanced. Then enjoy the pleasures, the benefits, and yourself. You have it coming.

> Enjoy the pleasures, the benefits, and yourself.
> You have it coming.

CHAPTER 22

A Second Chance

You have chosen wisely.
—The Knight, *Indiana Jones and the Last Crusade*

It happens to almost all of us. When things go well, we tend to take them for granted. When things go poorly, we want one thing and one thing only: a second chance.

Oh, what we wouldn't trade for another chance to do it "right," to enjoy what we have, or perhaps, this time, to try harder. Now that we know how much we have taken for granted, all we ask is a second chance.

So, right now, take some time to sit alone and think about all that you have and how easily it can be taken away. The Chinese say that you own all that you cannot lose in a shipwreck. Therefore, you own nothing. It may be gone tomorrow. Today is all that you have.

Use it wisely. Do not let the little inconveniences or excuses of the day keep you from your goals. Make wise choices for your health, your happiness, and a long life.

This moment is the only chance of which you can be assured.

CHAPTER 23

Sample Daily Meal Plans

This Program has been designed for the vegetarian
as well as the meat-eater,
for the finest cook and for those who can't even boil water.

The Profactor-H Program has been designed to be a livable, enjoyable plan that will, at the same time, help reduce your risk for Profactor-H and the many diseases and risk factors associated with it.
Each day, your meals and snacks will be divided into two types:

Risk-Reducing Meals and Snacks
Essential Balance Meals and Snacks

Risk-Reducing Foods have been shown to significantly decrease
your Profactor-H risk and are therefore included in *all* meals. Risk-
Reducing Meals and Snacks contain Risk-Reducing Foods *only*.

Essential Balance Foods are vital in complementing and balancing
the Risk-Reducing Foods in your program. Essential Balance Meals
and Snacks contain not just Essential Balance Foods but, rather,
both Essential Balance Foods *and* Risk-Reducing Foods.

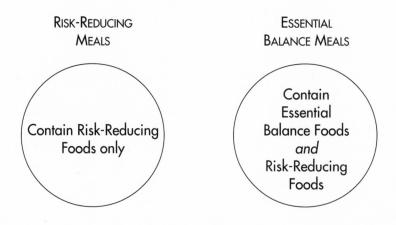

RISK-REDUCING
MEALS

Contain Risk-Reducing
Foods only

ESSENTIAL
BALANCE MEALS

Contain
Essential
Balance Foods
and
Risk-Reducing
Foods

Both Risk-Reducing Foods and Essential Balance Foods must be included, each day, as part of your program—even though there may be some meals that are made up of Risk-Reducing Foods only.

Although Essential Balance Foods can increase your insulin levels if they are eaten *frequently* throughout the day, on the Profactor-H Program you will eat them less frequently but in satisfying amounts; therefore, you can enjoy them every single day while continuing to reduce your Profactor-H risk.

For more details on the kinds of foods included in each food group, see the lists in chapter 16, "Options, Options, Options," on pages 220 to 223.

In the two chapters that follow, you will find many of our favorite and exciting Risk-Reducing and Essential Balance Recipes. They will offer you some new and different meal ideas, though you are always free to enjoy your personal favorites at home or while dining out.

Remember:

Risk-Reducing Meals and Snacks contain Risk-Reducing Foods only.

Essential Balance Meals contain Essential Balance Foods *in combination with* Risk-Reducing Foods.

The Question of Quantity

No matter what, the question of quantity always rears its ugly head. Most of us have been led into thinking that to be healthy or slim or both we must weigh and measure our food. It makes no sense. Healthy animals don't do it. Neither do most healthy humans.

Weighing and measuring your food does nothing to correct the problems that may be making you unhealthy or overweight to begin with, and holding yourself in check with such artificial means will not correct the cause of your difficulties.

This Program is designed to correct your Profactor-H imbalance. Measuring and weighing, counting and making exchanges, are not necessary. Changing *how often* you eat insulin-releasing foods during the day, and balancing your meals, however, are important in reducing your Profactor-H risk.

With your Options to guide you, the meal plans that follow will give you concrete (and delicious) examples, so that you can relax and enjoy yourself. Within your physician's recommendations, eat quantities that satisfy you. Eating without concern regarding amounts may seem unusual at first, but as you continue on the Program you will find that any excess appetite and cravings you might have will most likely normalize, and soon you will eat heartily, without overindulging, naturally.

If you still want a guide, choose "average-size" portions for all meals, make snacks equivalent to about one half an average lunch, and see pages 294 to 296 for guidelines for balancing your meals.

Health Agency Recommendations

As part of the Profactor-H Program, you will be able to easily incorporate low-fat and/or low-salt alternatives. If appropriate, choose low-fat and/or low-salt alternatives as part of your daily meal plan.

We have included suggestions for substituting low-fat and low-salt alternatives in all recipes and detailed recommendations on low-fat, low-cholesterol, and low-salt substitutions can be found in "Health Agency Recommendations," page 345. Dietary fat and salt recommendations should always be discussed with your physician.

Some Simple but Important Details

Two fourteen-day meal plans follow that will give you examples of planning meals for the Beginner, Intermediate, or Advanced Program. Since Nutrition Options A and B in each of these programs require only the addition of salads or vegetables to your regular meals, we have not judged it necessary to include examples of Options A or B. Instead, we have illustrated Nutrition Option C only in all of the meal plans that follow.

The first fourteen-day Sample Meal Plan provides examples of Nutrition Option C for either the Beginner or the Intermediate Program. Since Nutrition Option C selections in the Beginner and Intermediate Programs vary only as to the kinds of foods included in snacks—the same breakfast, lunch, and dinner Sample Meal Plans can apply to both. Examples of contents of snacks for each of these programs will, of course, differ and guidelines will be given.

The second fourteen-day Sample Meal Plan provides examples of Nutrition Option C for the Advanced Program. This Advanced Option provides the greatest relative risk reduction by far (12 points), and because it is more unusual than Advanced Nutrition Options A or B, which require only the addition of salads and/or vegetables to your regular meals, we wanted to provide you with some specific examples. In selecting Advanced Option C, you will eat only Risk-Reducing Foods at breakfast, lunch, and for all snacks. In this Option, you *must* include Essential Balance Foods (such as breads, potatoes, pasta, and other starches; fruit and juice; and snack foods and sweets if you like) in your evening meal—but include them in one meal a day only.

If you are a vegetarian, two special sections beginning on pages 317 and 338 have two seven-day meal plans. The first is for the Beginner's or Intermediate Program; the second, for the Advanced Program. These two-week meal plans will serve as models to help guide you in the selection of foods for each program's Option C. We have also included special vegetarian sections in the recipe chapters (chapters 24 and 25) that follow.

> You do not have to be a fine chef, a cook, or even know how
> to boil water to successfully follow the Profactor-H Program.

You do not have to be a fine chef, a cook, or even know how to boil water to follow the Profactor-H Program. You can eat all your meals at restaurants and still stay on the Program. You can never touch a stove and still be successful, but if you like to cook, regularly or on occasion, we have included our favorite recipes for your use.

The recipes for many of the Risk-Reducing and Essential Balance dishes that are listed in these meal plans can be found starting on pages 348 and 413, respectively. You may choose additional recipes for Essential Balance Meals from almost any cookbook that has ever been published. The choices will be literally unlimited. Just remember that your Essential Balance Meals must be balanced (see page 294) and should include, salad, protein, vegetables, and good complex carbohydrates. And, of course, add a nutritious and delicious dessert if you like.

The meal plans that follow are by no means all-inclusive.

You may mix and match Risk-Reducing Foods within Risk Reducing Meals as you like. You may include all foods (Essential Balance Foods *and* Risk-Reducing Foods) in your Essential Balance Meals. But *never*, no *never*, add Essential Balance Foods to your Risk-Reducing Meals. To do so would raise your Profactor-H levels and negate the effect of the Program.

A Sweet Reminder

Some of the meal plans that follow include recipes and beverage choices that contain artificial sweeteners. If you have selected a Bonus Option that calls for you to refrain from all artificial sweeteners, do not select these recipes or beverages.

Now, turn to the coming pages and see the wonderful meals that even the most advanced Options of each of the three Steps of the Program have to offer.

Sample Meal Plans

Fourteen-Day Meal Plan: Standard Choices

Beginner's and Intermediate Programs

DAY ONE

Essential Balance Breakfast
Any fruit or juice of your choice
Toast or bagel with butter, margarine, or jelly
Scrambled eggs (or egg substitute)
Sausage or bacon (or low-fat meat alternative)
Coffee or tea with milk and/or sugar or sugar substitute if desired

Risk-Reducing Lunch
Cream of Broccoli Soup (page 376)
Chef's Salad (page 368) with regular or low-fat dressing
Tea or coffee (with no sugar), diet soda, or carbonated water

Essential Balance Dinner
Shrimp with Herb Sauce (page 416)
or Zucchini Bisque (page 442)
Garden Salad (page 427)
Sweet and Pungent Pork (page 450)
Crescent rolls with butter or margarine
Wild rice
Steamed asparagus
Scottish Pecan Shortbread (page 487) with ice cream,*
ice milk,* or sherbet*
or fruit of your choice
Any beverage(s) of your choice

Snacks (if desired)
Beginner's Program: A balance of Risk-Reducing Foods alone
or in combination with Essential Balance Foods
Intermediate Program: A healthy choice of
Risk-Reducing Foods only

*Low-fat alternatives may be substituted.

Beginner's and Intermediate Programs
DAY TWO

Essential Balance Breakfast
Juice of your choice
Breakfast Crepes (page 351) or pancakes with fruit topping
Coffee or tea with milk and/or sugar or
sugar substitute if desired

Risk-Reducing Lunch
Shrimp Soup (page 380)
Spinach Salad (page 372)
Broiled, baked, roasted, or stir-fried chicken of your choice
Mixed vegetable stir-fry (cauliflower, mushroom, celery,
and green pepper)
Tea or coffee (with no sugar), diet soda, or carbonated water

Essential Balance Dinner
Barbecued Spare Ribs—Chinese Style (page 417)
or Cream of Avocado Soup (page 442)
Green-Goddess Salad (page 428)
Batter Fried Shrimp* (page 471)
Garlic sesame crisp bread
Baked potato with toppings of your choice
Green beans amandine
Pound Cake (page 487) with strawberries and whipped cream*
Any beverage(s) of your choice

Snacks (if desired)
Beginner's Program: A balance of Risk-Reducing Foods alone
or in combination with Essential Balance Foods
Intermediate Program: A healthy choice of
Risk-Reducing Foods only

*Low-fat alternatives may be substituted.

Beginner's and Intermediate Programs
DAY THREE

Essential Balance Breakfast
Tomato or orange juice
Bagel, roll, or toast with butter, margarine, or jam
Cheese and mushroom omelet (or egg substitute)
Coffee or tea with milk and/or sugar or
sugar substitute if desired

Risk-Reducing Lunch
Cool Cucumber Appetizer (page 358)
Asparagus Ham Delight (page 385)
Tea or coffee (with no sugar), diet soda, or carbonated water

Essential Balance Dinner
Minestrone Soup (page 441)
Kidney Bean Salad (page 429) or salad and
dressing of your choice
Golden-Fried Chicken* (page 463) and thick french fries*
Corn bread
Coleslaw
Steamed greens
Chocolate Chip Coffee Cake (page 486)
Any beverage(s) of your choice

Snacks (if desired)
Beginner's Program: A balance of Risk-Reducing Foods alone
or in combination with Essential Balance Foods
Intermediate Program: A healthy choice of
Risk-Reducing Foods only

*Low-fat alternatives may be substituted.

Beginner's and Intermediate Programs
DAY FOUR

Essential Balance Breakfast
One half grapefruit or melon
French toast* with fruit or syrup
Coffee or tea with milk and/or sugar or
sugar substitute if desired

Risk-Reducing Lunch
Tossed Green Salad (page 372) with regular or
low-fat dressing of your choice
Sole Delight (page 395)
Garlic stir-fried cauliflower
Tea or coffee (with no sugar), diet soda,
or carbonated water

Essential Balance Dinner
Cream of Asparagus Soup (page 440)
Italian Salad (page 429)
Veal with Peppers (page 456)
Italian bread with butter or margarine
Sautéed spinach
Pecan Pie (page 485) with regular or low-fat topping
Any beverage(s) of your choice

Snacks (if desired)
Beginner's Program: A balance of Risk-Reducing Foods alone
or in combination with Essential Balance Foods
Intermediate Program: A healthy choice of
Risk-Reducing Foods only

*Low-fat alternatives may be substituted.

Beginner's and Intermediate Programs
DAY FIVE

Essential Balance Breakfast
Fruit or juice of your choice
Ham and cheese omelet* (or egg substitute)
Home fries*
Bagel or biscuits with butter, margarine, or jam
Coffee or tea with milk and/or sugar or
sugar substitute if desired

Risk-Reducing Lunch
Any mixed green salad with dressing of your choice
Pork Tenderloin with Mushrooms, Green Peppers,
and Olives (page 390)
Garlic and Lemon Green Beans (page 371)
Tea or coffee (with no sugar), diet soda,
or carbonated water

Essential Balance Dinner
Mushroom Delights (page 419)
or Old-Fashioned Split-Pea Soup (page 440)
Baked Pork Chops and Apples (page 451)
Hot biscuits with butter or margarine
Steamed broccoli or asparagus
Crème Brûlée* (page 481)
Any beverage(s) of your choice

Snacks (if desired)
Beginner's Program: A balance of Risk-Reducing Foods alone
or in combination with Essential Balance Foods
Intermediate Program: A healthy choice of
Risk-Reducing Foods only

*Low-fat alternatives may be substituted.

Beginner's and Intermediate Programs
DAY SIX

Essential Balance Breakfast
Hot or cold cereal of your choice with regular or
low-fat milk
Fruit and/or juice of your choice
Coffee or tea with milk and/or sugar or
sugar substitute if desired

Risk-Reducing Lunch
Clam Soup (page 377)
Caesar Salad (page 365)
Broiled or baked fish
Spinach topped with regular or low-fat cheese
Tea or coffee (with no sugar), diet soda, or
carbonated water

Essential Balance Dinner
Tuna and Cheese Canapes* (page 420)
or Cream of Cauliflower Soup* (page 436)
Breaded Fish Fillets (page 473) or broiled flounder
Dinner rolls with butter or margarine
Steamed mixed vegetables
Chocolate Rugelach (page 480) with
fruit of your choice
Any beverage(s) of your choice

Snacks (if desired)
Beginner's Program: A balance of Risk-Reducing Foods alone
or in combination with Essential Balance Foods
Intermediate Program: A healthy choice of
Risk-Reducing Foods only

*Low-fat alternatives may be substituted.

Beginner's and Intermediate Programs
DAY SEVEN

Essential Balance Breakfast
Bran or corn muffin, bagel, or low-fat Danish of your choice
Butter, margarine, cream cheese,* or jam
Coffee or tea with milk and/or sugar or
sugar substitute if desired

Risk-Reducing Lunch
Spinach Salad (page 372)
Baked Bluefish (page 394)
Sautéed green peppers
Tea or coffee (with no sugar), diet soda,
or carbonated water

Essential Balance Dinner
Spinach Raita (page 420)
or Pumpkin Soup (page 437)
Finger salad with dressing of your choice
Stuffed Chicken Breasts (page 466)
Baked new potatoes with parsley and butter (or margarine)
Green beans topped with cheese*
Apple Cream Pie* (page 479)
Any beverage(s) of your choice

Snacks (if desired)
Beginner's Program: A balance of Risk-Reducing Foods alone
or in combination with Essential Balance Foods
Intermediate Program: A healthy choice of
Risk-Reducing Foods only

*Low-fat alternatives may be substituted.

Beginner's and Intermediate Programs

DAY EIGHT

Essential Balance Breakfast
Juice or fruit of your choice
Bagel, toast, or biscuits with margarine, butter,
cream cheese,* or jam
Mushroom omelet (or egg substitute)
Coffee or tea with milk and/or sugar or
sugar substitute if desired

Risk-Reducing Lunch
Celery Stuffed with Tuna (page 358)
Broiled cheeseburger (beef or turkey), no bun
Coleslaw (no sugar)
Tea or coffee (with no sugar), diet soda,
or carbonated water

Essential Balance Dinner
Shrimp with Herb Sauce (page 416)
or Corn Chowder (page 437)
Lamb Curry (page 461)
Saffron rice
Steamed green beans
Whole-grain bread or rolls
Iced Lemon Soufflé (page 478) and chocolate-chip cookies
Any beverage(s) of your choice

Snacks (if desired)
Beginner's Program: A balance of Risk-Reducing Foods alone
or in combination with Essential Balance Foods
Intermediate Program: A healthy choice of
Risk-Reducing Foods only

*Low-fat alternatives may be substituted.

Beginner's and Intermediate Programs
DAY NINE

Essential Balance Breakfast
Juice of your choice
Poached or smoked salmon or whitefish
Bagel with cream cheese*
Tomatoes, onions
Coffee or tea with milk and/or sugar or
sugar substitute if desired

Risk-Reducing Lunch
Tossed Green Salad (page 372) with regular or
low-fat dressing of your choice
Beef and Celery Ragout (page 391)
Tea or coffee (with no sugar), diet soda,
or carbonated water

Essential Balance Dinner
Marinated Pork (page 421)
or French Onion Soup (page 438)
Broiled Lobster Tails (page 471)
Baked potato or buttered rice*
French bread with margarine or butter
Sautéed green peppers with onions
Apple Cobbler (page 477)
Any beverage(s) of your choice

Snacks (if desired)
Beginner's Program: A balance of Risk-Reducing Foods alone
or in combination with Essential Balance Foods
Intermediate Program: A healthy choice of
Risk-Reducing Foods only

*Low-fat alternatives may be substituted.

Beginner's and Intermediate Programs

DAY TEN

Essential Balance Breakfast
Juice or fruit of your choice
Breakfast Cinnamon Bread (page 352), muffin, or Danish
Butter, margarine, cream cheese,* or jam
Coffee or tea with milk and/or sugar or
sugar substitute if desired

Risk-Reducing Lunch
Tossed Green Salad (page 372) with dressing of your choice
Italian Shrimp (page 398)
Steamed asparagus
Tea or coffee (with no sugar), diet soda,
or carbonated water

Essential Balance Dinner
Spinach-Egg Pie* (page 418)
or Cream of Asparagus Soup* (page 440)
Yogurt Chicken Breasts (page 468)
Scalloped potatoes
Italian garlic bread with butter or margarine
Mixed steamed green vegetables
Fresh Pears in Wine (page 478)
Any beverage(s) of your choice

Snacks (if desired)
Beginner's Program: A balance of Risk-Reducing Foods alone
or in combination with Essential Balance Foods
Intermediate Program: A healthy choice of
Risk-Reducing Foods only

*Low-fat alternatives may be substituted.

Beginner's and Intermediate Programs
DAY ELEVEN

Essential Balance Breakfast
Juice or fruit of your choice
Scrambled eggs (or egg substitute)
Corned beef hash*
Coffee or tea with milk and/or sugar or
sugar substitute if desired

Risk-Reducing Lunch
Tossed Green Salad (page 372) with dressing of your choice
Broiled Swordfish (page 397) or Italian Shrimp (page 398)
Sautéed mushrooms
Tea or coffee (with no sugar), diet soda,
or carbonated water

Essential Balance Dinner
Cream of Avocado* Soup (page 442)
Any mixed green salad with dressing of your choice
Beef-Vegetable Stew (page 447)
Coleslaw
Broccoli, bean, and mushroom medley
Homemade biscuits with butter or margarine
Lemon-Lime Meringue Pie (page 481)
Any beverage(s) of your choice

Snacks (if desired)
Beginner's Program: A balance of Risk-Reducing Foods alone
or in combination with Essential Balance Foods
Intermediate Program: A healthy choice of
Risk-Reducing Foods only

*Low-fat alternatives may be substituted.

Beginner's and Intermediate Programs
DAY TWELVE

Essential Balance Breakfast
Hot or cold cereal of your choice
Regular or low-fat milk
Banana or other fruit
Whole-grain bread or muffin with margarine, butter, or jam
Coffee or tea with milk and/or sugar or
sugar substitute if desired

Risk-Reducing Lunch
Shrimp Cheese Asparagus Soup (page 381)
Finger salad including raw celery, olives, green beans,
cauliflower, and/or mushrooms with regular or low-fat dressing
Roast Lamb with Herbs (page 389)
Tea or coffee (with no sugar), diet soda, or carbonated water

Essential Balance Dinner
California Avocado Halves (page 425)
or Minestrone Soup (page 441)
Any mixed green salad or salad of your choice with
dressing of your choice
Skewered Spiced Lamb (page 459)
Skewered new potatoes and chunks of vegetables
Rye bread with butter or margarine
Quick and Easy Mocha Pie* (page 482)
Any beverage(s) of your choice

Snacks (if desired)
Beginner's Program: A balance of Risk-Reducing Foods alone
or in combination with Essential Balance Foods
Intermediate Program: A healthy choice of
Risk-Reducing Foods only

*Low-fat alternatives may be substituted.

Beginner's and Intermediate Programs
DAY THIRTEEN

Essential Balance Breakfast
Juice or fruit of your choice
Breakfast Pancakes (page 353)
Syrup or fruit topping
Sausage or bacon (regular or low-fat)
Coffee or tea with milk and/or sugar or
sugar substitute if desired

Risk-Reducing Lunch
Tossed Green Salad (page 372) with regular or
low-fat dressing
Barbecued Lemon Chicken (page 392)
Stir-fried mushrooms, green peppers, and celery
Tea or coffee (with no sugar), diet soda,
or carbonated water

Essential Balance Dinner
Swedish Meatballs (page 424)
or Zucchini Bisque (page 442)
Any mixed green salad with dressing of your choice
Shrimp in Wine Sauce (page 469)
Bread sticks or fresh, warm French bread
Green beans amandine
Rum Cake Delight (page 483)
Any beverage(s) of your choice

Snacks (if desired)
Beginner's Program: A balance of Risk-Reducing Foods alone
or in combination with Essential Balance Foods
Intermediate Program: A healthy choice of
Risk-Reducing Foods only

Low-fat alternatives may be substituted.

Beginner's and Intermediate Programs
DAY FOURTEEN

Essential Balance Breakfast
Juice or fruit of your choice
Eggs Benedict*
Coffee or tea with milk and/or sugar or
sugar substitute if desired

Risk-Reducing Lunch
Fresh Seafood Salad (page 370)
Garlic and Lemon Green Beans (page 371)
Tea or coffee (with no sugar), diet soda,
or carbonated water

Essential Balance Dinner
Cream of Cauliflower Soup (page 436)
Any mixed green salad with dressing of your choice
Beef-and-Potatoes Casserole (page 443)
Sautéed spinach or green vegetable of your choice
Whole grain rolls
Chilled Cranberry Cake (page 484) with ice cream,
ice milk, or sherbet
Any beverage(s) of your choice

Snacks (if desired)
Beginner's Program: A balance of Risk-Reducing Foods alone
or in combination with Essential Balance Foods
Intermediate Program: A healthy choice of
Risk-Reducing Foods only

*Low-fat alternatives may be substituted.

SEVEN-DAY MEAL PLAN: VEGETARIAN CHOICES

Vegetarian Beginner's and Intermediate Programs

DAY ONE

Vegetarian Essential Balance Breakfast
Eggs Mayonnaise* (page 425) or egg substitute
Vegetarian "bacon"
Whole-grain bread or roll with jam or spread of your choice
Coffee or tea with milk, nondairy creamer,
and/or sweetener of your choice if desired

Vegetarian Risk-Reducing Lunch
Spinach Salad (page 372)
Asparagus and Egg Casserole (page 400)
Tea or coffee (with no sugar), diet soda,
or carbonated water

Vegetarian Essential Balance Dinner
Cream of Asparagus Soup (page 440)
Green-Goddess Salad (page 428)
Vegetarian "Beef" Casserole (page 488)
Wild rice
Whole-grain bread and butter or margarine
Green beans amandine
Cream Cheese Cake* (page 474) or nondairy substitute
Any beverage(s) of your choice

Vegetarian Snacks (if desired)
Beginner's Program: A balance of Risk-Reducing Foods alone
or in combination with Essential Balance Foods
Intermediate Program: A healthy choice of
Risk-Reducing Foods only

*Low-fat alternatives may be substituted.

Vegetarian Beginner's and Intermediate Programs

DAY TWO

Vegetarian Essential Balance Breakfast
Breakfast Soufflé (page 350)
Vegetarian "ham" or "bacon"
Toast, roll, or bagel with jam or spread of your choice
Coffee or tea with milk, nondairy creamer,
and/or sweetener of your choice if desired

Vegetarian Risk-Reducing Lunch
Romaine Lettuce Soup (page 377)
Stir-fried mushrooms and green peppers
Vegetarian Parsley Butter "Burgers" (page 401)
Tea or coffee (with no sugar), diet soda, or carbonated water

Vegetarian Essential Balance Dinner
Cream of Avocado Soup (page 442)
Garden Salad (page 427)
Flounder with Wild Rice and Water Chestnuts (page 490)
Steamed Broccoli
Fresh Pears in Wine (page 478)
Any beverage(s)

Vegetarian Snacks (if desired)
Beginner's Program: A balance of Risk-Reducing Foods alone
or in combination with Essential Balance Foods
Intermediate Program: A healthy choice of
Risk-Reducing Foods only

Low-fat alternatives may be substituted.

Vegetarian Beginner's and Intermediate Programs

DAY THREE

Vegetarian Essential Balance Breakfast
Juice or fruit of your choice
Scrambled eggs or egg substitute
Vegetarian corned beef hash
Breakfast Muffins (page 352) or muffins of your choice
Jam, jelly, nut butter, or spread of your choice
Coffee or tea with milk, nondairy creamer,
and/or sweetener of your choice if desired

Vegetarian Risk-Reducing Lunch
Curried Eggs (page 402)
Chef's Salad (you may use meat substitutes) (page 368)
Dressing of your choice (regular or low-fat)
Tea or coffee (with no sugar), diet soda, or carbonated water

Vegetarian Essential Balance Dinner
Minestrone Soup (page 441)
Italian Salad (page 429)
Fried Lemon Vegetarian "Chicken"* (page 489)
Brown rice with mushrooms
Whole-grain rolls with butter or margarine
Sautéed spinach
Banana Fritters* (page 475)
Any beverage(s) of your choice

Vegetarian Snacks (if desired)
Beginner's Program: A balance of Risk-Reducing Foods alone
or in combination with Essential Balance Foods
Intermediate Program: A healthy choice of
Risk-Reducing Foods only

*Low-fat alternatives may be substituted.

Vegetarian Beginner's and Intermediate Programs

DAY FOUR

Vegetarian Essential Balance Breakfast
Fruit or juice of your choice
Breakfast Crepes (page 351) with topping of your choice
Vegetarian "sausage"
Coffee or tea with milk, nondairy creamer,
and/or sweetener of your choice if desired

Vegetarian Risk-Reducing Lunch
Tossed Green Salad (page 372) with dressing of your choice
Vegetarian Oriental "Steak" Casserole (page 404)
or vegetarian "burger"
Sliced cucumbers, dill pickle, olives
Tea or coffee (with no sugar), diet soda, or carbonated water

Vegetarian Essential Balance Dinner
Zucchini Bisque (page 442)
Kidney Bean Salad (page 429) or salad of your choice
Seafood-Vegetable Delight (page 491)
Paprika baked new potatoes
Vegetable Joy (492)
Apple Cream Pie* (page 479)
or fruit of your choice
Any beverage(s) of your choice

Vegetarian Snacks (if desired)
Beginner's Program: A balance of Risk-Reducing Foods alone
or in combination with Essential Balance Foods
Intermediate Program: A healthy choice of
Risk-Reducing Foods only

*Low-fat alternatives may be substituted.

Vegetarian Beginner's and Intermediate Programs

DAY FIVE

Vegetarian Essential Balance Breakfast

Breakfast Cinnamon Bread (page 352)
with butter, margarine, or spread of your choice
Breakfast "sausage" or "ham"
Coffee or tea with milk, nondairy creamer, and/or
sweetener of your choice if desired

Vegetarian Risk-Reducing Lunch

Tossed Green Salad (page 372) with
dressing of your choice
Vegetarian Marinated "Burgers" (page 408)
Coleslaw (no sugar)
Dill pickle, olives
Tea or coffee (with no sugar), diet soda, or carbonated water

Vegetarian Essential Balance Dinner

Pumpkin Soup (page 437)
Hungarian Beet Salad (page 430)
Tofu stir-fry
Dark pumpernickel bread with spread of your choice
Steamed asparagus
Chocolate Rugelach (page 480) and fruit of your choice
Any beverage(s) of your choice

Vegetarian Snacks (if desired)

Beginner's Program: A balance of Risk-Reducing Foods alone
or in combination with Essential Balance Foods
Intermediate Program: A healthy choice of
Risk-Reducing Foods only

Low-fat alternatives may be substituted.

Vegetarian Beginner's and Intermediate Programs

DAY SIX

Vegetarian Essential Balance Breakfast
Fruit or juice of your choice
Breakfast Pancakes (page 353)
with real fruit topping
Coffee or tea with milk, nondairy creamer, and/or
sweetener of your choice if desired

Vegetarian Risk-Reducing Lunch
Tossed Green Salad (page 372) with
dressing of your choice
Fresh Seafood Salad (page 370)
Tea or coffee (with no sugar), diet soda, or carbonated water

Vegetarian Essential Balance Dinner
Mixed finger salad with dressing of your choice
Cream of Cauliflower Soup (page 436)
German Potato Salad (page 426)
Pacific Island Vegetarian "Chicken" (page 495)
Buttered noodles*
Mixed vegetables
Rye rolls
Apple Cobbler (page 477)
Any beverage(s) of your choice

Vegetarian Snacks (if desired)
Beginner's Program: A balance of Risk-Reducing Foods alone
or in combination with Essential Balance Foods
Intermediate Program: A healthy choice of
Risk-Reducing Foods only

---

*Low-fat alternatives may be substituted.

Vegetarian Beginner's and Intermediate Programs

DAY SEVEN

Vegetarian Essential Balance Breakfast
Hot or cold cereal
Regular or low-fat milk or nondairy creamer
Fruit of your choice
Coffee or tea with milk, nondairy creamer, and/or
sweetener of your choice if desired

Vegetarian Risk-Reducing Lunch
Spinach Salad (page 372)
Cauliflower Cheese Casserole with Sour Cream (page 411)
Tea or coffee (with no sugar), diet soda, or carbonated water

Vegetarian Essential Balance Dinner
French Onion Soup (page 438)
Garden Salad (page 427) with Mustard Vinaigrette (page 427)
Fettuccine with Avocados and Vegetarian "Sausage" (page 493)
Garlic stir-fried green beans
Sesame bread sticks
Lemon-Lime Meringue Pie (page 481)
or fruit of your choice
Any beverage(s) of your choice

Vegetarian Snacks (if desired)
Beginner's Program: A Balance of Risk-Reducing Foods alone
or in combination with Essential Balance Foods
Intermediate Program: A healthy choice of
Risk-Reducing Foods only

Low-fat alternatives may be substituted.

Advanced Program
DAY ONE

Risk-Reducing Breakfast
Scrambled eggs (or egg substitute)
Sausage or bacon (or low-fat meat substitute)
Coffee or tea

Risk-Reducing Lunch
Cream of Broccoli Soup (page 376)
Chef's Salad (page 368) with dressing of your choice
Tea or coffee (with no sugar), diet soda,
or carbonated water

Essential Balance Dinner
Zucchini Bisque (page 442)
or Shrimp with Herb Sauce (page 416)
Garden Salad (page 427) with
Mustard Vinaigrette (page 427)
Sweet and Pungent Pork (page 450)
Crescent rolls
Wild rice
Steamed asparagus
Scottish Pecan Shortbread (page 487) with
ice cream,* ice milk,* or sherbet*
or fruit of your choice
Any beverage(s) of your choice

Snacks (if desired)
A healthy choice of Risk-Reducing Foods only

*Low-fat alternatives may be substituted.

Advanced Program
DAY TWO

Risk-Reducing Breakfast
Breakfast Crepes* (page 351)
Coffee or tea

Risk-Reducing Lunch
Shrimp Soup (page 380)
Spinach Salad (page 372)
Broiled, baked, roasted, or stir-fried chicken
Mixed vegetable stir-fry (cauliflower, mushrooms,
celery, and green pepper)
Tea or coffee (with no sugar), diet soda, or carbonated water

Essential Balance Dinner
Barbecued Spare Ribs—Chinese Style (page 417)
or Cream of Avocado Soup** (page 442)
Green-Goddess Salad (page 428)
Batter Fried Shrimp** (page 471)
Garlic sesame crisp bread
Baked potato with toppings of your choice**
Green beans amandine
Pound Cake (page 487) with strawberries and whipped cream**
Any beverage(s) of your choice

Snacks (if desired)
A healthy choice of Risk-Reducing Foods only

---

*This is a specially designed Risk-Reducing recipe. *Do not* substitute regular varieties of this food in place of this recipe during Risk-Reducing breakfasts.
**Low-fat alternatives may be substituted.

Advanced Program
DAY THREE

Risk-Reducing Breakfast
Cheese and mushroom omelet (or egg substitute)
Coffee or tea

Risk-Reducing Lunch
Cool Cucumber Appetizer (page 358)
Asparagus Ham Delight (page 385)
Tea or coffee (with no sugar), diet soda,
or carbonated water

Essential Balance Dinner
Minestrone Soup (page 441)
Kidney Bean Salad (page 429) or salad of your choice
Golden-Fried Chicken* (page 463) and thick french fries*
Corn bread
Coleslaw
Steamed greens
Chocolate Chip Coffee Cake (page 486)
Fruit of your choice
Any beverage(s) of your choice

Snacks (if desired)
A healthy choice of Risk-Reducing Foods only

*Low-fat alternatives may be substituted.

Advanced Program

DAY FOUR

Risk-Reducing Breakfast
Breakfast Soufflé* (page 350)
Coffee or tea

Risk-Reducing Lunch
Tossed Green Salad (page 372) with
dressing of your choice
Sole Delight (page 395)
Garlic stir-fried green beans
Tea or coffee (with no sugar), diet soda,
or carbonated water

Essential Balance Dinner
Cream of Asparagus Soup (page 440)
Italian Salad (page 429)
Veal with Peppers (page 456)
Italian bread with butter or margarine
Sautéed spinach
Pecan Pie (page 485)
Fruit of your choice
Any beverage(s) of your choice

Snacks (if desired)
A healthy choice of Risk-Reducing Foods only

---

*This is a specially designed Risk-Reducing recipe. *Do not* substitute regular varieties of this food in place of this recipe during Risk-Reducing breakfasts.
Low-fat alternatives may be substituted.

Advanced Program

DAY FIVE

Risk-Reducing Breakfast
Ham and cheese omelet (or egg substitute)
Coffee or tea or diet soda

Risk-Reducing Lunch
Any mixed green salad with dressing of your choice
Pork Tenderloin with Mushrooms, Green Peppers,
and Olives (page 390)
Garlic and Lemon Green Beans (page 371)
Tea or coffee (with no sugar), diet soda,
or carbonated water

Essential Balance Dinner
Mushroom Delights (page 419)
Old-Fashioned Split-Pea Soup (page 440)
Baked Pork Chops and Apples (page 451)
Hot biscuits with butter or margarine
Steamed broccoli or asparagus
Crème Brûlée* (page 481)
Any beverage(s) of your choice

Snacks (if desired)
A healthy choice of Risk-Reducing Foods only

*Low-fat alternatives may be substituted.

Advanced Program

DAY SIX

Risk-Reducing Breakfast
Western omelet (or egg substitute)
Bacon or sausage (or low-fat meat substitute)
Coffee or tea

Risk-Reducing Lunch
Clam Soup (page 377)
Caesar Salad (page 365)
Broiled salisbury steak or turkey burger
Tea or coffee (with no sugar), diet soda,
or carbonated water

Essential Balance Dinner
Tuna and Cheese Canapes* (page 420)
Cream of Cauliflower Soup (page 436)
Breaded Fish Fillets (page 473) or broiled flounder
Dinner rolls with butter or margarine
Steamed mixed vegetables
Chocolate Rugelach (page 480) with
fruit of your choice
Any beverage(s) of your choice

Snacks (if desired)
A healthy choice of Risk-Reducing Foods only

*Low-fat alternatives may be substituted.

Advanced Program
DAY SEVEN

Risk-Reducing Breakfast
Breakfast Muffins* (page 352)
Coffee or tea

Risk-Reducing Lunch
Spinach Salad (page 372)
Baked Bluefish (page 394)
Tea or coffee (with no sugar), diet soda,
or carbonated water

Essential Balance Dinner
Spinach Raita (page 420)
or Pumpkin Soup (page 437)
Finger salad with dressing of your choice
Stuffed Chicken Breasts (page 466)
Baked new potatoes with parsley and butter or margarine
Green beans topped with cheese**
Apple Cream Pie** (page 479)
or fruit of your choice
Any beverage(s) of your choice

Snacks (if desired)
A healthy choice of Risk-Reducing Foods only

*This is a specially designed Risk-Reducing recipe. *Do not* substitute regular varieties of this food in place of this recipe during Risk-Reducing breakfasts.
**Low-fat alternatives may be substituted.

Advanced Program
DAY EIGHT

Risk-Reducing Breakfast
Mushroom omelet (or egg substitute)
Sausage or bacon (or low-fat meat substitute)
Coffee or tea

Risk-Reducing Lunch
Celery Stuffed with Tuna (page 358)
Broiled cheeseburger (beef or turkey), no bun
Tea or coffee (with no sugar), diet soda,
or carbonated water

Essential Balance Dinner
Shrimp with Herb Sauce (page 416)
or Corn Chowder (page 437)
Lamb Curry (page 461)
Saffron rice
Steamed green beans
Iced Lemon Soufflé (page 478) and cookies
or fruit of your choice
Any beverage(s) of your choice

Snacks (if desired)
A healthy choice of Risk-Reducing Foods only

Low-fat alternatives may be substituted.

Advanced Program
DAY NINE

Risk-Reducing Breakfast
Celery stuffed with cream cheese (regular or low-fat)
Poached or smoked salmon
¼ tomato, olives, radishes
Coffee or tea

Risk-Reducing Lunch
Tossed Green Salad (page 372) with
dressing of your choice
Beef and Celery Ragout (page 391)
Tea or coffee (with no sugar), diet soda,
or carbonated water

Essential Balance Dinner
Marinated Pork (page 421)
French Onion Soup (page 438)
Broiled Lobster Tails (page 471)
Baked potato or buttered rice
French bread
Sautéed green peppers with onions
Apple Cobbler (page 477)
Any beverage(s) of your choice

Snacks (if desired)
A healthy choice of Risk-Reducing Foods only

Low-fat alternatives may be substituted.

Advanced Program
DAY TEN

Risk-Reducing Breakfast
Breakfast Cinnamon Bread* (page 352)
Coffee or tea

Risk-Reducing Lunch
Tossed Green Salad (page 372) with
dressing of your choice
Italian Shrimp (page 398)
Tea or coffee (with no sugar), diet soda,
or carbonated water

Essential Balance Dinner
Spinach-Egg Pie (page 418)
or Cream of Asparagus Soup (page 440)
Yogurt Chicken Breasts (page 468)
Scalloped potatoes
Whole-grain bread with butter or margarine
Mixed steamed green vegetables
Fresh Pears in Wine (page 478)
Any beverage(s) of your choice

Snacks (if desired)
A healthy choice of Risk-Reducing Foods only

*This is a specially designed Risk-Reducing recipe. *Do not* substitute regular varieties of this food in place of this recipe during Risk-Reducing breakfasts.
Low-fat alternatives may be substituted.

Advanced Program
DAY ELEVEN

Risk-Reducing Breakfast
Crustless Breakfast Quiche* (page 354)
Coffee or tea

Risk-Reducing Lunch
Tossed Green Salad (page 372) with dressing of your choice
Broiled Swordfish (page 397) or Italian Shrimp (page 398)
Tea or coffee (with no sugar), diet soda,
or carbonated water

Essential Balance Dinner
Cream of Avocado Soup** (page 442)
Any mixed green salad with dressing of your choice
Beef-Vegetable Stew (page 447)
Coleslaw
Broccoli, bean, and mushroom medley
Homemade biscuits with butter or margarine
Lemon-Lime Meringue Pie (page 481)
or fruit of your choice
Any beverage(s) of your choice

Snacks (if desired)
A healthy choice of Risk-Reducing Foods only

*This is a specially designed Risk-Reducing recipe. *Do not* substitute regular varieties of this food in place of this recipe during Risk-Reducing breakfasts.
**Low-fat alternatives may be substituted.

Advanced Program
DAY TWELVE

Risk-Reducing Breakfast
Crustless Breakfast Quiche* (page 354)
Sliced cucumbers and celery
Coffee or tea

Risk-Reducing Lunch
Shrimp Cheese Asparagus Soup (page 381)
Roast Lamb with Herbs (page 389)
Finger salad (bite-size bits of raw cucumber, celery,
cauliflower, broccoli, mushrooms, radishes, etc.)
with dressing of your choice
Tea or coffee (with no sugar), diet soda,
or carbonated water

Essential Balance Dinner
California Avocado Halves (page 425)
or Minestrone Soup (page 441)
Any mixed green salad with dressing of your choice
Skewered Spiced Lamb (page 459)
Skewered new potatoes and chunks of vegetables
Rye bread with butter or margarine
Quick and Easy Mocha Pie** (page 482)
or fruit of your choice
Any beverage(s) of your choice

Snacks (if desired)
A healthy choice of Risk-Reducing Foods only

---

*This is a specially designed Risk-Reducing recipe. *Do not* substitute regular varieties of this food in place of this recipe during Risk-Reducing breakfasts.
**Low-fat alternatives may be substituted.

Advanced Program
DAY THIRTEEN

Risk-Reducing Breakfast
Breakfast Pancakes* (page 353)
Turkey sausage or turkey bacon
Coffee or tea

Risk-Reducing Lunch
Tossed Green Salad (page 372) with
dressing of your choice
Barbecued Lemon Chicken (page 392)
Tea or coffee (with no sugar), diet soda,
or carbonated water

Essential Balance Dinner
Swedish Meatballs (page 424)
or Zucchini Bisque (page 442)
Any mixed green salad with dressing of your choice
Shrimp in Wine Sauce (page 469)
Bread sticks or fresh, warm French bread
Green beans amandine
Rum Cake Delight (page 483)
or fruit of your choice
Any beverage(s) of your choice

Snacks (if desired)
A healthy choice of Risk-Reducing Foods only

*This is a specially designed Risk-Reducing recipe. *Do not* substitute regular varieties of this food in place of this recipe during Risk-Reducing breakfasts.
Low-fat alternatives may be substituted.

Advanced Program
DAY FOURTEEN

Risk-Reducing Breakfast
Ham and cheese omelet (or egg substitute)
Coffee or tea

Risk-Reducing Lunch
Garlic and Lemon Green Beans (page 371)
Fresh Seafood Salad (page 370)
Tea or coffee (with no sugar), diet soda,
or carbonated water

Essential Balance Dinner
Sesame noodles
or Cream of Cauliflower Soup (page 436)
Any mixed green salad with dressing of your choice
Beef-and-Potatoes Casserole (page 443)
Sautéed spinach or green vegetable of your choice
Chilled Cranberry Cake (page 484) with ice cream,*
ice milk,* or sherbet*
Any beverage(s) of your choice

Snacks (if desired)
A healthy choice of Risk-Reducing Foods only

*Low-fat alternatives may be substituted.

Vegetarian Advanced Program

DAY ONE

Vegetarian Risk-Reducing Breakfast
Eggs Mayonnaise* (page 425)
Coffee or tea

Vegetarian Risk-Reducing Lunch
Spinach Salad (page 372)
Asparagus and Egg Casserole (page 400)
Tea or coffee (with no sugar), diet soda,
or carbonated water

Vegetarian Essential Balance Dinner
Cream of Asparagus Soup (page 440)
Green-Goddess Salad (page 428)
Vegetarian "Beef" Casserole (page 488)
Wild rice
Whole-grain bread and butter or margarine
Green beans amandine
Cream Cheese Cake** (page 474)
or fruit of your choice
Any beverage(s) of your choice

Snacks (if desired)
A healthy choice of Risk-Reducing Foods only

*This is a specially designed Risk-Reducing recipe. *Do not* substitute regular varieties of this food in place of this recipe during Risk-Reducing breakfasts.
**Low-fat alternatives may be substituted.

Vegetarian Advanced Program
DAY TWO

Vegetarian Risk-Reducing Breakfast
Breakfast Soufflé* (page 350)
Coffee or tea

Vegetarian Risk-Reducing Lunch
Romaine Lettuce Soup (page 377)
Any mixed green salad with dressing of your choice
Vegetarian Parsley Butter "Burgers" (page 401)
Olives, celery, dill pickle, sugarless coleslaw
Tea or coffee (with no sugar), diet soda,
or carbonated water

Vegetarian Essential Balance Dinner
Cream of Avocado Soup** (page 442)
Garden Salad (page 427) with
Cucumber Yogurt Dressing (page 431)
Flounder with Wild Rice and Water Chestnuts (page 490)
Steamed broccoli
Fresh Pears in Wine (page 478)
Any beverage(s)

Snacks (if desired)
A healthy choice of Risk-Reducing Foods only

*This is a specially designed Risk-Reducing recipe. *Do not* substitute regular varieties of this food in place of this recipe during Risk-Reducing breakfasts.
**Low-fat alternatives may be substituted.

Vegetarian Advanced Program
DAY THREE

Vegetarian Risk-Reducing Breakfast
Breakfast Muffins* (page 352)
Coffee or tea

Vegetarian Risk-Reducing Lunch
Chef's Salad (use meat and/or dairy substitutes)
(page 368) with dressing of your choice
Vegetable stir-fry
Tea or coffee (with no sugar), diet soda,
or carbonated water

Vegetarian Essential Balance Dinner
Minestrone Soup (page 441)
Italian Salad (page 429)
Fried Lemon Vegetarian "Chicken" (page 489)
Fried brown rice with mushrooms
Whole-grain rolls with butter or margarine
Sautéed spinach
Banana Fritters** (page 475)
or fruit of your choice
Any beverage(s) of your choice

Snacks (if desired)
A healthy choice of Risk-Reducing Foods only

---

*This is a specially designed Risk-Reducing recipe. *Do not* substitute regular varieties of this food in place of this recipe during Risk-Reducing breakfasts.
**Low-fat alternatives may be substituted.

Vegetarian Advanced Program

DAY FOUR

Vegetarian Risk-Reducing Breakfast
Breakfast Crepes* (page 351)
Coffee or tea

Vegetarian Risk-Reducing Lunch
Tossed Green Salad (page 372) with
dressing of your choice
Vegetarian Oriental "Steak" Casserole (page 404)
Sliced cucumbers
Vegetable Joy (page 492)
Tea or coffee (with no sugar), diet soda,
or carbonated water

Vegetarian Essential Balance Dinner
Zucchini Bisque (page 442)
Kidney Bean Salad (page 429) or salad and
dressing of your choice
Seafood-Vegetable Delight (page 491)
Paprika baked new potatoes
Steamed parsley cauliflower
Apple Cream Pie** (page 479)
or fruit of your choice
Any beverage(s) of your choice

Snacks (if desired)
A healthy choice of Risk-Reducing Foods only

*This is a specially designed Risk-Reducing recipe. *Do not* substitute regular varieties of this food in place of this recipe during Risk-Reducing breakfasts.
**Low-fat alternatives may be substituted.

Vegetarian Advanced Program

DAY FIVE

Vegetarian Risk-Reducing Breakfast
Breakfast Cinnamon Bread* (page 352)
Coffee or tea

Vegetarian Risk-Reducing Lunch
Tossed Green Salad (page 372)
Vegetarian Marinated "Steaklets" (page 408)
Sautéed mushrooms and green peppers
Coffee or tea

Vegetarian Essential Balance Dinner
Pumpkin Soup (page 437)
Hungarian Beet Salad (page 430)
Vegetable Joy (page 492)
Tofu stir-fry
Dark pumpernickel bread with butter or margarine
Steamed asparagus
Chocolate Rugelach (page 480) and fruit of your choice
Any beverage(s) of your choice

Snacks (if desired)
A healthy choice of Risk-Reducing Foods only

---

*This is a specially designed Risk-Reducing recipe. *Do not* substitute regular varieties of this food in place of this recipe during Risk-Reducing breakfasts. Low-fat alternatives may be substituted.

Vegetarian Advanced Program
DAY SIX

Vegetarian Risk-Reducing Breakfast
Breakfast Pancakes* (page 353)
Coffee or tea

Vegetarian Risk-Reducing Lunch
Tossed Green Salad (page 372) with regular or
low-fat dressing
Fresh Seafood Salad (page 370)
Tea or coffee (with no sugar), diet soda,
or carbonated water

Vegetarian Essential Balance Dinner
Cream of Cauliflower Soup (page 436)
Mixed finger salad with dressing of your choice
German Potato Salad (page 426)
Pacific Island Vegetarian "Chicken" (page 495)
Buttered noodles**
Mixed vegetables
Rye rolls
Apple Cobbler (page 477)
Any beverage(s) of your choice

Snacks (if desired)
A healthy choice of Risk-Reducing Foods only

---

*This is a specially designed Risk-Reducing recipe. *Do not* substitute regular varieties of this food in place of this recipe during Risk-Reducing breakfasts.
**Low-fat alternatives may be substituted.

Vegetarian Advanced Program
DAY SEVEN

Vegetarian Risk-Reducing Breakfast
Crustless Breakfast Quiche* (page 354)
Coffee or tea

Vegetarian Risk-Reducing Lunch
Spinach Salad (page 372) with regular or
low-fat dressing
Cauliflower Cheese Casserole with Sour Cream** (page 411)
Tea or coffee (with no sugar), diet soda, or carbonated water

Vegetarian Essential Balance Dinner
French Onion Soup (page 438)
Garden Salad (page 427) with
Mustard Vinaigrette (page 427)
Fettuccine with Avocados and
Vegetarian "Sausage" (page 493)
Garlic stir-fried green beans
Sesame bread sticks
Lemon-Lime Meringue Pie (page 481)
or fruit of your choice
Any beverage(s) of your choice

Snacks (if desired)
A healthy choice of Risk-Reducing Foods only

---

*This is a specially designed Risk-Reducing recipe. *Do not* substitute regular varieties of this food in place of this recipe during Risk-Reducing breakfasts.
**Low-fat alternatives may be substituted.

Before incorporating any dietary guideline into your program, you should consult with your physician. Only your doctor can determine which recommendations are appropriate to you and your individual health needs.

HEALTH AGENCY RECOMMENDATIONS*

Health Agency Recommendation #1

Eat a variety of foods.

To Include Recommendation #1 in Your Program

Vary your Risk-Reducing Foods by choosing from an assortment of salad items, vegetables, proteins, and dairy items. For Essential Balance Foods, choose a variety of grains, starches, additional dairy items, fruit, juices, and desserts.

Health Agency Recommendation #2

Reduce consumption of fat (especially saturated fat) and cholesterol.

To Include Recommendation #2 in Your Program

When appropriate, choose low-fat or skim milk; low-fat or low-cholesterol cheeses, sour cream, and cream cheese; and whipped cream substitutes. Replace eggs with egg substitutes and use low-cholesterol margarine and cooking sprays in place of butter. Choose very lean cuts of meat, trimmed of all fat. Select fish or chicken or turkey without skin. Substitute turkey for beef and pork in burgers and sausage. Use low-cholesterol mayonnaise. When you use oil, choose olive oil instead of heavy tropical or other saturated oils.

For additional information on the impact of dietary fat on your Profactor-H risk, see chapter 7, "Fats and Fiber: Fears, Facts, and Fallacies."

For comparisons of saturated, monounsaturated, and polyunsaturated fats, see chapter 20, "Personalizing Your Program."

*Adapted from *The Surgeon General's Report on Nutrition and Health*; the U. S. Department of Agriculture and the Department of Health and Human Services' *Report on Dietary Guidelines for Americans*; the American Heart Association's diet, *Eating Plan for Healthy Americans*; and the American Cancer Society's *Eat to Live*.

Health Agency Recommendation #3

Add foods rich in vitamins A and C.

To Include Recommendation #3 in Your Program

For the appropriate meals, choose citrus fruits and juices, strawberries, and cantaloupe, as well as dark green leafy vegetables and tomatoes.

Include cruciferous vegetables (those from the cabbage family). Select foods such as bok choy, broccoli, brussels sprouts, cabbage, cauliflower, collards, kale, kohlrabi, mustard greens, rutabagas, turnips, and their greens.

Health Agency Recommendation #4

Achieve and maintain a desirable body weight.

To Include Recommendation #4 in Your Program

By selecting Nutrition and Activity Options in the Profactor-H Program, you will be well on your way to your ideal weight level, and in so doing, reducing many of the health risks often associated with excess weight.

Health Agency Recommendation #5

Increase consumption of complex carbohydrates and fiber by choosing whole-grain foods and cereal products, vegetables, and fruits. Avoid too much sugar.

To Incorporate Recommendation #5 in Your Program

Select Essential Balance Foods that include whole-grain breads, cereal products, rice, pasta, fruits, potatoes, and other vegetables, and include in your Risk-Reducing Foods lots of fresh vegetables. Keep your intake of sugar low by choosing desserts made of complex carbohydrates such as whole-grain breads or popcorn or low-fat whole-grain snacks rather than candy.

Health Agency Recommendation #6

Limit the amount of salt-cured, smoked, and nitrate-cured foods.

To Include Recommendation #6 in Your Program

Choose ham, bacon, hot dogs, sausages, pastrami, corned beef, salami, and other cold cuts only on rare occasions.

Health Agency Recommendation #7

Reduce intake of sodium by choosing foods relatively low in sodium and by limiting the amount of salt added in food preparation and at the table.

To Include Recommendation #7 in Your Program

At all meals, choose low-salt varieties of canned and packaged foods, as well as low-salt cheeses and other dairy products. Limit the amount of salt you add while cooking or at the table. At restaurants, ask for low-salt alternatives. Avoid smoked and salted products.

Health Agency Recommendation #8

If you drink alcoholic beverages, do so in moderation.

To Include Recommendation #8 in Your Program

Several of your Profactor-H Program Options will ask you to at times limit, reduce, or eliminate alcoholic beverages. If you do not select these Options, you may include Recommendation #8 by keeping amounts of alcoholic beverages at moderate levels.

Health Agency Recommendation #9

Women should increase consumption of foods high in calcium, including low-fat dairy products. Women of childbearing age should consume foods that are good sources of iron.

To Include Recommendation #9 in Your Program

Include calcium-rich canned fish (such as mackerel, salmon, sardines, and water-packed tuna), as well as spinach and greens, oysters, tofu, and low-fat cheese, along with iron-rich foods such as lamb, chicken, turkey, green beans, and mushrooms, at any meal. Essential Balance Foods may include iron-rich popcorn, potatoes, pasta, rice, and fresh and dried fruit, especially raisins.

CHAPTER 24

Risk-Reducing Recipes

Cooking is not a requirement of the Profactor-H Program; you are free to prepare quick meals or to eat as many of your meals as you like at restaurants. The Risk-Reducing recipes that follow are offered solely as an option for your use and enjoyment.

Just remember, whether you are using these recipes or enjoying your old favorites at home or out, Risk-Reducing Meals should contain *only* foods that are included in the Risk-Reducing Foods chart on pages 220 to 221. (More about your Essential Balance Meals in the chapter that follows.)

> Cooking is *never* a requirement of the Profactor-H Program. If you prefer, you are free to prepare quick meals of your choosing or to eat your meals at restaurants.

The Risk-Reducing Meal recipes that we have included are only a few examples of the many foods that you can include in your Risk-Reducing Meals. You will find an even wider variety of Risk-Reducing Foods listed in chapter 16. For some examples of daily meal plans, turn to chapter 23, "Sample Daily Meal Plans."

Risk-Reducing Meal recipes are designed, primarily, to provide you with exciting and satisfying ideas for your Risk-Reducing Meals. If you like, you can, in addition, combine these recipes with some Essential Balance Foods and enjoy them as part of your Essential Balance Meals, as well.

In general, Risk-Reducing Meals should *not* include any foods that are high in carbohydrates (such as starches, snack foods, fruit, and sweets—you can save them for Essential Balance Meals). For your Risk-Reducing Meals, foods should be baked, boiled, broiled, poached, roasted, sautéed, or stir-fried. Never include breading or batter of any kind in your Risk-Reducing Meals.

Adjust recipes to fit the number of servings you prefer. If you are eating alone, for example, you may wish to reduce a recipe by half or three quarters, or you may choose to make the full recipe and refrigerate or freeze the remainder for another Risk-Reducing Meal. You can also add some Essential Balance Foods to a Risk-Reducing Meal leftover to produce a future Essential Balance Meal.

The advent of the microwave has been a boon to all of us who enjoy an instant pre-frozen homemade meal for lunch or dinner, at home or at work, at a moment's notice. Lunches no longer have to be the same old cold meals; they can warm, nourish, and rejuvenate you for the rest of the day to come.

To enjoy homemade frozen meals, simply make several portions of a recipe at a time and freeze them in single-serving sealable bags. Then you can be sure the food you need and enjoy is always there when you want it. It takes very little time and effort to take good care of yourself. Do it.

Individual, Low-Fat, and Low-Salt Choices

For your information, in all of our recipes we have included low-fat and low-salt alternatives. For additional details on low-fat, low-cholesterol, and low-salt alternatives, see "Health Agency Recommendations," page 345. Dietary fat recommendations should always be discussed with your physician.

Some of the recipes that follow include artificial sweeteners as an ingredient. If you choose to, or have been told to, avoid artificial sweeteners, or if you have selected the Bonus Option that calls for you to refrain from all artificial sweeteners, do not select these recipes.

Our rewarding Risk-Reducing Meal recipes have been organized for your convenience:

Risk-Reducing Meals

To complement your Risk-Reducing Meals, Essential Balance Meal recipes follow in chapter 25.

Risk-Reducing Meals: Breakfasts

BREAKFAST SOUFFLÉ   *Serves 4*

This breakfast delight is light, airy, and delicious.

1 teaspoon butter (or low-fat substitute)	2 cups cottage cheese (regular or low-fat)
4 egg whites	2 egg yolks
1 teaspoon cream of tartar	½ package artificial sweetener

Preheat oven to 300°F.
Butter 9-inch round baking pan.

Beat egg whites until frothy but not stiff. Add cream of tartar and continue to beat until you can form high peaks.

In a medium bowl, combine cottage cheese, egg yolks, and sweetener and mix well. Gently fold in egg whites.

Pour mixture into baking pan and place into oven. Bake for 25–30 minutes. Turn up heat to broil and bake for 2–3 minutes. Be careful not to burn soufflé.

BREAKFAST CREPES   *Serves 4–6*

This unusually tasty breakfast treat will quickly disappear from the serving plate. Serve it hot and keep it coming.

6 egg whites	1 package artificial sweetener
1 teaspoon cream of tartar	1 tablespoon butter
½ cup cottage cheese	(or low-fat substitute)
(regular or low-fat)	¼ cup sour cream
½ teaspoon vanilla extract	(or low-fat substitute)

In a mixing bowl, combine egg whites and cream of tartar. Beat until stiff and set aside.

In another bowl, combine cottage cheese, vanilla extract, and sweetener. Mix well.

Add cottage cheese mixture to bowl containing beaten egg whites and gently fold into egg whites.

Add butter to small frying pan over moderate heat and melt.

Add 2 tablespoons of batter to pan and spread until it covers entire bottom of pan (forming a 4-inch-diameter crepe). Cook over moderate heat until crepe sets and appears brown on bottom.

Turn and brown on other side.

Repeat until all of the batter is used.

Spread 1 teaspoon sour cream on each crepe, roll into cylinder, and serve.

BREAKFAST MUFFINS   *Serves 4–6*

A light and airy muffin to help you start the day without feeling "heavy."

½ tablespoon sweet butter
  (or low-fat substitute)
4 eggs
½ teaspoon cream of
  tartar

¼ cup cottage cheese
  (regular or low-fat)
2 tablespoons soy flour
  (found in health food stores)
1 package artificial sweetener

Preheat oven to 300°F.

Coat muffin cups with room-temperature butter.

Separate egg whites and egg yolks.

Beat egg whites until frothy. Add cream of tartar and continue to beat until stiff peaks form.

In a medium bowl, combine egg yolks, cottage cheese, soy flour, and sweetener, and mix well.

Add flour mixture to beaten egg whites and fold in gently.

Fill each muffin cup two thirds full with batter.

Bake muffins until golden brown and they spring back when touched with the back of a fork (25–30 minutes).

Remove and serve.

BREAKFAST CINNAMON BREAD   *Serves 4–6*

A light and unusually tasty bread that is low in carbohydrates and fat and high in protein.

½ teaspoon butter
  (or low-fat substitute)
3 eggs
½ teaspoon cream of tartar
¼ cup cottage cheese
  (regular or low-fat)

½ teaspoon powdered
  cinnamon
2 tablespoons soy flour
  (found in health food stores)
1 package artificial sweetener

Preheat oven to 300°F.

Butter the sides and bottom of a 4-×-7-inch loaf pan.

Beat egg whites until frothy. Add cream of tartar and continue to beat until stiff but moist peaks form.

In a medium bowl, combine egg yolks, cottage cheese, cinnamon, soy flour, and sweetener. Mix well but do not overmix.

Add flour mixture to beaten egg whites and fold in gently.

Pour mixture into prepared pan and bake until loaf is brown and springs back when touched with the back of a fork (40–45 minutes).

BREAKFAST PANCAKES   *Serves 2–4*

An unusually tasty breakfast dish that is low in carbohydrates and fat and high in protein.

2 eggs
½ teaspoon cream of
   tartar
1 cup cottage cheese
   (regular or low-fat)

1 tablespoon soy flour
   (found in health food stores)
½ package artificial sweetener
1 teaspoon butter
   (or low-fat substitute)

Separate egg whites and yolks. Beat whites until frothy. Add cream of tartar and continue to beat until stiff, dry peaks form.

In a medium bowl, combine egg yolk, cottage cheese, soy flour, and sweetener. Mix well.

Place a square griddle over moderate to high heat, and melt butter. Do not burn.

Pour enough batter to form four 3-inch pancakes on hot griddle. Cook until brown on one side (about 2 minutes). Turn and brown on other side.

Stack and serve hot.

CRUSTLESS BREAKFAST QUICHE   *Serves 5–6*

A tasty breakfast dish that can be made ahead of time and served hot or cold.

1 teaspoon butter (or low-fat substitute)	2 teaspoons chopped onion or scallion
2 cups light cream (or milk or low-fat substitute)	¾ teaspoon paprika
1 cup grated cheese (cheddar, Gruyère, Parmesan, or Swiss, regular or low-fat varieties)	¼ teaspoon garlic powder
	4 eggs
	Salt
2 teaspoons dried sweet basil	Ground black pepper

Preheat oven to 325°F.

Butter bottom and sides of a 9-inch pie pan.

Add cream to a medium saucepan and heat until scalded. Reduce heat and stir in grated cheese.

When cheese is melted, add basil, onion, paprika, and garlic powder.

Remove from heat and cool for 5 minutes. Then add one egg at a time and mix in thoroughly until all eggs are used. Salt and pepper to taste and mix well.

Pour mixture into pie pan, place in oven, and bake until custard is set (45–50 minutes).

Serve hot or cold.

Risk-Reducing Meals:
Appetizers and Snacks

BROCCOLI-SCALLION DIP *Serves 6*

This creamy dip will get your party off on the right foot. Serve this dip in a bowl and surround with crisp, fresh vegetables such as cauliflower, celery, green peppers, green beans, and raw mushrooms.

2 medium stalks fresh broccoli
1 cup cottage cheese
(regular or low-fat)
1 tablespoon white or wine
vinegar
½ cup plain sour cream
(or low-fat substitute)

¼ cup chopped scallion
1 teaspoon salt
(or salt substitute)
½ teaspoon garlic powder
Coarsely ground black
pepper

Rinse broccoli and cut stems about three inches below the top of the stalk, discarding bottoms. Coarsely chop and set aside.

In a blender or food processor, blend cottage cheese with vinegar. Add broccoli, sour cream, scallion, salt, garlic powder, and pepper to taste; blend until mixed.

Cover and chill overnight.

SHRIMP WITH LEMON AND
BASIL SAUCE
Serves 6

A lemony treat that is always a hit.

½ cup sweet butter
(or low-fat substitute)
2 pounds raw shrimp, shelled
and deveined
1 tablespoon chopped fresh
basil or 2 teaspoons dried
sweet basil

Juice of 1 lemon
½ teaspoon low-salt Teriyaki
sauce
Salt (or salt substitute)
Ground black pepper
Toothpicks
Lettuce leaves

In a skillet, melt butter. Add shrimp and cook, stirring occasionally, until shrimp are red in color and thoroughly cooked, about 3–4 minutes.

Combine basil, lemon juice, and Teriyaki sauce and sprinkle on hot shrimp. Salt and pepper (to taste). Let sit for 2 minutes.

Place a toothpick through each shrimp and serve on a bed of lettuce.

BACON-WRAPPED SCALLOPS
Serves 8–10

This unusually tasty appetizer will quickly disappear from the serving plate. Serve it hot and keep it coming.

¼ cup Teriyaki sauce
(or low-salt substitute)
¼ cup water
20 medium scallops

10 strips bacon
(or low-fat substitute)
20 toothpicks
Paprika

Preheat oven to 400°F. In a small bowl, combine Teriyaki and water. Dip each scallop into mixture and allow to sit on a plate while you cut each bacon strip in half crosswise.

Cook bacon strips in a skillet until half done. Drain on paper towel and allow to cool for 3 minutes. Wrap a half slice of bacon around each scallop and secure each with a toothpick.

Line a shallow baking pan with aluminum foil, distribute scallops evenly on pan, sprinkle with a dash of paprika, and bake in oven until the bacon is crisp (about 5 minutes). Drain on paper towel and cool slightly before serving. This appetizer may be microwaved if you prefer.

GREEK MUSHROOMS   Serves 6

Add an international flavor to your meal. Start your guests off with this tasty surprise.

1 ½ pounds small mushrooms
2 cups water
1 cup virgin olive oil
Juice of 1 lemon
1 tablespoon white vinegar
1 stalk celery
1 clove garlic, peeled and quartered
1 teaspoon fresh or dried basil

½ teaspoon dried thyme
1 bay leaf
10 black peppercorns
½ teaspoon salt (or salt substitute)
Toothpicks
Lettuce leaves

Remove mushroom stalks and discard. Wash the caps and dry with paper towel.

Combine all ingredients except toothpicks and lettuce leaves in large saucepan and bring to a boil. Turn down heat and simmer for 5 minutes, occasionally stirring mixture.

Pour into bowl and marinate overnight in refrigerator.

Place a toothpick through each mushroom and serve them on a bed of lettuce.

COOL CUCUMBER APPETIZER   *Serves 6*

A refreshing taste tickler for the wonderful meal to follow.

4 medium cucumbers, peeled
  and sliced
Salt (or salt substitute)
6 scallions, chopped fine
Ground black pepper
½ teaspoon fresh or chopped
  basil

⅓ teaspoon chili powder
¼ teaspoon powdered
  cloves
1½ cups sour cream
  (or low-fat substitute)

Lightly salt cucumber slices and let stand 20 minutes. Place double layer of paper towel on plate, and lay slices on paper towel. Press out excess moisture from slices by covering with another plate and topping with a heavy object such as a large book or an iron.

Add scallions, pepper (to taste), basil, chili powder, and powdered cloves to the sour cream. Blend well. Sprinkle chili on both sauce and cucumbers as well. Serve cucumbers in individual dishes, topped with sour cream sauce.

CELERY STUFFED WITH TUNA   *Serves 6*

A real delight.

12 stalks celery
1 cup grated cheddar cheese
  (regular or low-fat)
1 can (6½ ounces) tuna fish
1 hard-boiled egg, chopped

2 tablespoons mayonnaise
  (regular or low-fat)
2 tablespoons dry white
  vermouth
Ground black pepper

Trim leaves and wash celery stalks, setting them aside to drain.

Combine remaining ingredients and blend well. Fill celery stalks with mixture and serve.

HUNGARIAN CHEESE
Serves 6–8

A refreshing snack or luncheon starter.

1 cup cottage cheese
(regular or low-fat)
½ cup mayonnaise
(regular or low-fat)
1 tablespoon poppy seeds
(caraway seeds may be
substituted)

1 tablespoon capers,
minced
1 tablespoon minced chives
1 tablespoon dry mustard
1 sardine, chopped
Paprika
Lettuce leaves

Put cheese through fine sieve or ricer.

Combine mayonnaise, poppy seeds, capers, chives, mustard, and sardine, and gradually blend into cottage cheese.

Form mixture into a mound, sprinkle with paprika, place on a bed of lettuce, and garnish with salad greens.

DEVILED EGGS
Serves 6

This little treat can be a snack or an appetizer that will satisfy.

12 eggs
¼ cup mayonnaise
(regular or low-fat)
2 tablespoons chopped
green pepper

2 tablespoons mild
prepared mustard
Paprika
Lettuce leaves

Hard-boil eggs (10 minutes in boiling water), remove shells, and slice in half lengthwise.

Scoop out yolks and mash them. In a mixing bowl, combine them with mayonnaise, green pepper, and mustard.

When blended thoroughly, spoon the mixture into the egg white halves.

Sprinkle with paprika and serve on a bed of lettuce.

SEA CLAM DIP   *Serves 6*

A quick and easy preparation. Serve this dip in a bowl and surround with crisp, fresh vegetables such as cauliflower, celery, green peppers, green beans, and raw mushrooms.

2 cans (7½ ounces each)
  minced clams, drained
2 cups sour cream
  (or low-fat substitute)
2 tablespoons chopped parsley
¼ teaspoon garlic powder
1 teaspoon Teriyaki sauce
  (or low-salt substitute)

2 tablespoons lemon juice
½ tablespoon salt
  (or salt substitute)
1 teaspoon hot sauce, or to
  taste
Paprika
Parsley sprigs

Blend drained clams, sour cream, chopped parsley, garlic powder, Teriyaki sauce, lemon juice, salt, and hot sauce.

Place in serving bowl, sprinkle lightly with paprika, and garnish with parsley sprigs.

STUFFED MUSHROOMS   *Serves 5–8*

A delectable appetizer or snack that can be prepared the day before.

15 medium-size mushrooms
2 tablespoons butter
  (or low-fat substitute)
4 ounces cream cheese
  (or low-fat substitute)
1 tablespoon heavy cream
  (or milk)
1 teaspoon Teriyaki sauce
  (or low-salt substitute)

1 teaspoon minced chives
1 teaspoon lemon juice
⅛ teaspoon salt
  (or salt substitute)
Ground black pepper
Paprika
Parsley sprigs

Preheat oven to 350°F. Remove mushroom stems and discard; wash caps and dry.

Put butter in a shallow baking pan that is big enough to hold all the mushroom caps in one layer, and place in oven to melt butter.

Combine cream cheese, cream, Teriyaki sauce, chives, lemon juice, salt, and pepper to taste.

Using a fork, mix until smooth.

Spoon generous amounts of mixture into each inverted mushroom cap and sprinkle lightly with paprika.

Place caps into the baking pan with butter and return to oven to bake for 10–15 minutes.

Place on serving tray, garnish with parsley, and set out toothpicks.

This recipe may be microwaved if you prefer.

LIVER MUSHROOMS
Serves 6

An unusual twist on a delicious appetizer or snack that can be prepared the day before.

1 pound large mushrooms	1 small package (3 ounces) cream cheese (or low-fat substitute), at room temperature
5 tablespoons butter (or low-fat substitute)	
½ pound chicken livers	¼ teaspoon dried sweet basil
1 tablespoon minced onion	Salt
	Ground black pepper
	Lettuce leaves

Wash mushrooms and dry well. Remove mushroom stems and chop them up. Place 3 tablespoons of butter in a skillet and heat.

Add washed mushroom caps and sauté (turning frequently) 5 minutes. Remove and set aside.

Melt remaining butter in the heated skillet, add chopped mushroom stems, onion, and livers, and sauté until the livers are browned.

Chop livers finely and set aside to cool.

Combine cream cheese, liver mixture, basil, and salt and pepper to taste.

Spoon the mixture into the mushroom caps, placing them on a bed of lettuce, and chill well before serving.

CREAM CHEESE AND HERBS   *Serves 6–8*

A tasty appetizer or snack that can be prepared beforehand.

2 cloves garlic, minced
1 tablespoon minced onion
¼ teaspoon salt
(or salt substitute)
Dry mustard
1 large package (8 ounces)
cream cheese (or low-fat
substitute)
½ cup mayonnaise
(regular or low-fat)

2 tablespoons lemon juice
1 tablespoon chopped pitted
green olives
1 tablespoon chopped pitted
black olives
½ teaspoon dried sweet basil
½ teaspoon Teriyaki sauce
(or low-salt substitute)
Chopped chives
(or scallions, or parsley)

In a medium mixing bowl, blend garlic, onion, and salt. Add dry mustard to taste.

Add cream cheese and mix until smooth.

Add mayonnaise, lemon juice, olives (green and black), basil, and Teriyaki sauce, and blend well.

Place in serving bowl, sprinkle with chopped chives, and chill. Serve with raw sliced or cut-up vegetables such as cauliflower or broccoli florets, celery stalks, green pepper slices, and fennel.

Risk-Reducing Meals: Salads, Dressings, and Vegetables

BASIL CHICKEN SALAD
Serves 6

This easy-to-make salad favorite is nice for leftover chicken

3 cups cooked, cubed chicken	1 cup sour cream (or low-fat substitute)
1½ cup diced celery	1½ cups chopped fresh basil
¼ cup chopped chives or scallion	Ground black pepper
	Salt (or salt substitute)

In a large bowl, combine chicken, celery, chives, sour cream, and basil; mix lightly with a fork.

Cover and refrigerate for at least 2 hours.

Just before serving, add pepper and salt to taste.

CREAMY HERBAL DRESSING
Makes about 1 cup

This light, creamy dressing will perk up any kind of salad.

½ cup cottage cheese (regular or low-fat)	¼ teaspoon dried tarragon
½ cup sour cream (or low-fat substitute)	½ tablespoon dried sweet basil
½ teaspoon spicy prepared mustard	Salt (or salt substitute) Ground black pepper

In blender, food processor, or mixing bowl, process cottage cheese until smooth.

Add sour cream, mustard, tarragon, and basil.

Salt and pepper to taste.

Refrigerate overnight.

CLASSIC ITALIAN MOZZARELLA SALAD

Serves 6

This delightfully refreshing salad is fun to make and eat. You can vary the recipe to taste.

1 cup diced celery	1 tablespoon mayonnaise
1 cup diced green peppers	(regular or low-fat)
1 cup diced mozzarella	¼ teaspoon dried thyme
3 tablespoons cider vinegar	¼ teaspoon dried sweet
2 tablespoons olive oil or	basil
vegetable oil	¼ teaspoon dried oregano
2 tablespoons lemon juice	Ground black pepper

In large salad bowl, combine celery, peppers, and mozzarella; set aside.

In small bowl, combine vinegar, olive oil, lemon juice, mayonnaise, thyme, basil, and oregano; mix thoroughly.

Pour mixture over salad and toss until mixture is uniformly distributed. Pepper to taste.

MUSTARD-GARLIC VINAIGRETTE

Makes about 1 cup

A tangy addition to any salad.

2 cloves garlic, minced	1 teaspoon grated imported
2 teaspoons Dijon mustard	Swiss cheese
2 tablespoons lemon juice	(or any other regular
⅓ cup water	or low-fat cheese)
¼ cup vegetable oil	Ground black pepper
(or walnut oil)	

In blender, food processor, or mixing bowl, combine garlic, mustard, lemon juice, and water until well mixed.
Continue mixing while oil is gradually added.
Add cheese and ground pepper to taste.
Let sit for at least 2 minutes before adding to salad.

CAESAR SALAD
Serves 6

One of the all-time favorite salads with a twist. It can be revisited again and again.

Salt (or salt substitute)
1 clove garlic, peeled and halved
1 teaspoon dry mustard
2 tablespoons lemon juice
Hot sauce
3 tablespoons olive oil

3 heads Boston lettuce
1 tablespoon grated Swiss cheese (regular or low-fat)
1 can (2 ounces) anchovies, drained
1 egg boiled 60 seconds (or egg substitute)

Sprinkle salt on bottom of large wooden bowl and generously rub bottom and sides of bowl with garlic clove.

Add mustard, lemon juice, and hot sauce (to taste) and stir with wooden spoon until salt dissolves.

Rinse lettuce until all traces of sand are removed. Dry with paper towel and tear lettuce into bite-size pieces; place in bowl.

Sprinkle with grated Swiss cheese; add anchovies; break egg (or egg substitute) and empty contents over salad.

Thoroughly mix by tossing gently until ingredients are distributed uniformly.

GREEN SALSA   *Makes about 1 cup*

Tangy but not hot.

3 tablespoons vinegar
½ cup olive oil
1 teaspoon spicy mustard
1 tablespoon chopped parsley
1 tablespoon chopped scallion

1 tablespoon chopped spinach
1 tablespoon chopped
watercress
1 medium green pepper, finely
chopped

In bowl, combine all ingredients and mix well. Refrigerate until thoroughly chilled.

GARLIC DRESSING   *Makes about 1 cup*

A salad delight.

½ teaspoon mild dry mustard
(or spicy, if you wish)
Salt (or salt substitute)
Coarsely ground black
pepper

2 cloves garlic, minced finely
1 tablespoon tarragon
vinegar
3 tablespoons lemon juice
1 cup olive oil

In a bowl or large jar, combine and mix mustard, and salt and black pepper to taste.

Add the remaining ingredients to the mixture and stir until thoroughly mixed.

Let sit for an hour and it is ready to use.

GREEN GARDEN MAYONNAISE

Makes about 2 cups

A tantalizing and unusual dressing

2 stalks celery and leaves
10 spinach leaves
10 scallions, chopped fine
2 tablespoons dried sweet
  basil

1 teaspoon lemon juice
1 cup mayonnaise
  (regular or low-fat)

In blender or food processor, chop celery, spinach, and scallions. Add basil, lemon juice, and mayonnaise. Blend well. Use on vegetable, fish, or chicken salads.

CUCUMBER SALAD

Serves 6

A quick and easy salad that people always find a delightful change of pace.

1 cup sour cream
  (or low-fat substitute)
1 teaspoon chopped chives
½ teaspoon salt
  (or salt substitute)
  Ground black pepper

2 tablespoons wine vinegar
2 large cucumbers, peeled and
  sliced thinly
6 large lettuce leaves
  (or cabbage leaves)
  Paprika

Mix sour cream, chives, salt, pepper (to taste), and vinegar.
Add cucumber slices and toss lightly.
Serve on lettuce or cabbage leaves.
Garnish with paprika.

SHRIMP SALAD AND DRESSING   *Serves 4*

Take advantage of the fruits of the sea to enjoy a satisfying salad for any meal of the day.

6 tablespoons virgin olive oil
1 tablespoon lemon juice
1 teaspoon Dijon mustard
¼ teaspoon salt
  (or salt substitute)
  Ground black pepper
1 teaspoon dried sweet
  basil

16 medium shrimp, peeled and
  deveined
½ cup peeled, sliced
  cucumbers
2 heads romaine lettuce
  (or other lettuce)
1 bunch watercress, large
  stems removed

First make dressing. In small bowl, combine olive oil, lemon juice, mustard, salt, and pepper to taste. Mix thoroughly.

In large pot, heat water and boil shrimp until red (about 5 minutes at a full boil).

In large bowl combine cucumber slices, lettuce, and watercress. Gently toss until thoroughly mixed.

Add shrimp, pour dressing over salad, and toss gently.

Chill for 1 hour and then serve.

CHEF'S SALAD   *Serves 4*

A wonderfully satisfying and filling meal that can be easily prepared.

3 cups lettuce (any type desired),
  plus 6–8 large leaves
1 cup thin strips of cooked
  chicken or turkey
1 cup thin strips of cooked ham
  (regular or low-fat)
1 cup thin strips of hard cheese
  (regular or low-fat)

1 can (2 ounces) anchovies,
  drained
4 hard-boiled eggs, cut in half
  lengthwise
8 radishes, cut in half
8 olives, black or green, pitted
  Coarse black pepper

In a large pot, combine 3 cups lettuce, poultry, ham, cheese, and anchovies. Toss gently.

Line a large bowl with the remaining lettuce leaves; add contents of pot and the eggs, cut side up.

Garnish with radishes and olives, pepper to taste, and serve with your favorite dressing.

BUTTERMILK DRESSING   *Makes about 1½ cups*

Take advantage of this simple but wonderful salad dressing.

1 cup buttermilk
  (or low-fat buttermilk)
¼ cup sour cream
  (or low-fat substitute)
¼ cup chopped fresh parsley
½ teaspoon dry mustard

¼ teaspoon sesame seeds
¼ teaspoon poppy seeds
½ teaspoon salt
  (or salt substitute)
¼ teaspoon coarse black
  pepper

Place all ingredients into a large bowl and combine with a whisk until smooth.

Cover and refrigerate.

CHICKEN OR TURKEY SALAD   *Serves 4*

An old standby that has weathered the tests of time and taste.

4 cups diced cooked chicken or turkey
4 cups diced celery
½ cup chopped green pepper
¼ cup mayonnaise (regular or low-fat)
¼ cup dried sweet basil
¼ cup chopped scallion

1 tablespoon dried dill weed
1 tablespoon chopped green olives
4 large lettuce leaves
Radishes and pitted whole olives
Coarse black pepper

In a large pot, combine poultry, celery, green pepper, mayonnaise, basil, scallion, dill, and olives. Toss gently.

Line a large bowl with lettuce leaves, spoon contents of pot over lettuce leaves. Garnish with radishes and olives, pepper to taste, and serve with your favorite dressing.

FRESH SEAFOOD SALAD   *Serves 6*

A cold seafood salad is a wonderful dish to serve for family or for friends.

1 pound medium shrimp, cleaned
½ pound sea scallops
½ pound fresh codfish
½ cup coarsely chopped cucumber

½ cup chopped celery
½ cup chopped scallion
Coarse black pepper
Your favorite dressing to taste
6 large lettuce leaves

Bring a large pot of water to a boil, add shrimp and scallops, and boil 1 minute. Turn off heat and let stand 1 more minute. Then drain and set aside.

In a large pan with a steamer over one inch of water, steam fish until fish flakes easily when separated by a fork (5–6 minutes).

In a large bowl, combine shrimp, scallops, and codfish. Add cucumber, celery, scallion, and pepper to taste. Add your favorite dressing and toss lightly. Cover and chill for 2 hours.

Line a plate with lettuce leaves, spoon salad into the center, and serve.

GARLIC AND LEMON GREEN BEANS   *Serves 4*

This recipe is one of those that is always simple to make and definitely tastes better a day or two after it has been prepared.

2 pounds green beans
¼ cup olive oil
1 clove garlic, chopped
1 teaspoon sesame oil

2 tablespoons lemon juice
Salt (or salt substitute)
Coarse black pepper

Wash and remove ends of beans.

In a large pan with a steamer over one inch of water, steam beans until tender (10–15 minutes).

Remove steamer with beans, drain the pan, and return beans to the hot pan.

Add olive oil, garlic, and sesame oil, and place over medium heat until hot. Stir several times while heating. Continue to heat 1 more minute while stirring continually.

Remove from heat. Toss with lemon juice; salt and pepper to taste. Serve hot or cold.

TOSSED GREEN SALAD   *Serves 4*

This salad is one of those that can be varied in so many different ways that what is presented below is merely a model. Use it as a foundation and then let your creative mind free. Just be sure to use only complementary (low-carbohydrate) vegetables.

4 cups torn lettuce leaves   ½ cup sliced mushrooms
  (any variety)   ¼ sprouts, alfalfa or bean
1 cup sliced celery   8 radishes, sliced
1 cup sliced cucumber   4 scallions, sliced
½ cup chopped broccoli   Coarse black pepper

In a large bowl, combine lettuce, celery, cucumber, broccoli, mushrooms, sprouts, radishes, and scallions. Toss lightly.

Add your favorite dressing and toss lightly again.

Pepper to taste and serve.

SPINACH SALAD   *Serves 4*

Even without "olive oil," Popeye would find this salad to be a wonderful change at the lunch or dinner table or in his favorite restaurant. Serve it to your family, guests, or Popeye with your favorite dressing.

1 pound spinach, raw   ½ cup chopped cauliflower
1 clove garlic, peeled   6 tablespoons thinly sliced
2 tablespoons olive oil   scallion
3 teaspoons lemon juice   2 hard-boiled eggs, sliced thick
¼ cup crumbled crisp cooked   across
  bacon (or bacon substitute)

Wash spinach several times, thoroughly. Remove tough stems, pat dry with paper towel, wrap in a damp paper towel, and refrigerate about 1 hour.

Cut garlic in half and rub cut surface over the inside surface of a large bowl. Coat inside of bowl with olive oil and lemon juice.

Tear chilled spinach into bite-size pieces and place into bowl prepared above.

Add bacon, cauliflower, and scallion. Toss lightly.

Arrange egg slices around edge of salad and serve with your favorite dressing.

TANGY SPINACH   *Serves 4*

One of Popeye's favorite vegetables served in a wonderful new way to tantalize family, guests, or Popeye.

1 tablespoon sesame seeds	1 tablespoon Teriyaki sauce
1½ pounds spinach, raw	(or low-salt substitute)
1 tablespoon sesame oil	1 teaspoon Dijon mustard
2 tablespoons red wine vinegar	Ground black pepper

In a dry, clean skillet over medium heat, add sesame seeds and gently shake and heat until several seeds take on color or some begin to pop. Remove from heat and set aside.

Wash spinach thoroughly and tear into large pieces.

Add spinach to a large deep skillet over medium heat, cover, and steam in water clinging to leaves, about 3–5 minutes. Immediately add cold water to pan to immerse spinach and stop cooking.

Drain and gently squeeze out as much moisture as possible.

Place spinach into medium bowl and set aside.

In a small bowl, combine sesame oil, vinegar, Teriyaki sauce, and mustard. Mix thoroughly.

Add mixture to spinach, toss gently, and sprinkle with toasted sesame seeds.

Serve hot, warm, or cold.

TANGY ASPARAGUS

Serves 6–8

Asparagus lovers and asparagus haters alike will love this "spicy" but not hot, nonpungent dish served along with the main course of the day. Wonderful served warm or cold.

1½ cups water
½ teaspoon salt
  (or salt substitute)
12 spears asparagus
2 small hot green chili
  peppers
⅛ teaspoon cumin

⅛ teaspoon dried oregano
⅛ teaspoon dried sweet basil
1 bay leaf
2 cloves garlic, quartered
  lengthwise
½ cup white vinegar

In a medium saucepan, combine all ingredients. Boil for 3 minutes exactly. Remove from heat and let cool. Drain off liquid and remove chilies, bay leaf, and garlic.

Serve with your favorite entrée.

GARLIC AND GREEN BEANS

Serves 4

Taking almost no time to prepare, this vegetable side dish will also disappear in no time once the family and guests get their first taste.

½ cup water
  Salt (or salt substitute)
1 pound fresh green beans,
  washed and trimmed

4 tablespoons butter
  (or low-fat substitute)
1 clove garlic, crushed
  Ground black pepper

In a deep skillet over high heat, add water, pinch of salt, and beans. Cover and cook until beans are barely tender.

Place beans into serving dish and cover to keep warm.

In a small saucepan over medium heat, add butter and garlic and mix well as butter melts. Pour mixture over beans, add salt and pepper to taste, and serve.

STEAMED BROCCOLI AND CHEESE   *Serves 4*

A very quick and simple dish to prepare, and very tasty to eat.

4 cups broccoli florets   1 cup shredded sharp cheddar
½ cup water   cheese (regular or low-fat)

In a deep skillet over high heat, combine broccoli and water. Cover and steam for 4 minutes.
Turn off heat, remove cover, and sprinkle cheese over broccoli. Return cover and let stand for 2 minutes.
Serve immediately with the main course.

Risk-Reducing Meals: Soups

CREAMY SPINACH-CHICKEN SOUP   *Serves 6*

This easy-to-make soup is a favorite and a nice use for leftover chicken.

2 pounds chicken backs and   6 white peppercorns
  wings   1 cup heavy cream
6 cups water   (or low-fat substitute)
3 cups frozen spinach   ½ cup sour cream
  (or fresh equivalent)   (or low-fat substitute)
1 stalk celery   3 tablespoons butter
1 small bay leaf   (or low-fat substitute)
1 teaspoon salt   Parsley sprigs
  (or salt substitute)

Fill medium pot with chicken parts and water. Add spinach, celery, bay leaf, salt, and peppercorns, and cover and cook over medium-low heat until tender (about 2 hours).

Strain and reserve broth and chicken meat. Discard chicken skin and bones and peppercorns.

Add heavy cream, sour cream, and butter to broth and heat just to simmer. Add chicken, stir until mixed, turn off heat, and serve with parsley garnish.

CREAM OF BROCCOLI SOUP   *Serves 6*

This delightfully refreshing soup is fun to make and eat hot or cold. You can vary the recipe to taste.

2 stalks celery with leaves
2 cups cauliflower florets
1 clove garlic
½ cup water
2 cups coarsely chopped cooked broccoli
1 teaspoon salt (or salt substitute)

1 dash cayenne pepper
1 cup chicken broth
½ cup heavy cream (or low-fat substitute)
Coarsely ground black pepper

Cut celery stalks crosswise into three parts.

In medium pot combine celery, cauliflower, garlic, and water. Simmer for 15 minutes.

Transfer contents of pot to blender and add broccoli, salt, and cayenne pepper. Cover and blend at high speed.

Uncover while blender is running and add broth and heavy cream.

Add black pepper to taste. Serve hot or chilled.

ROMAINE LETTUCE SOUP *Serves 8*

An unusual lunch soup.

2 tablespoons butter (or low-fat substitute)	Salt (or salt substitute) Ground black pepper
1 stalk celery, diced	4 egg yolks
1 quart chicken broth	1 cup heavy cream
2 quarts romaine lettuce, chopped	(or low-fat substitute)

In large saucepan, melt butter, add celery, and cook until tender (10 minutes).

Add broth and bring to boil.

Add lettuce and salt and pepper to taste; cook over low heat until lettuce is wilted (about 10 minutes).

Combine egg yolks and heavy cream and mix thoroughly. Stir into soup and cook, stirring until soup thickens (do not boil). Season to taste.

CLAM SOUP *Serves 6*

A nice change of pace for the cooler weather.

40 littleneck clams	1½ cups water
¼ cup olive oil	½ teaspoon salt
1 clove garlic, minced	(or salt substitute)
3 anchovy fillets, chopped	½ teaspoon ground black
1 tablespoon dried sweet basil	pepper
½ cup cooking sherry	¼ teaspoon dried oregano

Wash and scrub clams.

In large saucepan combine oil and garlic, and brown over medium heat. Add anchovies, basil, and sherry, and cook for 5 minutes.

Add water, salt, and pepper, and cook 3–4 minutes.

Add clams, cover pan, and cook until all shells open (or no more than 5 minutes). Discard any clams that did not open. Add oregano and cook 2 additional minutes. Serve immediately with any garnish.

LOBSTER BROCCOLI BISQUE   *Serves 6*

A tantalizing and unusual starter.

1 two-pound live lobster
5 tablespoons butter
  (or low-fat substitute)
1 cup chopped broccoli
½ teaspoon sweet basil
1 bay leaf
2 sprigs parsley

⅓ cup dry white wine
½ cup chicken broth
1 tablespoon sherry
½ cup sour cream
  (or low-fat substitute)
3 cups heavy cream
  (or low-fat substitute)

Split lobster and clean. Crack claws and cut body and tail in four to five pieces.

Melt 2 tablespoons butter in large skillet and sauté broccoli. Add bay leaf, parsley, and lobster. Sauté and stir occasionally until lobster turns red (about 5–6 minutes).

Add wine and chicken broth and simmer 20 minutes.

Remove lobster and cool. Set broth aside. Separate lobster meat from shells and set meat aside.

Melt 3 tablespoons butter in saucepan, add sherry, sour cream, and cream, and stir until just below boil. Immediately remove from heat. Grind shells and add to sauce; add sauce to broth, cover, and simmer for 20 minutes. Strain through fine sieve.

Bring strained sauce almost to boil, add lobster and any desired seasoning to taste.

CHICKEN AND CAULIFLOWER SOUP   *Serves 6*

One of the all-time favorite soups with a twist; can be revisited again and again.

2 stalks celery, chopped
½ head lettuce
2 tablespoons olive oil
1 quart chicken broth
½ cup cauliflower florets, chopped
1 large bay leaf

1 whole clove
Salt (or salt substitute)
Ground black pepper
¼ cup heavy cream, whipped (or low-fat substitute)
2 tablespoon chopped chives

Place celery and washed lettuce leaves into food chopper and grind with finest blade.

In large saucepan heat olive oil, add celery and lettuce, and sauté until soft, not browned. Add broth, cauliflower, bay leaf, clove, salt (to taste), and black pepper (to taste).

Strain broth. Puree strained vegetables in blender. Return puree to broth and serve either warm or cold, topped with whipped cream and garnished with chives.

CREAM OF SORREL SOUP   *Serves 6*

A wonderful change of pace that can be served either hot or cold.

1 teaspoon butter
(or low-fat substitute)
½ pound sorrel, chopped fine
5 cups chicken broth

4 egg yolks
2 cups heavy cream
(or low-fat substitute)
Coarsely ground black pepper

In saucepan melt butter, add sorrel, and sauté until wilted. Set pan aside.

In small pot heat broth to boiling, then keep on low heat.

In small bowl combine egg yolks and cream and mix with whisk. Add cream mixture to broth while constantly stirring. Do not allow mixture to boil.

Remove from heat, add sorrel, and mix. Serve hot topped with black pepper to taste, or refrigerate to be served cold.

SHRIMP SOUP   *Serves 4*

A wonderful lunchtime treat that will satisfy friends and family alike.

2 tablespoons olive oil
1 cup cauliflower florets, chopped
½ cup broccoli florets, chopped
¼ teaspoon thyme
1 bay leaf
1 tablespoon chopped parsley
1 tablespoon chopped scallion
1 tablespoon chopped spinach

1½ pounds shrimp, shelled and deveined
4½ cups chicken broth
½ cup dry white wine
Coarse black pepper
Salt (or salt substitute)
3 tablespoons butter (or low-fat substitute)

In a large saucepan, combine olive oil, cauliflower, broccoli, thyme, bay leaf, parsley, scallion, and chopped spinach. Heat until lightly browned. Set vegetables aside.

In another saucepan, combine shrimp, 1 cup broth, and wine. Cover and cook until shrimp are red (5–6 minutes). Set aside 8 shrimp for garnish and grind up remainder.

Combine remaining broth with sautéed vegetables and bring to a boil. Strain, remove bay leaf, and puree vegetables. Add ground shrimp to soup. Bring soup to a boil, turn off heat immediately, and add pepper, salt to taste, and butter. Garnish with remaining shrimp.

BEEF CONSOMMÉ

Serves 4

A quick, simple preparation that serves well on a cold winter's afternoon.

2 cans beef broth, 14 ounces each
1 soup can water
2 eggs (or egg substitute)
Ground black pepper
Salt (or salt substitute)

4 tablespoons grated Swiss cheese (regular or low-fat)
1 tablespoon lemon juice
4 thin lemon slices
2 tablespoons finely chopped parsley

In medium pot combine broth and water. Bring to boil over medium heat.

In bowl beat eggs (or egg substitute) thoroughly. Add salt and pepper to taste.

Combine egg mixture, grated cheese, and lemon juice. Add to boiling broth and whisk until smooth.

Garnish each bowl of soup with lemon slice and parsley.

SHRIMP CHEESE ASPARAGUS SOUP

Serves 4

Take advantage of this delightful and quick little bowl of soup.

12 spears asparagus, cut into bite-size chunks
1 can (14 ounces) chicken broth
4 ounces cheddar cheese (regular or low-fat), grated
½ cup heavy cream (or low-fat substitute)

Ground black pepper
1 teaspoon hot sauce
1 pound shrimp, peeled and deveined
4 sprigs parsley

In large pot, combine asparagus pieces and broth. Bring to boil and cook 5 minutes.

Reduce heat to medium-low and add cheese. Stir and heat until cheese is melted and blended with broth. Simmer while preparing shrimp.

In large pot of boiling water, add shrimp and cook until shrimp are red (5 minutes).

Add shrimp to broth and bring to a boil while stirring. Remove from heat and serve with a garnish of parsley.

Risk-Reducing Meals:
Beef, Veal, Pork, and Lamb

MINUTE STEAKS   *Serves 4*

This easy-to-make luncheon choice is a favorite for a wintery day.

½ cup olive oil
1 teaspoon Teriyaki sauce
(or low-salt substitute)
¼ cup finely chopped celery
(½ stalk and ½ leaves)

1 tablespoon butter
(or low-fat substitute)
8 cubed or minute steaks

In small bowl, combine olive oil, Teriyaki sauce, and celery. Set aside.

In large skillet, melt butter over moderate heat.

Over high heat, brown steaks on one side (about 2 minutes), turn and brown on other side (about 1 minute).

Immediately mix up olive oil, Teriyaki sauce, and celery, and pour mixture over steaks.

PORK ROAST

Serves 6

A wonderful taste treat that is not only delightful to the eye but also to the nose, tongue, and stomach.

4 pounds boneless pork roast
2 tablespoons Teriyaki sauce (or low-salt substitute)
Paprika

4 tablespoons olive oil
2 tablespoons sesame oil
3 cloves garlic, crushed

Preheat oven to 350°F.

Place meat thermometer in thickest part of pork roast and place roast on rack in deep baking pan that has 1 inch water on bottom.

Pour Teriyaki sauce over top of roast, then sprinkle with paprika (to taste).

Combine oils, pour over top of roast, and sprinkle on garlic.

Roast about 2½ hours (to desired temperature on meat thermometer).

HERBY LAMB LOIN CHOPS

Serves 4

This special treat is tasty and easy to prepare in advance.

1 pound boneless lamb loin chops
1 tablespoon ground black pepper
2 cloves garlic, minced
¼ teaspoon dried oregano

1 tablespoon dried sweet basil
½ cup chopped parsley
2 tablespoons Teriyaki sauce (or low-salt substitute)
4 spears broccoli or cauliflower

Place lamb chops in medium bowl.

In small bowl, combine remaining ingredients except broccoli and mix well. Immediately pour mixture over lamb.

Cover and refrigerate overnight.

In large, deep skillet place 1 inch water and broccoli spears (or cauliflower), cover, and turn on burner heat to full. Let heat and steam for 5 minutes and then shut off heat.

Remove lamb from marinade and broil (or grill over hot coals) 2–3 minutes on a side.

Slice thin and serve with steamed broccoli (or cauliflower).

CAULIFLOWER AND HAM   *Serves 4*

An unusual combination that is truly delicious.

½ head cauliflower
4 teaspoons butter
(or low-fat substitute)
1 cup sour cream
(or low-fat substitute)
½ cup grated Swiss cheese
(regular or low-fat)

¼ cup chopped parsley
Finely ground black pepper
1 cup fully cooked diced ham
(regular or low-fat variety)
1 cup chopped green pepper
Coarsely ground black
pepper

Preheat oven to 350°F.

Cut cauliflower into 2-inch florets.

Place 1 inch water in deep skillet, add cauliflower, and turn on burner heat to full. Cover and heat for 5 minutes. Turn off heat, pour off water, and keep covered.

In saucepan, melt butter; add sour cream, Swiss cheese, parsley, and pepper to taste. Stir until cheese is melted.

Lightly grease shallow baking pan.

Arrange ham and cauliflower in pan; sprinkle with chopped green pepper and pour sauce over all. Sprinkle all with coarse ground black pepper to taste.

Bake in 350°F oven for 20 minutes. Serve immediately.

This recipe may be microwaved if you prefer.

ASPARAGUS HAM DELIGHT   *Serves 4*

A quick recipe for using leftovers when some unexpected guests arrive around lunchtime.

12 fresh thick asparagus spears
4 fully cooked, deboned ham
    slices (regular or low-fat),
    ¼ pound each
2 tablespoons butter
    (or low-fat substitute)
4 tablespoons sour cream
    (or low-fat substitute)

1 cup grated cheddar cheese
    (regular or low-fat)
½ teaspoon salt
    (or salt substitute)
2 teaspoons lemon juice
1 tablespoon Dijon
    mustard

Place 1 inch water in deep skillet, add asparagus, cover, and cook over high heat for 5 minutes. Turn off heat, pour off water, and keep covered.

In oven-proof casserole dish, arrange ham slices and place 3 asparagus spears over each.

In small saucepan, melt butter, then reduce heat and add remaining ingredients, stirring until completely mixed.

Pour sauce over asparagus and ham.

Place in oven and cook until hot (8–10 minutes).

DOUBLE PEPPER FILLET OF BEEF   *Serves 6*

A tantalizing and delightful cut of beef.

1 beef fillet (about 3½ pounds),
    rolled and tied
2 cloves garlic, slivered
3 tablespoons Teriyaki sauce
    (or low-salt substitute)

1 tablespoon paprika
2 tablespoons coarse ground
    black pepper
1 teaspoon dried sweet basil

Preheat oven to 425°F.

Using sharp pointed knife tip, poke 1-inch slits into surface of fillet and insert a garlic sliver into each until all slivers are used. Try to distribute slivers evenly over surface.

Pour Teriyaki over surface and sprinkle with paprika, pepper, and basil.

Put fillet in shallow roasting pan, insert meat thermometer into thick part of roast, and place in oven. After 15 minutes reduce heat to 350°F, and cook until desired doneness (rare, medium, or well).

SAUCY SIRLOIN STEAK   *Serves 5–6*

A hearty steak with a saucy twist that should delight the palate.

4 tablespoons olive oil
1 tablespoon sesame oil
1 sirloin steak
   (2–2½ pounds)
½ cup chopped scallion

4 tablespoons chopped chives
1 tablespoon red wine vinegar
¾ cup dry red wine
   Coarse ground black pepper
   Parsley sprigs

In deep skillet combine olive oil and sesame oil and heat over medium heat.

When hot add steak and cook 8–10 minutes on each side depending on desired doneness (rare, medium, well).

When done, set steak on platter and keep warm. Raise burner heat to medium-high and add scallion, chives, and vinegar to oil at bottom of skillet; stir for 20 seconds.

Add wine and simmer on lower heat for 1 minute. Raise burner heat to medium-high and return steak to skillet. Cook 1 minute on each side and remove from heat.

Slice crosswise into thin slices and serve topped with sauce from bottom of skillet.

Garnish with parsley sprigs.

LEMONY VEAL   *Serves 4*

A wonderful contrast in flavors.

4 tablespoons olive oil
½ cup chopped scallion
1½ pounds cubed boneless
     veal
½ cup chicken broth
½ cup large green olives,
     pitted
2 stalks celery, diced

Grated lemon peel
4 tablespoons sour cream
     (or low-fat substitute)
2 teaspoons dried tarragon
1 tablespoon lemon juice
Ground black pepper
Salt (or salt substitute)

In flameproof casserole heat 2 tablespoons oil over low heat, add
scallion and sauté for 3 minutes.

Add veal cubes and quickly brown over medium-high heat. Turn
off heat and set aside.

In small bowl, combine broth, olives, celery, lemon peel, remaining 2 tablespoons olive oil, sour cream, tarragon, and lemon juice.

Add mixture to casserole, cover, and simmer until veal is tender
(about 1 hour).

Pepper and salt to taste.

BROILED LAMB CHOPS   *Serves 4*

A wonderfully tasty dish with a delicate flavor.

2 large cloves garlic, crushed
2 tablespoons dried sage
2 tablespoons dried rosemary
2 tablespoons dried thyme

Coarsely ground black
     pepper
8 thick loin lamb chops
Parsley sprigs

In small bowl, combine garlic, sage, rosemary, thyme, and pepper
(to taste). Mix well.

Coat both sides of chops with mixture and press mixture into chops. Cover and refrigerate overnight.

Broil chops about 4 minutes per side, and serve hot with a garnish of parsley sprigs.

HAMBURGERS WITH DILL   *Serves 6*

Another delectable form of ground beef.

3 pounds ground round steak (or other suitable low-fat cut)	Salt (or salt substitute)
	6 teaspoons butter
	(or low-fat substitute)
1½ tablespoons chopped fresh dill weed (or 1½ teaspoons dried dill)	Ground black pepper
	Teriyaki sauce
	(or low-salt substitute)

Combine meat with dill and divide into six equal parts; form burgers. Heat deep skillet over medium heat until quite hot (about 10 minutes). Sprinkle salt (to taste) on bottom of pan and add burgers.

Sear both sides of burgers, reduce heat, and continue to cook until desired doneness (rare, medium, well).

Top each burger with 1 teaspoon butter, black pepper (to taste), and Teriyaki (to taste).

PEPPERED STEAK   *Serves 6*

A spicy little treat for lunch.

Coarsely ground black pepper	1 teaspoon Teriyaki sauce
2 pounds sirloin strip steak	(or low-salt substitute)
2 teaspoons salt	Lemon juice to taste
(or salt substitute)	Parsley sprigs
¼ cup butter	
(or low-fat substitute)	

Sprinkle pepper on flat surface such as cutting board, press steak into pepper, and work into both sides using palms of hands.

Sprinkle large skillet with salt and heat. When salt begins to brown, place steaks in skillet and brown over high heat. Reduce heat and cook to desired doneness (rare, medium, well).

In small pan, combine remaining ingredients except parsley, and heat.

Remove steaks from pan and pour mixture over steaks.

Garnish with parsley sprigs

ROAST LAMB WITH HERBS   *Serves 6*

A savory recipe for lamb.

1 lamb roast (about 3 pounds)	1 bay leaf
1 clove garlic, crushed	½ teaspoon dried thyme
1 teaspoon salt	½ teaspoon dried sage
(or salt substitute)	½ teaspoon dried marjoram
2 tablespoons coarsely ground	1 tablespoon Teriyaki sauce
black pepper	(or low-salt substitute)
1 teaspoon dried sweet basil	1 tablespoon olive oil
½ teaspoon powdered ginger	

Preheat oven to 350°F.

Place meat on rack in roasting pan.

In small bowl combine remaining ingredients and mix thoroughly.

Make slits in lamb and rub mixture into slits and over entire surface of lamb.

Insert meat thermometer into thick part of roast; place pan in oven. After 10 minutes reduce heat to 300°F and cook until desired doneness (rare, medium, or well).

SPICED BEEF   *Serves 6–8*

This tasty hot dish is also delicious served cold.

4–5 pounds chuck roast	1 teaspoon powdered cloves
Cider vinegar	1 teaspoon ground black
Red wine	pepper
1 cup chopped scallion	1 ½ teaspoons salt
1 bay leaf	(or salt substitute)
1 teaspoon powdered	3 cups broccoli florets
cinnamon	4 stalks celery, trimmed
1 teaspoon powdered	2 tablespoons butter
allspice	(or low-fat substitute)

In medium pot, place roast and enough cider vinegar and wine in 1:1 proportions to cover roast 1 inch above top.

Add scallion, bay leaf, cinnamon, allspice, cloves, pepper, and salt. Cover pot and marinate in refrigerator overnight.

When ready, preheat oven to 275°F. Remove meat from marinade and set liquid aside.

Place meat into roasting pan and pour in half of marinade liquid. Add 2 cups of water, cover, and roast for about 3 hours.

Grind or mince broccoli and celery and sauté in butter until celery is golden brown. Add to roasting pan for the last ½ hour of cooking.

When ready, slice meat and serve hot.

PORK TENDERLOIN WITH MUSHROOMS, GREEN PEPPERS, AND OLIVES   *Serves 4*

A delicious and simple pork recipe.

1 ½ pounds pork tenderloin	1 medium green pepper, sliced
2 tablespoons butter	in strips
(or low-fat substitute)	½ cup dry white wine

½ pound mushrooms, sliced
1 tablespoon dried sweet
  basil
6 sliced green olives stuffed
  with pimentos

2 tablespoons lemon juice
Parsley

Cut pork into 1-inch crosswise slices.

Place butter in skillet and heat over medium heat. When hot, sauté pork slices until golden brown. Lower heat.

Add green pepper strips.

In small pot bring wine to boil and then pour over meat. Immediately add mushrooms and basil. Cover skillet and simmer for ½ hour.

When finished, add olives and lemon juice, and serve with parsley garnish.

BEEF AND CELERY RAGOUT   *Serves 4*

A simple but elegant dish that will always be a hit.

2 pounds boneless beef, lean
1 tablespoon garlic powder
6 stalks celery, cut in strips
3 cups beef bouillon
2 cups sliced mushrooms
2 cups broccoli florets
½ cup chopped parsley

3 cloves, gently crushed
1 teaspoon dried thyme
1 teaspoon salt
  (or salt substitute)
10 black peppercorns, gently
  crushed

Preheat broiler. Cut beef into 1-inch cubes and sprinkle with garlic powder.

Place beef on broiling rack and place in broiler about 4 inches below flame; brown all sides (about 15 minutes).

Transfer beef to Dutch oven. Add remaining ingredients and cover.

Bring to boil, reduce heat, and simmer on top of stove until beef is tender (1–1½ hours).
Serve hot.

Risk-Reducing Meals: Poultry and Seafood

BARBECUED LEMON CHICKEN   *Serves 6*

This easy-to-make, simple summer favorite is something that can be enjoyed even in the winter.

6 large boneless chicken breasts
2 tablespoon lemon juice
4 teaspoons olive oil
2 cloves garlic, minced

½ teaspoon dried sweet basil
½ teaspoon cayenne pepper
½ teaspoon Teriyaki sauce (or low-salt substitute)

Remove fat and skin from chicken breasts. Rinse breasts thoroughly. Arrange breasts in a single layer in a shallow baking dish.

In small bowl, combine remaining ingredients and mix well.

Pour mixture over chicken and turn to distribute mixture on both sides of chicken.

Cover and refrigerate overnight for best results.

(In nice weather) Cook chicken over hot coals of a greased grill.

(In bad weather) Broil chicken, 6 minutes per side.

CHICKEN WITH BROCCOLI AND CABBAGE   *Serves 8*

This stir-fry can be prepared in advance and served up as an "on the spot" dinner for the sheer delight of your guests. Makes a great all-in-one, easy lunch to carry with you, too.

2 pounds boneless skinned chicken breasts
2 tablespoons olive oil
2 tablespoons minced ginger root
6 cups broccoli florets and stems, chopped
¾ pound mushrooms, sliced
¾ cup chicken stock
2 tablespoons dry sherry (or cooking wine)

2 tablespoons Teriyaki sauce (or low-salt substitute)
2 tablespoons mayonnaise (regular or low-fat)
2 tablespoons water
4 cups sliced red or white cabbage
Ground black pepper

Cut chicken into thin strips (little-finger-size). Set aside.

In large heavy skillet, heat oil until very hot.

Slowly add chicken and half of ginger root to skillet. If sticking occurs, add a bit more oil. Stir continually and slowly for about 2 minutes. Remove from skillet and set aside.

In hot skillet, combine broccoli, mushrooms, and remaining ginger root, and stir continually for 2 minutes. Add a little water if sticking occurs.

Mix chicken stock, sherry, and Teriyaki sauce, and pour mixture over broccoli mixture in skillet. Cover, and let steam for 2 minutes.

Stir in chicken mixture, mayonnaise, water, and bring to boil.

Add cabbage; stir for 1 minute or until cabbage is coated with sauce. Serve hot.

LONG ISLAND DUCKLING   *Serves 4*

This succulent showstopper is an elegant choice for lunch or dinner.

1 large duckling (5–7 pounds)
2 tablespoons olive oil
1 tablespoon sesame oil
1 cup dry sherry
2 teaspoons lemon juice
2 tablespoons cognac
1 teaspoon Teriyaki sauce
   (or low-salt substitute)
½ teaspoon salt
   (or salt substitute)

Coarsely ground black
   pepper to taste
1 teaspoon hot sauce
Dash of allspice
1 teaspoon dried sweet basil
½ teaspoon dried sage
½ cup watercress
½ cup celery, cut into thin strips
   (about 2 inches long)

Carefully remove all skin possible from duck, being careful not to cut flesh. Quarter duck.

Combine olive oil and sesame oil in large skillet and heat. When oil is hot, add duck quarters and brown on all sides.

Add half the sherry to skillet, cover, and cook until duck is tender (40–50 minutes). Remove duck to hot plate and keep hot.

Combine remaining ingredients except watercress and celery in skillet and heat, stirring constantly.

Return duck to skillet and simmer over low heat 5 minutes. Serve with garnish of watercress and celery strips.

BAKED BLUEFISH   *Serves 5–6*

Simple but delectable. Ready anytime you need it.

2 tablespoons vegetable oil
1 bluefish (4–5 pounds),
   cleaned and split
2 teaspoons sesame oil

2 cloves garlic, minced fine
2 tablespoons lemon juice
½ cup chopped parsley
Lemon wedges

Preheat oven to 425°F.

Spread vegetable oil over surface of large, shallow baking pan. Place fish skin side down in baking pan and sprinkle surface uniformly with sesame oil, garlic, and lemon juice.

Bake, uncovered, until flesh flakes with fork (20–25 minutes).

Garnish with parsley and serve with lemon wedges.

This recipe may also be microwaved.

SOLE DELIGHT
Serves 4

Another quick and tantalizing way to prepare one of the best tasting fish.

1½ pounds sole fillets	2 tablespoons finely chopped
1 tablespoon lemon juice	broccoli florets
2 teaspoons olive oil	Coarsely ground black
½ teaspoon dried sweet basil	pepper

Preheat oven to 425°F.

Arrange fillets in a single layer in a suitable baking dish.

In small bowl, combine lemon juice, olive oil, basil, and broccoli. Mix thoroughly and sprinkle over fillets. Pepper to taste.

Bake, uncovered, for 10–12 minutes, or until the flesh flakes easily with a fork.

This recipe may be microwaved if you prefer.

ORIENTAL HALIBUT STEAKS   *Serves 6*

A hearty dish to satisfy the fussiest fish eater.

3 halibut steaks
(1½–1¾ inches thick)
Salt (or salt substitute)
¼ cup finely chopped
cauliflower florets
2 tablespoons Teriyaki sauce
(or low-salt substitute)

Ground black pepper
3 tablespoons toasted sesame
seeds
½ teaspoon dried crumbled
thyme leaves
⅓ cup melted butter
(or low-fat substitute)

Preheat oven to 350°F.
Arrange steaks in buttered shallow baking pan.
Salt to taste.
Combine remaining ingredients and sprinkle one third of mixture
on each steak.
Bake, uncovered, about 25–30 minutes, or until steaks flake easily
with fork.
This recipe may be microwaved if you prefer.

POACHED SALMON STEAK   *Serves 6*

From the Pacific Northwest to your table in a matter of 25–30 minutes of cooking time.

2 tablespoons butter
(or low-fat substitute)
⅓ cup chopped onion
⅓ cup chopped green
pepper
⅓ cup chopped celery

1–1½ quarts water
½ cup white vinegar
Salt (or salt substitute)
White peppercorns
Large salmon steak
(about 3 pounds)

In large skillet, melt butter; add onion, green pepper, and celery. Cook mixture 5–8 minutes. Add water, vinegar, salt (to taste), and peppercorns and simmer for 5 minutes.

Bring liquid to boil as you wrap steak in coarse cheesecloth.

Submerge steak in boiling liquid. Immediately lower heat; allow steak to simmer 25–30 minutes.

Remove steak, carefully unwrap, and serve hot with appropriate sauce (for example, Hollandaise sauce).

BROILED SWORDFISH   *Serves 4*

One of the all-time favorites with a twist; can be revisited again and again.

1½ pounds swordfish steaks	2 tablespoons dried sweet
Salt (or salt substitute)	basil
Ground black pepper	2 tablespoons lemon juice
⅛ teaspoon paprika	Watercress
¼ cup olive oil	

Grease broiler rack, turn on broiler, and place rack about 2 inches below flame.

Wash steaks and sprinkle with salt and pepper (to taste), and paprika.

Place steaks on preheated broiler rack. Coat top of steaks with half of the olive oil and broil for 3 minutes. Turn steaks and coat with remaining olive oil, sprinkle with basil, and broil for 4–5 more minutes.

Sprinkle with lemon juice and garnish with watercress.

CRABMEAT WITH HERBS   *Serves 6*

An unusual taste treat that can be prepared in short order.

1½ pounds crabmeat	2 tablespoons lemon juice
6 tablespoons olive oil	1 tablespoon dried sweet basil
Salt (or salt substitute)	1 tablespoon chopped scallion
Coarsely ground black	1 tablespoon dried tarragon
pepper	Parsley sprigs

Remove all bits of nonedible material from crabmeat.

In a skillet, heat olive oil until hot and add crabmeat; stir continually until cooked thoroughly (about 2 minutes).

Remove from heat and add salt and black pepper (to taste), lemon juice, basil, scallion, and tarragon; mix thoroughly.

Garnish with parsley sprigs and serve.

ITALIAN SHRIMP   *Serves 4*

Take advantage of the fruits of the sea to enjoy a satisfying dish for any day.

½ cup olive oil	1 tablespoon finely chopped
½ teaspoon salt	parsley
(or salt substitute)	2 pounds large shrimp, shelled
Ground black pepper	and deveined
2 tablespoons dried sweet	Lettuce leaves
basil	4 lemon wedges

In small bowl, combine olive oil, salt, black pepper (to taste), basil, and parsley; mix well.

Grease broiler rack, turn on broiler, and place rack about 2 inches below flame.

Dip shrimp in mixture and then place shrimp on heated broiler rack.

Broil 2 minutes per side.

Place broiled shrimp into baking dish, sprinkle with olive oil, and bake at 450°F for 10 minutes.

Serve on beds of lettuce with lemon wedges on the side.

This recipe may be microwaved, if you prefer.

CHICKEN WITH OLIVE SAUCE   *Serves 4*

A sure winner with any guest.

4 skinned, boneless chicken breasts	4 tablespoons sliced green olives
1 tablespoon olive oil	4 tablespoons chopped fresh basil
2 tablespoons lime juice	
1 tablespoon wine vinegar	4 green pepper rings
1 clove garlic, crushed	Ground black pepper
4 tablespoons sliced black olives	

In a large skillet, heat olive oil and brown chicken over medium-high heat. Lower heat, cover, and cook until tender (8–10 minutes).

Remove chicken to serving plate and keep warm.

Combine lime juice, vinegar, garlic, black and green olives, and basil in the skillet used for the chicken. Gently heat.

Slice the chicken and arrange on plates with pepper rings. Pepper to taste.

Risk-Reducing Meals:
Vegetarian Choices

ASPARAGUS AND EGG CASSEROLE   *Serves 4*

This elegant casserole dish is a delight by itself or with a salad of your choice.

1 tablespoon butter (or low-fat substitute) 1 large can asparagus spears 4 hard-boiled eggs, sliced Salt (or salt substitute) Ground black pepper 1 can mushrooms	2 cups heavy cream (or low-fat substitute) ½ cup cheddar cheese (regular or low-fat), grated 2 large slices Swiss cheese (regular or low-fat)

Preheat oven to 350°F.

Grease bottom and sides of medium casserole.

Arrange half of the asparagus spears on bottom of casserole.

Cover with half of the egg slices, salt and pepper to taste, and sprinkle with half of cheddar cheese. Add mushrooms.

Top with remainder of asparagus spears and cover with remainder of egg slices, salt and pepper to taste, and sprinkle with remainder of cheddar cheese. Cover with cream.

Place Swiss cheese slices over all and place in oven for 30 minutes.

Remove from oven and serve hot.

VEGETARIAN PARSLEY BUTTER "BURGERS"

Serves 6

A surefire taste delight that perks up any Risk-Reducing Meal.

6 tablespoons butter
(or low-fat substitute)
2 tablespoons chopped parsley

6 vegetable "burgers"*
1 clove garlic, crushed

In large mixing bowl, mix two thirds of butter with parsley. Chill until solid.

Place remaining butter in large frying pan and heat until melted. Add "burgers" and fry both sides until brown (4–5 minutes).

Spread garlic over both sides of "burgers" and serve each with a small scoop of parsley butter on top.

VEGETARIAN "BURGERS" DELIGHT

Serves 4

This tasty, easy-to-prepare dish can be served plain or with vegetables.

1 tablespoon sesame oil
6 tablespoons butter
(or low-fat substitute)
1 clove garlic, minced
6 vegetable "burgers"*
6 stalks celery, chopped
½ cup red wine
½ cup water
2 bay leaves

Salt (or salt substitute)
3 tablespoons chopped parsley
Ground black pepper
1 teaspoon dried thyme
1½ cups sour cream
(or low-fat substitute)
1 teaspoon paprika
2 tablespoons Teriyaki sauce
(or low-salt substitute)

Preheat oven to 375°F and oil a deep casserole dish with sesame oil. In small saucepan melt butter and sauté garlic. Add "burgers" and

*For Risk-Reducing Meals, nonmeat alternatives should contain 4 grams of carbohydrate or less per average serving.

brown on both sides (3 minutes per side). Remove "burgers" and place in the casserole dish.

Place celery in hot butter used to cook "burgers" and sauté 5 minutes. Add wine, water, bay leaves, salt, parsley, pepper (to taste), and thyme, and heat for 5 minutes, stirring continually.

Pour mixture over "burgers," cover, and bake for 1 hour.

Immediately before serving, add sour cream, paprika, and Teriyaki sauce to the casserole liquid, stirring as you do so. Spoon sauce over burgers and serve.

CURRIED EGGS *Serves 6*

An unusual combination that is truly delicious.

6 eggs
½ teaspoon curry powder
1 tablespoon chopped dill pickle
1 teaspoon mild prepared mustard
2 tablespoons sour cream (or low-fat substitute)

Finely ground black pepper
Salt (or salt substitute)
1 tablespoon capers
4 large iceberg lettuce leaves
Paprika

In a saucepan of boiling water, place eggs and hard-boil (10 minutes). Cool eggs, peel, and slice in half lengthwise. Remove yolks and set white halves aside.

Place yolks into mixing bowl with curry powder, chopped pickle, mustard, sour cream, black pepper (to taste), salt (to taste), and capers. Mix thoroughly and spoon equal portions back into egg white halves.

Place lettuce leaves on a platter, arrange filled halves, sprinkle with paprika, and serve.

SPICY OMELET   *Serves 4*

A quick recipe that will spark the palate and perk up any meal.

8 eggs (or egg substitute)
1 4-ounce can green chilies
  (peppers) in brine, drained
  and chopped fine
1 teaspoon butter
  (or low-fat substitute)

Salt (or salt substitute)
Ground black pepper
Sprigs of parsley

Thoroughly mix eggs in mixing bowl and add chilies.

In small saucepan melt butter, then reduce heat and add egg mixture; season to taste with salt and black pepper.

Turn heat to high and cook until done to desired consistency (1–3 minutes).

Garnish with parsley and serve.

VEGETARIAN SAUTÉED "CHICKEN"   *Serves 6*

A wonderful contrast in flavors.

2 tablespoons olive oil
6 vegetable "chicken" slices
  (3 inches diameter)*
⅔ cup white wine
1 teaspoon dried sweet basil

1 tablespoon lime juice
1 clove garlic, crushed
Ground black pepper
Salt (or salt substitute)
Sprigs of parsley

Place oil and "chicken" in a large frying pan. Brown "chicken" (3 minutes per side) and remove from pan.

*For Risk-Reducing Meals, nonmeat alternatives should contain 4 grams of carbohydrate or less per average serving.

To the frying pan, add white wine, basil, lime juice, and garlic; cook for 2 minutes.

Bring to slow boil for 3 minutes. Return chicken to pan and heat an additional 3 minutes.

Pepper and salt to taste. Garnish with parsley.

VEGETARIAN ORIENTAL "STEAK" CASSEROLE

Serves 6

A tantalizing and delightful meatless casserole.

1 tablespoon vegetable oil	6–8 vegetarian "steaklets"*
2 tablespoons butter	½ cup water
(or low-fat substitute)	1½ cups sour cream
1 large green pepper, chopped	(or low-fat substitute)
6 stalks celery, chopped	3 tablespoons Teriyaki sauce
3 cloves garlic, crushed	(or low-salt substitute)
2 teaspoons freshly grated	
ginger root	

Preheat oven to 350°F. Spread 1 tablespoon oil around bottom of deep casserole dish.

Add butter to saucepan and melt over medium heat. Add green pepper, celery, garlic, and ginger root; sauté until light brown.

Cut "steaklets" into small pieces (about 1 inch square) and add to saucepan, stirring together 4 minutes.

Pour mixture into casserole.

In small bowl, combine water, sour cream, and Teriyaki sauce and pour over casserole. Cover and bake for 30–35 minutes.

*For Risk-Reducing Meals, nonmeat alternatives should contain 4 grams of carbohydrate or less per average serving.

VEGETARIAN PEPPER "STEAKS"   *Serves 6*

A hearty vegetarian "steak" with a saucy twist that should delight the palate.

6 vegetable "steaklets"*
1 teaspoon sesame oil
4 tablespoons olive oil
2 tablespoons coarsely ground
  black pepper
½ cup red wine

2 tablespoons cognac
1 tablespoon butter
  (or low-fat substitute)
  Salt (or salt substitute)
  Ground black pepper
1 clove garlic, crushed

Set "steaklets" on plate, then combine both oils in small bowl. Quickly dip both sides of each "steaklet" into oil mixture and return to plate.

Pour remaining oil into large frying pan, heat pan over medium flame and, when oil is hot, brown "steaklets," 3 minutes per side.

Lower heat, cover pan, and cook for 6 minutes.

Remove "steaklets," place on platter, and keep warm.

In pan in which "steaklets" were browned, add wine, cognac, butter, salt (to taste), pepper (to taste), and garlic. Mix well.

Turn up heat and bring ingredients to just under a boil. Lower heat and cook for 4 minutes.

Immediately pour sauce over "steaklets" and serve.

VEGETARIAN "BURGERS" IN WHITE SAUCE   *Serves 6*

A delectable and spicy meal.

3 tablespoons olive oil
6 vegetable "burgers"*
¼ cup water
4 tablespoons white wine
1 clove garlic, crushed

⅔ cup mayonnaise
  (regular or low-fat)
1 tablespoon white
  horseradish

*For Risk-Reducing Meals, nonmeat alternatives should contain 4 grams of carbohydrate or less per average serving.

Place oil and "burgers" in a large frying pan. Brown "burgers" (3 minutes per side), remove from pan, and place on platter in warm oven.

To the frying pan, add water, wine, garlic, mayonnaise, and horseradish; bring to a boil.

Pour hot sauce over "burgers" and serve immediately.

EGGS INDIAN STYLE   *Serves 6*

A wonderful variation for the versatile egg.

6 eggs
3 tablespoons olive oil
1 tablespoon sesame oil
1 clove garlic, minced fine
2 tablespoons curry powder
3 tablespoons sour cream
(or low-fat substitute)
¾ cup water

1 tablespoon lemon juice
Salt (or salt substitute)
Coarsely ground black
pepper
3 tablespoons chopped parsley
2 tablespoons slivered lemon
peel

In a saucepan of boiling water, place eggs and hard-boil (10 minutes). Set aside to cool.

In medium frying pan combine olive oil and sesame oil. Heat oil over medium heat and, when hot, add garlic and sauté. Add curry powder, sour cream, water, lemon juice, salt (to taste), and pepper (to taste). Reduce heat and allow mixture to cook until just about to boil.

Peel eggs and slice lengthwise. Add egg slices to mixture in frying pan. Stir in gently.

Turn off heat, stir in lemon peel and parsley, and serve immediately.

VEGETARIAN BRANDIED "STEAK" *Serves 6*

A spicy, aromatic little treat.

4 tablespoons olive oil
6 vegetable "steaklets"*
2 tablespoons cognac
1 tablespoon crème de menthe
1 tablespoon finely chopped celery

1 tablespoon finely chopped chives
1 teaspoon coarsely ground black pepper

Coat bottom of a large frying pan with oil, heat over moderate heat, and brown "steaklets" (3 minutes per side).

Remove "steaklets" and keep warm.

In frying pan with the heated oil, combine the cognac, crème de menthe, celery, and chives. Mix thoroughly.

Return "steaklets" to pan and cook with sauce for 2 minutes. Serve immediately; pepper to taste.

HERBY EGGS *Serves 4*

A wonderfully tasty dish with a delicate flavor.

1 tablespoon butter (or low-fat substitute)
4 eggs
1½ cups heavy cream (or low-fat substitute)
1½ cups sour cream (or low-fat substitute)

2 tablespoons chopped fresh basil
1 tablespoon chopped fresh tarragon
Salt (or salt substitute)
Coarsely ground black pepper
Sprigs of parsley

Preheat oven to 350°F.

In small saucepan, melt butter. Brush melted butter on insides of individual custard cups. Place cups in baking pan half filled with hot water.

*For Risk-Reducing Meals, nonmeat alternatives should contain 4 grams of carbohydrate or less per average serving.

Break eggs into a small bowl and beat thoroughly.

In a saucepan, combine cream and sour cream and heat just to boiling.

Lower heat and add eggs, stirring constantly. Continue to stir, and add basil, tarragon, salt (to taste), and pepper (to taste).

Fill custard cups about three fourths full with egg mixture. Place cups in baking pan and fill pan with water halfway up cups. Put into oven and bake for 20 minutes. Insert knife into the contents of one custard cup. If it comes out clean, then the eggs are ready. If not, cook an additional 5 minutes.

Garnish with parsley and serve hot.

VEGETARIAN MARINATED "BURGERS" OR "STEAKLETS"
Serves 6

A delectable dish that can be enjoyed over and over again.

¼ cup water
2 stalks celery with leaves
1 cup chopped broccoli florets
⅓ cup olive oil
1 clove garlic, minced
1 teaspoon ground ginger

½ cup Teriyaki sauce
(or low-salt substitute)
1 tablespoon lemon juice
6 vegetable "steaklets" or "burgers"*

In a blender, combine water and celery. Blend until the mixture is a puree.

In a large, deep bowl, combine celery puree, broccoli, oil, garlic, ginger, Teriyaki sauce, and lemon juice.

Break up vegetable "steaklets" or "burgers" into bite-size pieces and add to the bowl. Mix gently, cover, and refrigerate overnight.

Drain marinade (sauce) into a saucepan. Heat sauce and let simmer. Place "burger" chunks or "steaklets" into shallow pan and broil until nicely brown (8–10 minutes).

*For Risk-Reducing Meals, nonmeat alternatives should contain 4 grams of carbohydrate or less per average serving.

Put "burger" chunks or "steaklets" on plates and serve sauce on the side.

VEGETARIAN "STEAK" SUPREME   *Serves 6*

A specialty that is easy to prepare.

2 tablespoons olive oil
6 vegetable "steaklets"*
2 tablespoons butter
  (or low-fat substitute)
½ green pepper, chopped
2 cloves garlic, minced fine
  Salt (or salt substitute)
  Ground black pepper
4 tablespoons white wine

4 tablespoons dry red wine
4 tablespoons water
2 egg yolks
⅓ cup heavy cream
  (or low-fat substitute)
⅓ cup sour cream
  (or low-fat substitute)
2 tablespoons chopped
  parsley

Coat bottom of a large frying pan with oil, heat over moderate heat, and brown "steaklets" (3 minutes per side). Remove from heat.

In the same frying pan, melt butter, add green pepper and garlic, and sauté. Then add salt and black pepper to taste.

Stir in the wines and water; simmer for 4 minutes.

In a small bowl, combine egg yolks, heavy cream, and sour cream. Mix thoroughly.

Pour the cream mixture into the frying pan with the wine mixture and stir well. Add parsley and the browned "steaklets." Bring to a simmer, turn off the heat, and serve hot.

*For Risk-Reducing Meals, nonmeat alternatives should contain 4 grams of carbohydrate or less per average serving.

VEGETARIAN "BURGERS" IN WINE

Serves 6

A simple but elegant dish that will always be a hit.

2 tablespoons olive oil
6 vegetable "burgers"*
½ cup chopped broccoli
  florets
½ cup chopped cauliflower
  florets

3 stalks celery, sliced thin
  Salt (or salt substitute)
  Ground black pepper
1 cup water
1 cup white wine

Preheat oven to 375°F.

Coat bottom of a large frying pan with oil, heat over moderate burner, and brown "burgers" (3 minutes per side).

In an oven-proof serving casserole combine broccoli, cauliflower, and celery. Place browned "burgers" on top of vegetables. Sprinkle with salt (to taste) and pepper (to taste). Pour water and white wine over everything.

Bake casserole uncovered until most of liquid is evaporated (about 50–60 minutes). Baste occasionally. Serve hot, straight from the casserole.

*For Risk-Reducing Meals, nonmeat alternatives should contain 4 grams of carbohydrate or less per average serving.

CAULIFLOWER CHEESE CASSEROLE
WITH SOUR CREAM
Serves 4

A delicious and simple change of pace that will delight any guests.

1 tablespoon olive oil
1½ cups coarsely chopped
cauliflower florets
Salt (or salt substitute)
Coarsely ground black
pepper
1 clove garlic, crushed
1½ cups sour cream
(or low-fat substitute)

½ pound cheddar cheese
(regular or low-fat),
grated
1 tablespoon dried sweet basil
1 teaspoon dried rosemary
2 tablespoons butter
(or low-fat substitute)

Preheat oven to 375°F and oil a deep casserole dish.

Wash cauliflower and place into skillet with ½ inch water at the bottom. Turn heat up to high and cook, uncovered, for 5 minutes. Remove from heat, drain off water, and arrange cauliflower in bottom of the casserole.

Sprinkle salt (to taste), pepper (to taste), and garlic over cauliflower.

Stir sour cream and cheese together and pour over cauliflower, spreading sauce to all sides of casserole.

Sprinkle surface with tarragon and basil. Dot with butter. Bake for 15–20 minutes.

VEGETARIAN "STEAK" SURPRISE   *Serves 6*

A delicious and surprisingly simple change of pace that will delight any guests for lunch.

3 tablespoons olive oil
6 vegetarian "steaklets"*
4 cloves garlic, crushed
1½ tablespoons pimento-stuffed olives, chopped coarsely
1 teaspoon spicy prepared mustard
1 teaspoon chopped scallion

½ pound cheddar cheese (regular or low fat), grated
1 pickled cauliflower floret (optional)
½ cup water
1 cup sour cream (or low-fat substitute)
Sprigs of parsley

Preheat oven to 350°F. Spread 1 tablespoon oil around bottom of deep casserole dish.

In large frying pan, heat remaining olive oil and add "steaklets." Brown them (3 minutes per side), then set aside on plate.

Spread garlic on both sides of "steaklets" and place them in bottom of casserole dish.

To frying pan used for the "steaklets," add olives, mustard, scallion, cheese, cauliflower, and water. Turn on medium heat and stir for 4 minutes.

Pour sauce over "steaklets" and bake (uncovered) for 50 minutes.

Remove casserole from oven, spread sour cream over steaklets, cover, and let stand 5–7 minutes. Garnish with parsley.

*For Risk-Reducing Meals, nonmeat alternatives should contain 4 grams of carbohydrate or less per average serving.

CHAPTER 25

Essential Balance Recipes

Your Essential Balance Meals insure that, each day, you include Essential Balance Foods in your eating program. Essential Balance Foods are those foods that contain moderate to high amounts of carbohydrate. Some examples of Essential Balance Foods are fruits, fruit juices, breads, pastas, potatoes, rice, and desserts.

It is important to understand that Essential Balance Meals are *not* made up of Essential Balance Foods totally. Essential Balance Meals must also include Risk-Reducing Foods as well. At your Essential Balance dinner, your pasta (Essential Balance Food), for instance, will also have some good ground turkey or beef (Risk-Reducing Food) meatballs on top. And along with your green vegetables and salad (Risk-Reducing Foods), you will also get to have some good bread and fruit and even some dessert (all Essential Balance Foods).

> Essential Balance Meals are *not* made up
> of Essential Balance Foods only.
> They include Risk-Reducing Foods as well.

For more details on the differences between Essential Balance Foods and Risk-Reducing Foods, see chapter 14, "The Profactor-H Program: How It Works." For help in balancing your Essential Balance Meals, see "A Question of Balance," page 294. Additional information can be found in the introduction to Risk-Reducing Recipes starting on page 348.

The recipes that follow are intended to be eaten during the Essential Balance Meals. These recipes are only offered as examples of the kinds of foods that can be eaten during these meals. You can also consult the Sample Meal Plans starting on page 303.

When you choose your Essential Balance Meal foods, make sure that you select foods that contain complex carbohydrates—foods such as pasta, rice, whole-grain breads, and potatoes. Choose less of the sweets and heavy desserts. Fruit is a simple sugar and you should check with your doctor regarding the appropriate amount for you. Also remember to include Risk-Reducing proteins, vegetables, and salad in your Essential Balance Meals as well.

Essential Balance Foods may be prepared in any way you desire. For low-fat or low-salt guidelines, see "Health Agency Recommendations" on page 345.

Please remember, extensive cooking and preparation are *not* required on this Program. You can choose your old-time favorite and quick meals, and they can be prepared and eaten at home; but also feel free to eat at restaurants whenever you like.

The recipes that follow have been included for those who enjoy cooking and those who are looking for something "special" or "new." They represent only a small portion of all the foods—for as long as your choices do not oppose your physician's recommendation, you can enjoy any foods you like at your Essential Balance Meals . . . as long as your Essential Balance Meals are well-rounded and correctly balanced.

We have arranged these recipes for your easy access:

ESSENTIAL BALANCE MEALS:

As with our Risk-Reducing Meal recipes, we have included low-fat and low-cholesterol alternatives.

Remember that Essential Balance Meal leftovers should *not* be included in your Risk-Reducing Meals unless they contain *only* Risk-Reducing ingredients.

Essential Balance Meals: Appetizers and Snacks

CHICKEN-LIVER PÂTÉ   *Serves 8*

This wonderful spread can perk up the appetite of any guest.

1 pound chicken livers
1 can (13½ ounces) chicken
  broth
4 hard-boiled eggs (optional)
4 tablespoons butter or
  rendered chicken fat
  (or low-fat substitute)

1 teaspoon chopped garlic
1 medium chopped onion
  Salt (or salt substitute)
  Coarse ground pepper

Place chicken livers in a large saucepan, add the broth, and simmer until done, 10–12 minutes.

Drain the cooked livers, reserving about ¼ cup of the liquid. In a blender, combine livers and a few tablespoons of the liquid in which the livers were cooked and puree. If using, chop the eggs finely and add to the pureed livers.

Add butter or fat to a deep frying pan and lightly brown the garlic and onion, and then blend all of the ingredients to make a paste, seasoning to taste with salt and pepper.

Serve this pâté in a bowl and surround with crisp, fresh vegetables such as cauliflower, celery, green peppers, green beans, and broccoli florets. An alternative is to serve the pâté on buttered (or low-fat substitute) toast quarters or in lettuce cups.

SHRIMP WITH HERB SAUCE   *Serves 8*

A tangy treat that is always a hit.

40 shrimp, shelled and deveined	1 tablespoon chopped chives
8 large lettuce leaves	1 tablespoon chopped cucumber
½ cup mayonnaise (regular or low-fat)	Juice of 1 lemon
1 tablespoon chopped fresh basil or 2 teaspoons dried sweet basil	

Add shrimp to a large pot of boiling water and cook, stirring occasionally, until shrimp are red in color and thoroughly cooked, about 3–4 minutes.

For each person, arrange 5 shrimp on a large lettuce leaf. Cover each with waxed paper or plastic wrap and chill.

Combine the remaining ingredients and chill for 1 hour. Place a toothpick through each shrimp, spoon the mayonnaise sauce over the shrimp, and serve.

BARBECUED SPARERIBS—CHINESE STYLE

Serves 8–10

This finger-lickin'-good appetizer will quickly disappear from the serving plate. Serve it hot and keep it coming.

4 pounds spareribs
1 cup Teriyaki sauce
  (or low-salt substitute)
½ cup water
3 tablespoons red wine
1 tablespoon sugar
  (or sugar substitute)

1 teaspoon salt
  (or salt substitute)
1 clove garlic, mashed
Lettuce leaves

Rinse the ribs well. Without cutting completely through the meat, score between each rib.

In a medium bowl, combine all of the remaining ingredients and set aside.

Place the ribs in a large bowl or pot and pour the wine mixture over the ribs. Let the ribs and liquid stand for 1 hour, turning the ribs every 20 minutes.

Remove the meat from the liquid and set the liquid aside.

Place the ribs on a grill preheated with medium coals (or gas grill equivalent) and cook for 1½ hours. Turn frequently and brush with the remaining liquid. (Optional—bake and baste in a roasting pan for 1½ hours at 350°F.)

Separate ribs and serve on a bed of lettuce.

DEVILED EGGS

Serves 6

Add spark to the start of your meal.

6 hard-boiled eggs
Chopped ham, chicken, or
tuna
1 teaspoon Teriyaki sauce
(or low-salt substitute)

2 tablespoons mayonnaise
(regular or low-fat)
Salt (or salt substitute)
Ground black pepper
Large lettuce leaves

Cut eggs lengthwise and remove yolks. Arrange the whites on a cake rack and add meat to each cavity.

Force yolks through a food mill or fine sieve. In a mixer, combine yolks with Teriyaki sauce and mayonnaise. Beat until smooth. Salt and pepper to taste. (Optional—also add anchovy paste, dry mustard, paprika, dried basil, or lemon juice.)

Use a pastry bag with a large star tube and spoon mixture into it. Hold pastry bag close to egg white cavity and force mixture through the tube, moving in a zigzag to form a pattern.

Place on a tray lined with large lettuce leaves and serve chilled.

SPINACH-EGG PIE

Serves 6–8

A satisfying taste tickler for the wonderful meal to follow.

Pastry for 1 eight-inch pie
crust
1 pound spinach washed,
cooked, and drained
4 eggs
1 cup sour cream
(or low-fat substitute)

¾ cup soft bread crumbs
1 tablespoon butter
(or low-fat substitute), melted
2 tablespoons grated Swiss
cheese (regular or low-fat)
Plain or flavored dry bread
crumbs

Preheat oven to 450°F.

Roll the pastry to ⅛-inch thickness and fit loosely into an 8-inch pie pan. Using a fork, prick sides and bottom of pastry well and bake until set but not brown (5 minutes).

Remove from oven and lower temperature to 350°F.

Coarsely chop the spinach, drain well, and spread spinach over the pastry.

Break the eggs over the spinach and cover them with the sour cream.

Combine the soft bread crumbs, butter, and cheese and sprinkle over the filling. Return to oven and bake until the eggs are set (15–20 minutes).

Remove from oven, sprinkle with the dry bread crumbs, and serve hot, or chill and serve cold.

MUSHROOM DELIGHTS   *Serves 10–15*

A special treat that will have your guests talking for weeks.

1 large package (8 ounces) cream cheese (or low-fat substitute)	1 large onion, minced
	¹₂ pound mushrooms, chopped
	¹₄ teaspoon dried sweet basil
¹₂ cup butter at room temperature (or low-fat substitute)	¹₂ teaspoon salt (or salt substitute)
	Ground black pepper
1¹₂ cups our	2 tablespoons our
3 tablespoons butter (or low-fat substitute)	¹₄ cup sweet or sour cream (or low-fat substitute)

Mix cream cheese and ½ cup butter thoroughly. Add 1½ cups flour and blend with fingers or pastry blender until smooth. Chill 30–45 minutes.

Preheat oven to 450°F. Lightly grease and flour a cookie sheet.

On a floured surface, roll out dough to a thickness of ⅛ inch. Use a 3-inch biscuit cutter to cut out rounds. Set aside and prepare mushroom filling.

In a skillet, combine 3 tablespoons butter and the minced onion, and heat until light brown. Add mushrooms, and stir and cook, without boiling, for 3–4 minutes.

Reduce heat and add the remaining ingredients to the skillet and cook, without boiling, until thickened.

Place a teaspoon of mushroom filling on each round and fold the dough over the filling. Press the edges together with a fork. Use the fork to prick the top crust for venting. Bake on the cookie sheet for 20 minutes or until crust is light brown.

TUNA AND CHEESE CANAPES   *Serves 6–8*

A simple but elegant snack or luncheon starter.

1 cup grated Swiss cheese
   (regular or low-fat)
½ cup canned tuna in oil
   (or in water), drained
2 tablespoons cooking sherry
   (or other dry wine)

Ground black pepper
12 slices toast
   (white or whole wheat)

Preheat oven to 350°F.

In a medium bowl, combine Swiss cheese, tuna, and wine. Add pepper to taste and blend the mixture well.

Toast bread lightly, spread mixture on the toasted slices, and bake for 5 minutes.

SPINACH RAITA   *Serves 6*

This little treat can be a cooling accompaniment to spiced foods, particularly dishes typical of India.

6 ounces fresh spinach,
   washed and trimmed
1 large cucumber, peeled,
   seeded, and chopped
4 cups plain yogurt
   (or low-fat substitute)

2 teaspoons ground cumin
½ teaspoon ground cardamon
   Salt (or salt substitute)
   Ground black pepper
   Paprika (mild or hot)

Dry spinach leaves and place in a large covered pot containing ⅛ cup of water.

Steam over medium heat until leaves are wilted, 3–4 minutes.

Remove from heat, drain spinach in a colander, and cool to room temperature.

Gently squeeze out remaining liquid and chop spinach fine.

Place cucumber on paper towels to drain excess liquid.

In a medium mixing bowl, combine yogurt, cumin, cardamon, salt (to taste), and pepper (to taste).

Add spinach and cucumber and mix until all ingredients are blended.

Cover and refrigerate for at least 2 hours.

Sprinkle with paprika (to taste) and serve.

MARINATED PORK   *Serves 8–10*

A delectable starter of Korean origin but satisfying to any ethnic taste.

2 thin-cut pork tenderloins	3 cloves garlic, minced
2 cups Teriyaki sauce	2 teaspoons ground ginger
(or low-salt substitute)	¾ cup sesame seeds
3 tablespoons sugar	2 tablespoons peanut oil
(or equivalent substitute)	(or olive oil)
2 tablespoons minced onion	Lettuce leaves

Trim fat from tenderloins.

In a medium bowl, combine Teriyaki sauce, sugar, onion, garlic, ginger, sesame seeds, and oil. Mix thoroughly.

Add pork and marinate in refrigerator, 3 hours. Turn and baste the pork frequently.

Preheat oven to 375°F.

Remove the pork from the liquid and set liquid aside.

Transfer the pork to an oiled roasting pan and roast, uncovered, for 45–50 minutes.

Simmer the liquid for 10 minutes, and place in a suitable serving dish.

Cut the cooked pork into thin slices, place on a bed of lettuce, and serve hot (with toothpicks to pick up the pieces) with the liquid for dipping.

FETTUCCINE WITH CREAM SAUCE   *Serves 6–8*

A delectable dish that has become a tradition since the time that Marco Polo brought pasta back to Italy.

1 pound fettuccine noodles	1 teaspoon Teriyaki sauce
16 cups water	1 teaspoon ground black
1½ teaspoons salt	pepper
(or salt substitute)	½ cup chopped scallion
2 sticks butter, softened	Freshly grated Parmesan
(or low-fat substitute)	cheese (regular or low-fat),
1 cup whipping cream	to be served with the dinner
(or low-fat substitute)	Hot garlic bread
1½ cups grated Parmesan	
cheese (regular or low-fat)	

Preheat oven to 300°F. Place large casserole dish into oven to warm.

In a large pot, combine water and salt and bring to a boil.

Add fettuccine to boiling water and gently stir until strands are well separated (about 1 minute). Once water has returned to a boil, cook until done (7–8 minutes).

Meanwhile, in a medium bowl, combine softened butter, cream, cheese, and Teriyaki sauce. Beat until ingredients are light and fluffy (well mixed).

Drain fettuccine well in a colander and transfer to the casserole dish that has been warming in the oven.

Pour butter-cream mixture over fettuccine, sprinkle top with pepper and chopped scallion, and toss until each strand is well coated.

Serve immediately with additional Parmesan cheese and garlic bread.

FRITTERS À LA SWISS CHEESE   *Serves 6–8*

An hors d'oeuvre that is sure to tantalize the appetite of any guest.

2 cups olive oil
1½ cups Swiss cheese (regular or low-fat), grated
3 tablespoons flour
1 tablespoon dried sweet basil

1 teaspoon coarsely ground black pepper
¼ teaspoon dry mustard
4 egg whites
½ cup plain dry bread crumbs
Lettuce leaves

Place oil into a deep skillet and slowly heat to 375°F (use deep-fry thermometer).

In a medium bowl, combine cheese, flour, basil, pepper, and mustard.

In a bowl with a mixer, beat egg whites until stiff.

Add whites to the bowl containing the other ingredients and mix well.

Make 1-inch fritters (balls) from the mixture and roll each fritter in the bread crumbs.

Deep-fry the fritters until golden brown (1–2 minutes). Do not crowd the fritters when frying.

Drain the fritters on a paper towel.

Before serving, heat fritters in a 375°F oven (5 minutes), place on a bed of lettuce, and serve hot with toothpicks and your favorite dipping sauce.

SWEDISH MEATBALLS   *Serves 8–10*

A standard that is always a taste primer.

2 eggs
1 cup milk (regular or low-fat)
½ cup dry bread crumbs
4 tablespoons butter
    (or low-fat substitute)
½ cup chopped onion
1 pound lean ground chuck
½ pound lean ground pork
½ teaspoon salt
    (or salt substitute)

⅛ teaspoon dried sweet basil
⅛ teaspoon ground allspice
⅛ teaspoon ground cardamon
⅛ teaspoon ground nutmeg
¼ cup flour
    Ground black pepper
1 can (10 ounces) condensed
    beef broth
1 cup heavy cream
    (or low-fat substitute)

In a large bowl, beat the eggs and then combine milk and dry bread crumbs.

Melt 2 tablespoons of the butter in a large skillet and sauté the onion until soft (4–5 minutes). Remove onion with a slotted spoon and add to mixture in the bowl. Add the chuck, pork, salt, basil, allspice, cardamon, and nutmeg. Mix well until all ingredients are blended.

Cover and refrigerate for 1 hour. When chilled, shape mixture into 25–30 meatballs and brown in the large skillet in which the remaining 2 tablespoons butter have been melted. Remove meatballs and place them into a 2-quart casserole.

Preheat oven to 350°F.

Pour off drippings from the skillet and return one fourth to the skillet. Stir in flour; salt and pepper to taste. Heat the skillet while gradually adding beef broth and stir constantly until it boils. Remove from heat, stir in cream until smooth. Pour mixture over meatballs in the casserole and bake covered for 30 minutes. Serve hot.

CALIFORNIA AVOCADO HALVES   *Serves 6*

A sheer delight that will please the palate and stimulate the appetite.

2 tablespoons chili sauce
2 tablespoons ketchup
1 tablespoon white vinegar
2 tablespoons brown sugar
1 teaspoon Worcestershire
  sauce

8 dashes Tabasco sauce
4 tablespoons lemon juice
3 large ripe avocados,
  chilled

In a medium bowl, combine chili sauce, ketchup, vinegar, brown sugar, Worcestershire sauce, Tabasco, and 2 tablespoons of the lemon juice.

Refrigerate 3–4 hours.

When ready to serve, peel avocados and cut them in half lengthwise. Remove the pits and brush the cut sides with the remaining lemon juice; fill the cavities with the sauce, and place on a serving tray.

EGGS MAYONNAISE   *Serves 6–8*

A delicious way to begin any meal.

1¼ cups mayonnaise
  (regular or low-fat)
⅓ cup chili sauce
1 teaspoon grated onion
1 tablespoon dried sweet
  basil
  Dash of cayenne pepper

2 tablespoons white vinegar
1 teaspoon Worcestershire
  sauce
1 teaspoon white horseradish
  (prepared)
10 eggs
3 cups shredded lettuce

In a medium bowl, combine mayonnaise, chili sauce, grated onion, basil, cayenne, vinegar, Worcestershire sauce, and horseradish. Blend well with rotary mixer.

Cover and refrigerate until ready to serve.

Hard-boil the eggs, peel, and refrigerate until ready to serve.

When ready to serve, arrange lettuce on salad plates, cut each egg lengthwise and place two or three halves on each lettuce bed.

Spoon 2 or 3 tablespoons of the mayonnaise mixture over the eggs on each salad plate.

Essential Balance Meals:
Salads, Dressings, and Vegetables

GERMAN POTATO SALAD   *Serves 8*

An old standard that is a complement to any meat meal.

6 large potatoes	¾ cup white vinegar
1 pound bacon (or low-fat substitute)	½ tablespoon dried sweet basil
2 teaspoons coarsely ground black pepper	1 large onion, chopped
	3 tablespoons celery seeds
½ cup sugar	

Place potatoes in a large pot of water heated to boiling and cook until able to be pierced with the tines of a fork. Remove from heat, cool, and peel.

Cut up bacon into 1-inch pieces and place into large skillet over medium heat. Sauté until crisp. Remove bacon and drain on several pieces of paper towel.

Heat bacon drippings while adding pepper, sugar, vinegar, and basil. Mix well and continue to heat until all sugar is dissolved.

Slice potatoes and place into large bowl. Add onion and bacon dripping mixture and blend well.

Add bacon and celery seeds and toss gently a couple of times.

Serve warm or cold.

MUSTARD VINAIGRETTE   *Makes about 1 cup*

Spruce up any salad with this tangy vinaigrette.

¼ cup wine vinegar
1 teaspoon dry red wine
2 tablespoons water
½ cup chicken broth
1 tablespoon Dijon mustard
½ tablespoon dried sweet
  basil

Salt (or salt substitute)
Ground black pepper
1 clove garlic, minced
1½ tablespoons olive oil

In a medium bowl, combine vinegar, wine, water, broth, mustard, basil, salt and pepper (to taste), and garlic. Add oil slowly and whisk continually. Just before serving, whisk thoroughly.

GARDEN SALAD   *Serves 6–8*

A fresh garden salad is a treat to enjoy when you let your imagination run free.

1 head Boston lettuce
½ pound spinach
  (medium leaves)
2 dozen large sorrel leaves
1 small cucumber
4 medium radishes
⅓ cup lemon juice
⅔ cup olive oil

1½ teaspoons salt
  (or salt substitute)
½ teaspoon coarsely ground
  black pepper
1 teaspoon sugar
1 clove garlic, cut in
  quarters

Wash all leafy vegetables well and drain. Break up lettuce leaves into bite-size pieces and place into large salad bowl. After removing midribs from spinach and sorrel leaves, repeat the process for them.

Peel cucumber and thin-slice cucumber and radishes, adding slices to bowl. Cover and refrigerate until ready to use.

In a medium jar with a tight lid, combine lemon juice, olive oil, salt, pepper, sugar, and garlic; shake well and refrigerate until ready to use.

When ready, remove salad bowl and jar from refrigerator, shake jar well, remove cover, and pour over salad. Toss salad until all parts are well coated.

GREEN-GODDESS SALAD   Serves 8

A marvelous blend of vegetables, herbs, spices, and other tasty ingredients.

6 anchovy fillets, chopped	¼ teaspoon salt
1 cup mayonnaise	(or salt substitute)
(regular or low-fat)	¼ teaspoon coarsely ground
¼ cup tarragon vinegar	black pepper
¼ cup chopped fresh basil	½ head Boston lettuce
¼ cup chopped parsley	½ head Romaine lettuce
2 tablespoons chopped onion	3 cups cubed cooked chicken
½ teaspoon dry mustard	4 medium tomato slices

In a small bowl, combine anchovies, mayonnaise, vinegar, basil, parsley, onion, mustard, salt, and pepper. Mix thoroughly and refrigerate for at least 3 hours.

When ready to serve, wash lettuce well and pat dry; break up all lettuce into bite-size pieces and place into large salad bowl.

Put chicken cubes into center of lettuce and pour anchovy dressing onto lettuce and toss lightly until all greens are coated.

Garnish with tomato slices.

KIDNEY BEAN SALAD   *Serves 6*

A tantalizing and unusual salad.

2 cans (16 ounces each) kidney   ¼ teaspoon dry mustard
   beans, drained   2 large sweet onions
⅓ cup wine vinegar   6 sprigs parsley
3 tablespoons olive oil   1 clove garlic
1 teaspoon salt   1 jar (8 ounces) pimentos,
1 teaspoon coarsely ground   drained
   black pepper

In large bowl, combine beans, vinegar, oil, salt, pepper, and mustard. Mix thoroughly.

On a cutting board, chop well the onions, parsley, garlic, and pimentos. Add these to the bowl and mix again.

Refrigerate for at least 1 hour before serving.

ITALIAN SALAD   *Serves 8–10*

Quick and easy to put together, and a delight to serve to family and guests alike.

2 medium cucumbers   2 tablespoons red wine vinegar
2 bunches radishes   1 teaspoon chopped chives
3 oranges, peeled   1 clove garlic, minced
3 tablespoons olive oil   8 large lettuce leaves

Peel cucumbers and slice thin, trim radishes and slice thin, and slice peeled oranges and then halve slices.

In bowl, combine cucumbers, radishes, and oranges. Mix gently.

In another bowl, combine oil, vinegar, chives, and garlic. Mix thoroughly and pour over salad.

Toss salad and serve over lettuce leaves.

HUNGARIAN BEET SALAD   *Serves 8*

This delightfully refreshing salad is a wonderful part of any Essential Balance Meal.

2 pounds red beets
2 tablespoons white vinegar
2 tablespoons water
1 teaspoon salt
(or salt substitute)

1 tablespoon sugar
½ teaspoon caraway seeds
1 teaspoon prepared red
horseradish
4 eggs, hard-boiled

In medium pot of water, cook beets until tender. Pour off water, peel and slice beets, and set aside.

In small bowl, combine vinegar, water, salt, sugar, caraway seeds, and horseradish.

Pour mixture over beets and refrigerate overnight.

Before serving, peel eggs, slice or cut into wedges, and serve as garnish to beets.

LEMON MAYONNAISE   *Serves 6–8*

A simple dressing that complements all green salads.

⅔ cup mayonnaise
(regular or low-fat)
2 teaspoons lemon juice

2 tablespoons heavy cream
(or low-fat substitute)

In small bowl, combine mayonnaise, lemon juice, and cream. Mix thoroughly, cover, and refrigerate until ready to use. Use for any mixed green salad.

THOUSAND ISLAND DRESSING   *Serves 6–8*

A dressing that is very popular.

2 tablespoons pickle relish, prepared

2 tablespoons finely chopped green pepper

2 tablespoons finely chopped red pepper

2 tablespoons finely chopped yellow pepper

2 tablespoons finely chopped onion

1 cup mayonnaise (regular or low-fat)

2 tablespoons chili sauce

2 tablespoons heavy cream (or low-fat substitute)

In small bowl, combine all ingredients, mix thoroughly, cover, and refrigerate until ready to use. Use for any mixed green salad.

CUCUMBER YOGURT DRESSING   *Serves 6–8*

Take advantage of this simple, cool, and satisfying dressing.

1 large cucumber

1 cup plain yogurt (regular or low-fat)

2 cups chopped fresh mint

½ teaspoon salt

¼ teaspoon ground black pepper

Skin cucumber and cut into lengthwise quarters, then cut into thin crosswise slices.

In medium bowl, combine cucumber, yogurt, mint, salt, and pepper. Mix thoroughly, cover, and refrigerate for at least 1 hour before use.

Use for any mixed green salad.

BROCCOLI-CAULIFLOWER SWEET DELIGHT

Serves 4–6

Take advantage of the wonderful combination of cancer-fighting cruciferous vegetables exploding with fiber and vitamins A and C in this savory and flavorful dish.

1 pound broccoli florets	¼ cup seedless raisins
1 pound cauliflower florets	Salt (or salt substitute)
2 tablespoons olive oil	Ground black pepper
3 tablespoons pine nuts	
3 cloves garlic, peeled and flattened	

In a large steamer, place broccoli and cauliflower florets and steam until tender (5 minutes).

Add oil to a large skillet and heat over medium heat. Add broccoli and cauliflower to hot oil and cook until vegetables start to brown (5–6 minutes).

Add nuts, garlic, and raisins, and cook until garlic and nuts are lightly golden and raisins are softened.

Salt and pepper to taste. Serve hot, at room temperature, or cold.

SCALLOPED SWEET POTATOES WITH RED ONIONS
Serves 4

This unusual dish, with its uncompromising nutrition, taste, and texture, will have your family and guests talking for weeks to come.

1 teaspoon olive oil
3 medium sweet potatoes, with skin
2 tablespoons unsalted butter (or low-fat substitute)
2 tablespoons whole-wheat flour
1 tablespoon dried sweet basil
1 tablespoon dried parsley

1 teaspoon dried rosemary
1 teaspoon dried thyme
Salt (or salt substitute)
Ground black pepper
1 cup milk (regular or low-fat)
2 medium onions, sliced thin
½ cup shredded Swiss cheese (regular or low-fat)

Preheat oven to 350°F.

Coat a baking dish with olive oil.

Cut potatoes into ¼-inch slices and place slices into a large pot with enough water to cover the slices. Bring to a boil, then reduce heat, cover, and cook until potatoes are just beginning to feel tender to the touch of fork tines (5–6 minutes). Remove from heat and set aside.

In a medium saucepan over low heat, melt butter, add flour, and stir until mixture is smooth. Add basil, parsley, rosemary, and thyme. Salt and pepper to taste. Slowly add milk and blend until mixture is smooth and thickened. Remove pan from heat.

Overlap one third of the potato slices in the bottom of a baking dish and cover with one third of the onion slices; spoon one third of the sauce over the onions. Repeat this procedure twice more, ending up with three layers of potatoes, onions, and sauce.

Bake uncovered for 20 minutes. Remove from oven, sprinkle with cheese, and return to oven for 10 minutes; serve piping hot.

HERBY GREEN BEANS   *Serves 4–6*

Take advantage of this simple but tasty vegetable dish.

2 tablespoons butter
(or low-fat substitute)
½ cup chopped scallions
1 pound green beans, washed
and trimmed
1 can (28-ounces) tomato puree

¼ teaspoon dried sweet basil
¼ teaspoon dried rosemary
½ teaspoon salt
(or salt substitute)
¼ teaspoon ground black
pepper

In a large skillet over medium heat, melt butter, and sauté scallions for 3 minutes.

Add green beans and sauté for 2 more minutes.

Add tomato puree, basil, rosemary, and salt and pepper.

Cover, reduce heat, and simmer until beans are tender (8–10 minutes).

Serve hot or cold.

STIR-FRIED VEGETABLES   *Serves 6*

This tangy, wonderful combination of nature's bounty is a memorable addition to any meal prepared for a gathering of family or friends.

¾ cup water
1 teaspoon Teriyaki sauce
(or low-salt substitute)
1 teaspoon sesame oil
2 teaspoons sugar
8 black Chinese mushrooms,
soaked and sliced
2 tablespoons olive oil
1 clove garlic, crushed
½ teaspoon minced ginger
root

4 cups bean sprouts
3 cups sliced Chinese cabbage
2 carrots, peeled and sliced
(½-inch pieces)
4 scallions, sliced
1 teaspoon cornstarch in
2 tablespoons water
Salt (or salt substitute)
Ground black pepper
3 cups cooked rice

Prepare all vegetables prior to cooking.

In a medium saucepan, combine ½ cup water, 1 teaspoon Teriyaki sauce, sesame oil, and sugar. Add mushrooms and simmer over low heat until liquid is almost absorbed.

In a wok over medium-high heat, add olive oil and briefly fry garlic and ginger. Quickly add bean sprouts, cabbage, carrots, and scallions, and stir-fry for 2–3 minutes.

Add mushroom mixture and remaining ¼ cup water to vegetable mixture in wok. Bring to a boil and add cornstarch dissolved in water. Stir until thickened. Season with salt and pepper (to taste).

Serve hot over rice. Embellish with your favorite garnish.

ORANGE-PECAN SQUASH   *Serves 6–8*

A wonderful dish for the fall or any time of the year.

4 small acorn squash, halved and seeded

1½ tablespoons brown sugar

1½ tablespoons butter (or low-fat substitute)

1 tablespoon grated orange peel

3 tablespoons fresh orange juice

¼ teaspoon salt (or salt substitute)

3 tablespoons pecans, chopped

Preheat oven to 350°F.

On a greased baking sheet, place squash halves cut face down and bake until tender (30–35 minutes).

Scoop out pulp into a medium bowl until only thin shell is left.

Combine pulp, brown sugar, butter, orange peel, orange juice, and salt. Stir until mixture is fluffy.

Spoon mixture into all of the shells and sprinkle with pecans.

Place in oven and bake until tops just begin to brown (10–12 minutes).

Essential Balance Meals: Soups

CREAM OF CAULIFLOWER SOUP   *Serves 6*

This easy-to-make and quick soup is just right as a warm-up for the main dish.

2 cups cauliflower florets
4 tablespoons butter
(or low-fat substitute)
½ cup sliced onion
2 large stalks celery, chopped
with leaves

3 cups chicken broth
2 cups heavy cream
(or low-fat substitute)
2 tablespoons chopped
parsley
Coarsely ground black pepper

In a medium pot of boiling water, cook cauliflower until soft (10 minutes). Remove cauliflower, pour off water, and set pot aside.

In a medium bowl, mash the cauliflower and set aside.

In the pot used for the cauliflower, melt butter over medium heat, then add onion and celery. Cook until onion is soft (4–5 minutes).

Add broth and cauliflower and heat to boiling. Reduce heat and add cream. Stir continually for 5 minutes without allowing soup to boil. Turn off heat and serve.

After soup has been spooned into each bowl, sprinkle with parsley and black pepper to taste.

PUMPKIN SOUP

Serves 6

This delightful soup is best served as a Halloween surprise but can be enjoyed any time of the year.

4 cups milk (regular or low-fat)
4 cups pumpkin, canned
2 tablespoons butter
 (or low-fat substitute)
3 tablespoons brown sugar

Salt (or salt substitute)
Coarsely ground black
 pepper
1 pinch ground nutmeg
1 cup diced lean cooked ham

In a medium pot, heat milk until scalded. Add pumpkin, butter, brown sugar, salt and pepper (to taste), nutmeg, and ham. Mix thoroughly and heat, but do not boil, for 3 minutes. Serve immediately.

CORN CHOWDER

Serves 6

An unusual soup that is tasty and filling.

1 tablespoon butter
 (or low-fat substitute)
½ cup chopped salt pork
4 tablespoons chopped
 onion
½ cup chopped celery
4 tablespoons chopped red
 pepper
1 cup peeled and diced
 potato
2½ cups water
¼ teaspoon salt
 (or salt substitute)

¼ teaspoon dried thyme
¼ teaspoon ground black
 pepper
¼ teaspoon Teriyaki sauce
 (or low-salt substitute)
½ bay leaf
3 teaspoons flour
2 cups milk
 (regular or low-fat)
2 cups whole-kernel corn,
 canned
Chopped parsley

In medium skillet, melt butter, add pork, and lightly brown all pieces. Add onion, celery, and red pepper, and sauté until golden brown.

Add potatoes, water, salt, thyme, pepper, Teriyaki sauce, and bay leaf. Simmer until potatoes are tender (45–50 minutes).

Mix until blended, turn up heat, and bring to boiling. Add flour, milk, and corn, and heat and stir 5 minutes, but do not boil.

Spoon into bowls, sprinkle with parsley, and serve.

FRENCH ONION SOUP   *Serves 6*

This restaurant classic can be easily prepared and enjoyed at home.

¼ cup butter
(or low-fat substitute)
4 cups thinly sliced onion
4 cans (10 ounces each)
condensed beef broth
1 teaspoon salt
(or salt substitute)

6 thick slices French bread
2 tablespoons grated Parmesan
cheese (regular or low-fat)
6 slices Swiss cheese
(regular or low-fat)

In a large pot or kettle, melt butter over medium heat. Add onion and sauté until golden (6–8 minutes).

Add broth and salt, raise the heat, and bring to a boil. Reduce heat, cover pot, and simmer for 30 minutes.

Preheat oven to broil.

Toast bread on both sides.

Place soup into individual ovenproof bowls. Float 1 piece of toast in each bowl, sprinkle Parmesan on top of each piece, and cover with a slice of Swiss cheese. Place bowls in broiler and heat until cheese is bubbly (3–5 minutes).

Handle bowls with pot holders and place each on its own plate to serve. Remember: The bowls just came out of a hot oven.

BEEF AND VEGETABLE SOUP   *Serves 10–12*

A hearty and robust soup that will not only fill the bowl but will help to fill an empty stomach.

2 pounds beef shin
2 large marrow bones
1 teaspoon salt
  (or salt substitute)
4 cups thinly sliced cabbage
8 carrots, peeled and cut into
  2-inch pieces
1 cup chopped celery
½ cup chopped green peppers
2 cups chopped onion
1 can (28 ounces) whole
  tomatoes, with liquid
1 can (12 ounces) whole-kernel
  corn

½ cup canned or frozen cut
  green beans
½ cup canned or frozen lima
  beans
½ cup canned or frozen peas
2 cups peeled and cubed
  potatoes
1 small can tomato paste
2 tablespoons chopped parsley
1 teaspoon sugar
½ teaspoon ground cloves
  Ground black pepper

Fill a large pot or kettle with 4 quarts of water and stir in salt. Place beef and marrow bone into pot, cover, and bring to boil. When boiling, skim surface.

Add cabbage, carrots, celery, peppers, onion, and tomatoes. Bring to boil, lower heat to simmer, and cover. Cook 30 minutes.

Add remaining ingredients and salt and pepper to taste; cover and simmer 3½ hours.

Remove pot from heat, remove meat and bones, and separate meat from bones. Discard bones.

When meat is cool, cut into cubes, return to the pot with the broth and vegetables, and refrigerate pot overnight.

Skim fat from surface and discard. Place pot over low-medium heat and bring soup slowly to boil. Remove from heat and serve piping hot.

A good crusty bread makes a nice addition to the meal.

OLD-FASHIONED SPLIT-PEA SOUP *Serves 4*

A wonderful lunchtime or dinnertime soup that will satisfy friends and family alike.

1½ cups split green peas, quick cooking	½ teaspoon sugar
	⅛ teaspoon dried thyme
2½ pounds cooked ham shank	2 cloves garlic, split
4 cups chicken broth	1 bay leaf
1 cup chopped onion	¼ teaspoon salt
½ cup chopped celery	(or salt substitute)
½ cup peeled carrot, cut into coins	¼ teaspoon coarse black pepper

Fill a large pot or kettle with 1 quart of water, add peas, and bring to a boil. Reduce heat, cover, and simmer for 45 minutes.

Add all remaining ingredients, cover, and simmer for 1½ hours.

Remove pot from heat, take out ham shank and cool, and then cut meat from the bone. Dice meat and set aside.

Remove vegetables and liquid from pot, press though coarse sieve, and return to pot. Add diced ham to pot and slowly reheat, uncovered, until soup is hot (15–20 minutes).

Serve plain or with a garnish.

CREAM OF ASPARAGUS SOUP *Serves 6*

A wonderful change of pace that can be served either hot or cold.

2 cups canned asparagus, chopped	½ cup sour cream (or low-fat substitute)
1 large can cream of asparagus soup	¼ teaspoon dried thyme
	Salt (or salt substitute)
1½ cups heavy cream (or low-fat substitute)	Ground black pepper
	½ cup water
½ teaspoon dried sweet basil	Additional sour cream or cut asparagus spears

In a large blender, add all ingredients (except the ½ cup of water) and blend at high speed until mixture is smooth (2–3 minutes).

Pour into refrigerator container and refrigerate overnight. Add water. Serve cold or hot.

Garnish with sour cream or cut asparagus spears.

MINESTRONE SOUP
Serves 8–10

A rich and hearty Italian soup that always satisfies the appetite.

1 cup dried large white beans	1 small zucchini, sliced
½ cup dried lentils	1 bay leaf
1 quart water	1 cup peeled and diced
½ pound salt pork, chopped	potatoes
8 cups beef broth	Salt (or salt substitute)
1 medium onion, chopped	Ground black pepper
1 cup tomato puree	1 cup peas, fresh or frozen
½ cup garbanzo beans,	¼ cup pasta elbows
canned, drained	Parmesan cheese
1 cup diced carrots	(regular or low-fat)
2 stalks celery, diced	

In small bowl with enough water to cover, add beans and lentils, and soak overnight.

When ready to begin cooking, to a large pot or kettle, add 1 quart water and pork, and heat to boiling. Reduce heat immediately and simmer 10–15 minutes.

Drain beans and lentils and add to pot; simmer until all beans are tender to touch of fork tines (1 hour).

Add broth, onion, tomato puree, garbanzos, carrots, celery, zucchini, and bay leaf. Simmer for 20 minutes.

Add potatoes, salt and pepper (to taste). Simmer until potatoes are beginning to be tender to the touch of fork tines.

Add peas and pasta and cook until pasta is tender (10–12 minutes). Add water if soup is too thick.

Serve hot or cold. Sprinkle Parmesan cheese over top of soup in each bowl when serving.

CREAM OF AVOCADO SOUP   *Serves 4–6*

A delicious and wonderful use for what is left over when you wish to grow an avocado plant from an avocado seed.

2–3 avocados, peeled and seeded
2 cups heavy cream (or low-fat substitute)
2 cups chicken broth

1 tablespoon lemon juice
Salt (or salt substitute)
Coarsely ground black pepper
Dill weed, fresh or dried

To a food processor or blender, add avocados, cream, broth, lemon juice, and salt and pepper (to taste). Blend until smooth.

Place in container and refrigerate for at least 3 hours. Serve hot or cold with dill weed garnish.

ZUCCHINI BISQUE   *Serves 10–12*

An especially good use of one of the most productive plants in your (or your neighbor's) garden in late summer.

2 cups chicken broth
2½ pounds unpeeled zucchini
1 medium onion, chopped
Salt (or salt substitute)
Ground black pepper

¼ pound butter (or low-fat substitute)
⅛ teaspoon ground nutmeg
½ cup heavy cream (or low-fat substitute)

To large saucepan, add broth.

Slice zucchini and add to saucepan along with onion, salt and pepper (to taste), butter, and nutmeg. Simmer 10 minutes.

In two batches, puree in food processor or blender.

Place puree into large saucepan and add cream, mixing thoroughly. Serve hot or cold.

Essential Balance Meals:
Beef, Veal, Pork, and Lamb

BEEF-AND-POTATOES CASSEROLE   *Serves 12*

A satisfying dish for the hearty and light eater alike.

Butter (or low-fat substitute)
2 medium turnips
2 medium potatoes
¾ pound lean chopped beef
(or low-fat substitute)
1 large onion
1½ cups sliced mushrooms
¼ teaspoon dried sweet basil
¼ teaspoon dried rosemary
1 cup green peas
(fresh or frozen)

¼ cup chopped fresh
parsley
Salt (or salt substitute)
Ground black pepper
1 tablespoon unsalted butter
(or low-fat substitute)
2 tablespoons flour
1 cup beef broth or bouillon
¼ cup flavored dry bread
crumbs

Coat a baking dish with butter. Set aside.

Peel turnips and potatoes, cut each in half, and place in a large pot of water. Boil turnips and potatoes until soft. Drain, cool, and cut into ¼-inch slices. Set aside.

Coat a large skillet with butter, heat; add beef and cook until lightly brown. Remove beef and set aside in medium bowl. Pour off excess fat and return 2 teaspoons to the skillet.

Preheat oven to 350°F.

Thin-slice onion and add all but 6 slices of onion to skillet. Cook over medium heat until onion is tender. Add mushrooms, basil, and rosemary, and cook until mushrooms are tender. Add salt and pepper (to taste).

Line bottom of the baking dish with turnip and potato slices. Cover with beef-onion mixture. Repeat layering until you end up with a layer of turnips and potatoes on top.

In a small saucepan, melt unsalted butter, mix in flour until blended, then add broth and over low-medium heat stir until thickened.

Pour thickened sauce over the top of the casserole, top with remaining onion slices, cover, and bake for 40 minutes.

Remove cover, sprinkle with flavored bread crumbs, and bake 10 more minutes.

Serve piping hot.

STEAK AND WINE   *Serves 6–8*

This simple gourmet dish adds good hearty taste to fine cooking.

5 pounds thick, lean sirloin steak

1 clove garlic, cut in half

⅓ cup olive oil

1½ teaspoons salt (or salt substitute)

½ teaspoon coarsely ground black pepper

1¼ teaspoons dried sweet basil

½ cup dry red wine

1 tablespoon butter (or low-fat substitute)

Preheat oven to 350°F.

Dry steak with paper towel and rub each side with garlic. Set remaining garlic aside.

Put oil in a large skillet and place over high heat until very hot.

Brown steak very well on both sides, 3–5 minutes each side.

Remove from heat and place steak in a shallow roasting pan; add salt, pepper, and basil; add reserved garlic.

Using top third of oven, bake for 25 minutes. Remove steak from pan and keep warm in oven.

Pour off excess fat from pan, remove garlic, add wine, and bring to a brief boil, stirring to loosen brown particles.

Remove from heat, stir in butter, and use as sauce.

Cut steak into thinly sliced diagonals and serve with sauce on the side.

BRISKET POT ROAST   *Serves 10*

This good old standard never loses its appeal to the nose and the palate.

Salt (or low-salt substitute)
Ground black pepper
5–6 pounds brisket of beef
1 large onion
2 large carrots

4 stalks celery
1 large green pepper
1 large tomato
1 cup water (or more, as needed)

Preheat oven to 350°F.

Salt and pepper beef to taste. Place beef in large skillet and, over high heat, brown fat side.

Slice onion thin, cut peeled carrots and celery into 1-inch pieces, and quarter each carrot piece. Seed and slice green pepper. Peel tomato and cut into moderate-size chunks.

Placed browned meat into a large roasting pan. Add remaining ingredients.

Place in oven, cover, and roast until tender (2½–3 hours). Check occasionally to see that water has not cooked away.

Remove from oven and place meat on serving platter and keep warm.

Prepare gravy by straining pan juice, removing vegetables from the juice, and pressing the vegetables through a food mill.

Combine pan juice and pressed vegetables, heat thoroughly, and serve with roast.

VEAL SURPRISE   *Serves 6*

Meat loaf is meat loaf, but veal loaf is always a welcome change and a taste delight.

2 tablespoons olive oil	1½ pounds finely ground
1 large onion	veal
1 large green pepper, chopped	2 large egg whites
3 large carrots, peeled	1 cup plain dry bread crumbs
2 cloves garlic, minced	Salt (or salt substitute)
2 large ripe plum tomatoes	Ground black pepper
2 tablespoons dried sweet basil	¼ cup flavored dry bread
4 tablespoons cooking sherry	crumbs

Preheat oven to 350°F.

Using 1 tablespoon olive oil, coat a loaf pan or small casserole.

Chop onion and green pepper and cut carrots into ⅛-inch coins and set each aside.

In saucepan, heat remaining 1 tablespoon olive oil. Add garlic, chopped onion, and green pepper, and cook over low-medium heat for 3–4 minutes. Add tomatoes (and any residual juice), carrots, basil, and sherry. Simmer and stir for 10 minutes.

In a large bowl, combine veal, egg whites, heated vegetable mixture, and plain bread crumbs; salt and pepper (to taste), and thoroughly mix.

Transfer contents of bowl to loaf pan or casserole, pat gently down uniformly, sprinkle with flavored bread crumbs, and bake 1 hour.

BEEF-VEGETABLE STEW   *Serves 6*

A rich, hearty main course that will satisfy the fussiest tastes.

3 pounds lean stew beef
8 tablespoons olive oil
1 large onion, chopped
1 large green pepper, chopped
1 cup sliced celery
½ cup water
1 can (10 ounces) condensed beef broth
1 can (8 ounces) tomato sauce
4 tablespoons chopped chives
2 cloves garlic, finely chopped
1 tablespoon salt (or salt substitute)

¼ teaspoon ground black pepper
1 tablespoon dried sweet basil
2 bay leaves
3 large potatoes, peeled and quartered
12 baby carrots, peeled and cut in half lengthwise
6 small white onions, peeled
2 tablespoons water
2 tablespoons flour

Cut beef into 1-inch cubes.

Place oil and one third of meat into a large Dutch oven and brown meat on all sides over medium heat. Remove browned meat and, with no additional oil, repeat process for each succeeding one third of meat.

After all meat is browned and removed from pan, add onion, pepper, and celery to the pan and sauté about 6–8 minutes.

Return all of the beef to the pan, add water, broth, tomato sauce, chives, garlic, salt, pepper, basil, and bay leaves. Bring to a boil, reduce heat, cover, and simmer for 1 hour.

Add potatoes, carrots, and onions. Cover and continue to simmer for another 1–1½ hours (until meat and vegetables are tender to the touch with a fork).

Mix water with flour, stir into beef mixture, cover, and simmer for 10 minutes.

CLASSIC NEW ENGLAND BEEF DINNER

Serves 8

A remarkably simple dinner to prepare but a joy to the taste.

5 pounds corned beef brisket	8 medium carrots, peeled
1 clove garlic	6 large potatoes, peeled and
2 whole cloves	quartered
12 black peppercorns, whole	12 small white onions, peeled
2 bay leaves	1 medium head cabbage

Rinse corned beef and place into a kettle of cold water, just enough to cover the meat. Add garlic, cloves, peppercorns, and bay leaves.

Bring to a boil, reduce heat, and simmer for 5–6 minutes. Skim off surface, cover, and continue to simmer (3–3½ hours).

Add carrots, potatoes, onions. Cut cabbage into 8 wedges and add to the pot; cover and simmer for an additional ½ hour.

Remove meat from pot, slice thinly across the grain. Remove vegetables and serve along with the meat.

A nice mustard sauce is a fine addition.

STUFFED CABBAGE ROLLS *Serves 5–6*

A mainstay for Hungarians and Romanians alike, this seldom-made delight is both easy to prepare and wonderful to eat.

4 quarts water
1 large head green cabbage
1 pound lean ground chuck
½ cup raw white rice
1 medium onion, grated
2 medium eggs, beaten
1 teaspoon salt (or salt substitute)
⅛ teaspoon ground allspice
¼ cup water
1 large onion, sliced

Sauce:
2 cans (8 ounces each) tomato sauce
1 can (12 ounces) tomatoes
⅓ cup lemon juice
¼ cup water
1 teaspoon salt (or salt substitute)
⅛ teaspoon ground black pepper
¼ cup light brown sugar

Place water into a large pot and bring to a boil. Add cabbage and simmer until leaves are pliable (3–4 minutes). Remove cabbage and drain.

Without damaging them, remove 12 large leaves from cabbage and trim the thick rib of each leaf.

Preheat oven to 375°F.

In a large bowl, combine meat, rice, grated onion, eggs, salt, pepper, allspice, and water. Blend well with fork.

Place about ¼ cup of the meat mixture into the hollow of each cabbage leaf. Fold sides of leaf over filling, rolling up leaf from the thick end, and hold each leaf together with a wooden toothpick.

In the bottom of a Dutch oven or in a large pot, place several extra cabbage leaves. Add cabbage rolls, seam side down. Top with onion slices.

In a large bowl, combine tomato sauce, tomatoes, lemon juice, ¼ cup water, salt, and pepper. Pour over cabbage rolls.

Bring to boil over medium heat.

Sprinkle with sugar, cover, and bake 1½ hours covered and 1½ hours uncovered.

VEAL CHOPS AND OLIVES

Serves 8

A simple, quick dish to prepare, tender, and with a delicate texture and flavor that are sure to be long remembered.

8 tablespoons butter
(or low-fat substitute)
8 thick loin veal chops
2 tablespoons chopped onion
1 clove garlic, chopped

½ cup finely diced lean ham
¼ cup pitted and chopped
green olives
1 teaspoon Teriyaki sauce
(or low-salt substitute)

In a large skillet, heat butter; add chops and brown both sides over medium heat.

Add onion, garlic, and ham and stir over medium heat until onion is transparent.

Turn chops, cover, and cook over low heat for 20 minutes. Remove chops to a platter and keep warm.

Add olives and Teriyaki sauce to the skillet and heat for 1 minute. Serve chops and pour ingredients of skillet over the chops.

SWEET AND PUNGENT PORK

Serves 6

A new twist on an Oriental cuisine favorite that is a wonderful contrast in flavors, complementing white rice and Chinese tea.

1½ pounds lean pork, cut into
1-inch cubes
2 cups water
1 teaspoon salt
(or salt substitute)
¼ cup Teriyaki sauce
(or low-salt substitute)
1 clove garlic, quartered
⅓ cup sugar

¼ cup cornstarch
1 cup wine vinegar
½ cup apricot syrup (drained
from following ingredient)
⅔ cup apricot halves in heavy
syrup
½ teaspoon coarsely ground
black pepper

In a large saucepan combine pork, water, salt, Teriyaki sauce, and garlic. Bring to a boil, reduce heat, cover, and simmer gently (50–60 minutes). Remove garlic and discard. Remove meat and set pan with broth aside.

In a clean saucepan, combine sugar, cornstarch, vinegar, and syrup until well mixed.

Add broth from the original saucepan, and cook and stir over medium heat until sauce becomes semiclear and thick.

Add pork cubes, apricots, and black pepper, and mix thoroughly. Heat thoroughly. Serve over white rice.

BAKED PORK CHOPS AND APPLES　*Serves 6*

This simple recipe highlights the delightful taste of pork.

6 thick lean pork chops
1½ teaspoons dried sweet basil
Salt (or salt substitute)
Ground black pepper
1 pound carrots, peeled and cut into coins

2 cups sliced onion
1 pound Granny Smith apples
¼ cup light-brown sugar

Preheat oven to 350°F.

Rinse off pork chops.

On a nonabsorbent surface like waxed paper, combine basil and salt and pepper (to taste). Dip both sides of chops into the seasoning.

In a baking dish or medium casserole, arrange a layer of carrot coins. Cover with half the onion slices.

In a slightly overlapping pattern, arrange chops and sprinkle with remaining seasoning. Cover everything with remaining onion slices.

Peel and quarter apples, being sure to remove core. Distribute apple quarters uniformly over chops and sprinkle with brown sugar.

Cover and bake for 2½ hours. Remove cover, baste, and bake 30 minutes uncovered.

Cool for 5–10 minutes and serve with a garnish.

ROAST PORK WITH HERBS   *Serves 6–8*

A hearty dish that satisfies the fussiest meat eaters.

3½ pounds lean loin of pork
1 tablespoon chopped chives
1 tablespoon chopped onion
1 teaspoon chopped garlic
2 tablespoons flour
1 teaspoon salt
  (or salt substitute)
⅛ teaspoon ground black
  pepper

1 teaspoon dried sweet basil
1 teaspoon dried sage
¼ teaspoon dried thyme
¼ teaspoon dried oregano
¼ teaspoon Teriyaki sauce
  (or low-salt substitute)
1½ cups water

Preheat oven to 375°F.

Rinse off pork, insert meat thermometer near but not on the bone in meaty part, and place meat, fat side up, in shallow roasting pan.

Roast uncovered until thermometer reads 185°F (2½–3 hours). Remove meat and keep warm.

Pour off drippings from pan, returning all meat juice and 1 tablespoon of the fat.

Add chives, onion, and garlic and sauté over medium heat (3 minutes). Remove from heat, stir in flour until smooth; add salt, pepper, basil, sage, thyme, oregano, and Teriyaki sauce.

Slowly add the water, mixing continuously. Bring to a boil and mix until gravy is thick and smooth. Reduce heat and simmer (2 minutes). Place gravy in server and pass around with the pork.

PORK CHINESE STYLE   *Serves 4*

An interesting pork dish using leftover pork roast that will highlight
a festive meal.

3 tablespoons olive oil
½ cup chopped onion
1½ cups cooked lean pork, cut
 into small thin strips
1½ cups chicken broth
½ cup thinly sliced celery
1 cup sliced mushrooms
1 cup bean sprouts

2 tablespoons cornstarch
¼ teaspoon sugar
 Salt (or salt substitute)
 Ground black pepper
2 tablespoons Teriyaki sauce
 (or low-salt substitute)
2 tablespoons water
 Chinese noodles

In a skillet heat oil. Cook onion until transparent.
Add pork, broth, celery, mushrooms, and sprouts. Simmer 5 minutes.
In small bowl combine cornstarch, sugar, salt and pepper (to taste),
Teriyaki sauce, and water. Add to skillet with simmering pork and
stir over medium heat until thickened.
Serve over a bed of Chinese noodles.

STUFFED PORK CHOPS   *Serves 4*

A pork delight with an imaginative twist that will surprise your guests.

4 double-rib lean pork chops
2 tablespoons olive oil
1 teaspoon sesame oil
1 medium onion, chopped
2 cups mushrooms, chopped
1 cup dry flavored bread
 crumbs

 Salt (or salt substitute)
 Ground black pepper
¼ teaspoon dried sage
2 tablespoons sour cream
 (or low-fat substitute)
¼ cup water

Preheat oven to 350°F.
Cut pockets in the pork chops.

Add olive and sesame oil to a deep skillet and heat. Add onion and sauté until soft.

Stir in mushrooms and cook for 2 minutes. Add bread crumbs, salt and pepper (to taste), and sage. Mix thoroughly. Add sour cream to moisten mixture.

With a spoon fill the pocket in each chop with the stuffing mixture. Seal each opening with a wooden toothpick. Add water to a baking pan and arrange the chops in the pan.

Bake, covered, for 30 minutes, remove cover, and continue baking for 30–45 more minutes. Serve with your favorite sauce or a garnish of parsley.

GLAZED SMOKED SHOULDER BUTT   *Serves 6–8*

A holiday favorite that will brighten the spirits and fill the belly.

3 pounds lean smoked pork
  shoulder butt, fully cooked
½ cup water
1 can (9 ounces) crushed
  pineapple
¼ cup brown sugar, packed
  firmly

¼ teaspoon ground cinnamon
⅛ teaspoon ground cloves
¼ teaspoon dry mustard
2 tablespoons white vinegar
4 canned apricot halves cut in
  half

Preheat oven to 375°F.

Cut the pork into 1-inch-thick slices and place, in an overlapping fashion, in a deep, large baking dish.

Add water and bake 30 minutes. Remove from oven and discard liquid.

In a small saucepan, combine remaining ingredients and stir continually while bringing to a boil. Reduce heat and simmer for 3 minutes.

Pour mixture over pork slices and bake for 30 minutes.

Pour excess sauce into a serving dish, and serve along with the meat. If desired, garnish with sprigs of parsley.

BAKED VIRGINIA HAM
Serves 20–24

This holiday tradition can be enjoyed at any time of the year, festive occasion or not.

10–12 pounds lean Virginia ham
Whole cloves
1 cup dark brown sugar, firmly packed
1 teaspoon dry mustard
3 tablespoons fresh orange juice
1 tablespoon white vinegar

In a large pot of water, soak ham for 24 hours.

Remove ham, scrub surface with stiff brush, and rinse well in cold water.

Place ham in a large pot and cover with water to 1 inch above ham. Bring water to boil and reduce heat. Cover and simmer 4–5 hours.

Remove from heat and allow to cool in liquid.

Preheat oven to 325°F.

Remove ham from liquid and remove excess fat and skin.

Using a small sharp knife, cut ¼-inch-deep parallel lines, 1 inch apart, diagonally across the long axis of the ham. Repeat the cuts perpendicular to the first set of cuts. This should form a pattern of diamonds on the surface of the ham. Insert one clove, pronged end up, in the center of each diamond.

Insert meat thermometer in center, away from the bone, and place ham on rack in a shallow roasting pan.

Place in oven, uncovered, for 2½ hours.

In a mixing bowl, combine remaining ingredients, remove ham from oven, and spread mixture over ham surface. Bake until thermometer reads 155–160°F. Let stand for 20 minutes, then slice and serve.

VEAL WITH PEPPERS
Serves 4

The delicate flavor of veal with peppers is a wonderful and surprising change for the palate.

4 large green peppers, cut in
  eighths
1 tablespoon olive oil
½ pound veal, cut into thin
  strips
2 teaspoons sugar
  Salt (or salt substitute)

1 cup chicken broth
1 teaspoon cornstarch
1 teaspoon Teriyaki sauce
  (or low-salt substitute)
1 teaspoon dried sweet basil
2 tablespoons water

Place peppers in a saucepan of boiling water, cover, and parboil (3 minutes). Drain immediately and set aside.

In a large skillet heat oil, add veal, stir often, and sauté for 2 minutes.

Add peppers, sugar, salt (to taste), and broth. Cover and simmer for 10 minutes.

In a small mixing bowl, combine cornstarch, Teriyaki sauce, basil, and water. Add to veal and stir until thickened (2–3 minutes). Serve over rice or pasta.

ROAST LEG OF LAMB   *Serves 6*

A light and tender dish that is right all year long.

5 pounds lean leg of lamb, trimmed	Lemon juice
	Sesame oil
1 clove garlic, slivered	Salt (or salt substitute)
1 teaspoon dried rosemary	Ground black pepper

Preheat oven to 300°F.

Cut small slits in surface of lamb and insert slivers of garlic. Rub surface of meat with rosemary, lemon juice, and oil. Salt and pepper to taste.

Insert meat thermometer in center of roast.

Place a rack in a roasting pan and set meat on rack; roast until desired temperature is reached for rare (140°F—about 1 hour), medium (160°F—about 1¼ hours), or well done (175°F—about 1½ hours).

Remove meat and set on warming tray for 20 minutes.

Carve and serve with pan gravy.

SWEDISH LEG OF LAMB   *Serves 8*

A delicious main course that goes well with many of your favorite side dishes.

4 pounds lean leg of lamb	2 tablespoons sugar
1 teaspoon salt	1 teaspoon dried thyme
¼ teaspoon ground black pepper	2 tablespoons flour
¾ cup black coffee	1½ cups milk (regular or low-fat)
1 tablespoon heavy cream (or low-fat substitute)	2 teaspoons currant jelly

Preheat oven to 350°F.

Place a rack in a shallow roasting pan.

Insert meat thermometer in meat away from the bone. Place meat into the roasting pan, place in oven, uncovered, and roast (½ hour).

In a medium mixing bowl, combine salt, coffee, cream, sugar, and thyme, and mix well. Pour over the meat and continue to roast until the thermometer reaches 175°F (about 1 more hour).

Remove meat, let stand in warm place for 20 minutes, and then slice and serve hot.

For gravy, brown flour and combine with drippings, milk, and currant jelly. Stir over low heat until blended.

STUFFED SHOULDER OF LAMB   *Serves 6*

An elegant main course that delights the eye, the nose, and the palate.

3 teaspoons butter	Peel of 1 lemon, grated
(or low-fat substitute)	Salt (or salt substitute)
1 cup mushrooms, diced	Ground black pepper
1 clove garlic, minced	¼ cup soft bread crumbs, fresh
½ pound ham, minced	2 eggs, lightly beaten
1 tablespoon chopped fresh dill	1 lean boned shoulder of lamb,
¼ cup onion, chopped	pocketed for stuffing

Preheat oven to 300°F.

Place butter in a large skillet and melt. Add mushrooms and sauté.

Add garlic, ham, dill, onion, lemon peel, salt and pepper (to taste), bread crumbs, and eggs and mix thoroughly.

Stuff meat pocket with mixture and tie string around meat to hold pocket closed.

Place a rack in a roasting pan, place meat on the rack, and place pan into the oven. Roasting time will be about 20 minutes per pound.

SKEWERED SPICED LAMB   *Serves 4*

A simple but wonderful kebab that can be done in almost no time at all but will receive rave reviews from your diners.

1 pound boneless lamb	½ teaspoon ground cinnamon
1 small onion, chopped fine	1 tablespoon hot paprika
3 cloves garlic, chopped fine	¼ cup beef broth
1 teaspoon ginger root, grated	Salt (or salt substitute)
1 teaspoon finely chopped	Ground black pepper
parsley	2 tablespoons sesame oil
2 tablespoons red wine vinegar	

Cut lamb into 1½-inch cubes and place in a medium mixing bowl.

In another medium mixing bowl, combine the remaining ingredients and mix thoroughly.

Transfer lamb to bowl containing liquid mixture and make sure all of the meat is covered with liquid. Refrigerate overnight. Turn at least once while in the refrigerator.

Heat broiler or grill, remove bowl from refrigerator, thread meat on metal skewers, and place 4–5 inches away from source of heat; cook for 10 minutes. Baste meat several times with the remaining liquid.

Serve hot on a bed of rice or lettuce.

BROILED LAMB CHOPS   *Serves 8*

Known mostly as a meat used in Middle Eastern cooking, lamb can be a wonderful meat prepared in "Western" fashion.

8 lean lamb chops, double thick	Ground black pepper
6 tablespoons olive oil	1 teaspoon paprika
2 cloves garlic, sliced	8 pats of butter
2 teaspoons dried sweet basil	(or low-fat substitute)
1 teaspoon dried thyme	2 tablespoons lemon juice
Salt (or salt substitute)	8 parsley sprigs

Rinse chops and set aside.

In a large bowl combine oil, garlic, basil, and thyme; mix well. Add chops and marinate. Refrigerate for 2 hours.

Remove chops and place on a broiling rack. Place the rack about 2 inches from the heat source. Brown each side for 5 minutes (10 minutes total). Transfer chops to heated serving dish, salt and pepper to taste, put one pat of butter in the center of each chop, sprinkle with lemon juice, and place a sprig of parsley on top of each pat of butter.

Serve with your favorite vegetables and potatoes or rice.

LAMB CURRY

Serves 4

An all-time favorite in the Mideast and always a change of pace at home for either the family or guests.

¼ cup butter
  (or low-fat substitute)
1 teaspoon sesame oil
4 medium scallions, chopped
1 clove garlic, chopped
1 pound cubed boneless lamb shoulder
1 cup plain yogurt
  (regular or low-fat)

1 teaspoon grated ginger
1 tablespoon dried sweet basil
2 teaspoons ground coriander
¼ teaspoon ground cinnamon
½ teaspoon ground cardamon
¼ teaspoon ground cloves
½ teaspoon ground curry

Place butter and oil into a medium pot and melt butter over moderate heat.

Add scallions and garlic and sauté until scallions are soft. Remove scallions and garlic and set aside.

Add the lamb to heated pot and brown on all sides.

Return scallions and garlic and add all remaining ingredients. Mix thoroughly and coat all sides of lamb. Cover and continue to simmer for 30 minutes.

Serve with rice or couscous.

RACK OF LAMB

Serves 5–6

Almost any cut of lamb can be prepared well, but one of the all-time favorites is the simple but tasty Rack of Lamb.

3 pounds rack of lean lamb
1 teaspoon salt
  (or salt substitute)
1 clove garlic, sliced in half

½ cup apricot preserves
¼ cup lemon juice
  Ground black pepper

Preheat oven to 300°F.

Cover end of each rib with aluminum foil to avoid burning. Rub lamb with salt and garlic. Avoiding the bone and the fat, insert a meat thermometer into the approximate center of the rack.

In a shallow roasting pan place a roasting rack and then the lamb, fat side up.

Do not cover. Place in oven and roast 30 minutes.

In the meantime, in a medium bowl combine apricot preserves, lemon juice, and pepper (to taste).

Remove pan from oven and spoon half of the glaze on the lamb. Without covering, return the pan to the oven and continue to roast the lamb for 30 more minutes.

Remove the pan from the oven and repeat the glaze process with the remainder of the glaze. Return the pan to the oven and roast until desired temperature is reached (175°F for medium and 185°F for well done).

Serve with your favorite vegetables and mint jelly.

Essential Balance Meals:
Poultry and Seafood

SWEET AND SOUR CHICKEN   *Serves 4*

This Chinese delight is always welcome.

2 whole chicken breasts	1 cup sugar
2 whole chicken legs	2 tablespoons cornstarch
⅓ cup flour	¾ tablespoon white vinegar
½ cup olive oil	1 tablespoon Teriyaki sauce
Salt (or salt substitute)	(or low-salt substitute)
Ground black pepper	¼ teaspoon ground ginger
1 can (8 ounces) pineapple	1 chicken bouillon cube
chunks	1 large green pepper

Preheat oven to 350°F.

Wash and pat dry chicken parts. Roll each piece in the flour.

Heat oil in large skillet, add a few chicken pieces, and brown both sides. Remove to shallow roasting pan and repeat the process for the remaining pieces of chicken.

Arrange the chicken pieces skin side up, or if skin is removed, skinned side up. Salt and pepper (to taste). Set aside.

Drain liquid from pineapple chunks into 2-cup measure and add enough water to make 1½ cups of liquid.

In a medium saucepan, combine pineapple liquid, sugar, cornstarch, vinegar, Teriyaki sauce, ginger, and bouillon cube.

Over high heat, bring to a boil and continue heating (2 minutes). Remove from heat and pour contents over chicken in pan.

Bake uncovered for 20 minutes.

Clean and slice the pepper into ½-inch-wide strips. Add pineapple chunks and pepper strips to the chicken and bake until chicken is tender (an additional 30–40 minutes).

Serve over a bed of white rice.

GOLDEN-FRIED CHICKEN   *Serves 4*

A main course that is right at any time of the year.

3½ pounds broiler-fryer, cut in eighths	Ground black pepper
¼ cup flour	2 cups vegetable oil (or shortening)
¼ cup flavored bread crumbs	Parsley sprigs
Salt (or salt substitute)	

Wash chicken pieces and damp-dry with paper towel.

In a 1-gallon plastic bag combine flour, bread crumbs, and salt and pepper (to taste). Add two pieces chicken at a time, shake to coat evenly with mixture, and remove to plate. Repeat process until all pieces of chicken have been coated.

To an electric skillet, add oil and heat to 375°F.

Add chicken, a few pieces at a time, and brown all sides. Remove to a clean plate. Repeat process until all pieces have been browned.

Carefully drain all fat from skillet and then return 2 tablespoons fat to skillet. Reduce heat to 300°F and add all chicken pieces, skin side down (if skinned, that side down).

Cover and cook 30 minutes. Uncover, turn all pieces over, and cook uncovered for 15 minutes.

Remove chicken and place on serving platter. Garnish with parsley sprigs and serve hot.

GOLDEN ROAST TURKEY   *Serves 12–15*

You need no special occasion for this holiday favorite that can also be enjoyed at other times of the year.

12 cups white bread cubes	13–16 pound turkey, ready to cook
¼ cup dried sweet basil	1 tablespoon butter
½ cup chopped parsley	(or low-fat substitute),
2 teaspoons salt	melted
(or salt substitute)	Powdered garlic
½ cup butter	Paprika
(or low-fat substitute)	Coarsely ground black
3 cups chopped celery	pepper
1 cup chopped onion	Salt (or salt substitute)

Preheat oven to 325°F.

In a large bowl, combine bread cubes, basil, parsley and salt. Mix well.

In medium skillet add butter and heat. When butter is hot, add celery and onion, and sauté until golden (8–10 minutes).

Add contents of skillet to bread mixture and blend well. Set dressing aside.

Remove all excess parts, wash turkey inside and out, dry well, and set aside.

Spoon dressing into neck cavity until filled and then spoon remaining dressing into body cavity. Using poultry pins and twine, lace up body cavity opening. Tie leg ends together and secure wing tips. Insert meat thermometer into thickest part of inner thigh.

Place the turkey on a roasting rack and the rack into a shallow roasting pan. Brush outside of turkey with butter and sprinkle on garlic powder (to taste), paprika (to taste), pepper (to taste), and salt (to taste).

Place open pan into oven and roast turkey until thermometer reaches 185°F (4½ hours). A loose tent of foil placed over turkey 2–3 hours into roasting process will reduce the amount of browning.

Remove from oven and place turkey on a large serving platter. Remove any poultry pins, twine, and foil. Remove all stuffing and place into a large bowl. Place bowl into warm oven that has been turned off. Let turkey stand for 20–30 minutes and then carve.

Serve with stuffing and any gravy and relishes that you desire.

CHICKEN PAPRIKA   *Serves 4–6*

A simple but wonderful recipe of Hungarian origin that is now enjoyed by people of many nationalities.

6 pound roaster chicken
3 tablespoons butter
  (or low-fat substitute)
3 tablespoons olive oil
2 cups chopped onion
2 cloves garlic, minced
3 tablespoons mild paprika

2 teaspoons salt
  (or salt substitute)
2 cups chicken broth
2 teaspoons flour
2 cups sour cream
  (or low-fat substitute)

Cut chicken into eighths and wash all parts. Set aside.

To a large, heavy pot add butter and olive oil, and heat until butter is melted.

Add onion, garlic, and paprika. Simmer until onion is golden brown.

Add salt and broth and bring contents of pot to a boil. Reduce heat to a simmer, add chicken, cover, and cook until chicken is tender (1 hour).

In a small bowl, combine flour and sour cream.

Reduce heat to just below boiling and slowly stir mixture into the pot containing the chicken. Heat, but do not boil, for 5 more minutes.

Served traditionally on wide noodles, but tastes just as wonderful on a bed of rice.

STUFFED CHICKEN BREASTS   *Serves 6*

This dish is for those times that you would like something elegant but simple and quick to prepare.

6 large chicken breasts, boned and skinned	½ cup minced shallots
8 tablespoons butter (or low-fat substitute)	12 medium mushroom caps
	1½ cups dry wine
6 thin slices Virginia ham	1 cup chopped tomato
6 small and thin pieces of Swiss cheese (regular or low-fat)	⅓ cup heavy cream (or low-fat substitute)
	⅓ cup chopped parsley

Rinse chicken breasts and beat with mallet or cleaver until very thin.

In a large skillet heat butter until hot but not browning. Take one piece of chicken, move it around in the hot butter until no longer pink (2–3 minutes), and immediately place on a large, flat dish.

On one half of the top of the breast place a piece of ham and a piece of cheese. Fold other half over first half and secure with a toothpick.

Repeat process for each breast.

To drippings in the skillet add shallots and mushrooms and sauté about 3 minutes.

Add wine and tomato and simmer for 3 more minutes, then add cream.

Without boiling, add stuffed chicken breast to sauce and simmer for 3 minutes, turning the pieces once or twice.

Sprinkle with parsley and serve over noodles or rice.

CHICKEN CACCIATORE   *Serves 6*

A marvelous dish with tomato sauce and mushroom base that delights the nose and tickles the palate.

2-pound broiler-fryer, cut into eighths
3 tablespoons olive oil
2 tablespoons butter (or low-fat substitute)
1 large can (15 ounces) tomato sauce
1 large can (2 pounds) whole tomatoes
Salt (or salt substitutte)
Ground black pepper
¾ cup dry red wine
1 teaspoon dried oregano
1 teaspoon dried sweet basil
2 tablespoons chopped parsley
½ teaspoon minced garlic
4 tablespoons flour
3 tablespoons water
12 medium mushrooms

Wash and pat dry all chicken parts.

In a 6-quart pan, combine oil and butter, and heat.

Place 4 pieces of chicken on bottom of pan, brown well on both sides, and remove from the pan. Repeat for the remaining pieces of chicken.

Return all browned chicken parts to the pan and add tomato sauce, whole tomatoes, salt and pepper (to taste), wine, oregano, basil, and parsley. Cover and simmer until chicken is tender (45–50 minutes).

In a small bowl, combine flour and water, then pour into pan and stir.

Add mushrooms and cook until sauce is thickened (10–15 minutes).

YOGURT CHICKEN BREASTS
Serves 6

A tradition among Mideast, Russian, and Indian cultures, yogurt is used to give chicken a succulent flavor that allows blended spices to penetrate the meat, making the eating a joy.

3 whole chicken breasts, with bone but skinned
1½ cups plain yogurt (regular or low-fat)
3 cloves garlic, minced
3 teaspoons dried tarragon
Salt (or salt substitute)

Pepper
3 teaspoons olive oil
1 medium onion, sliced thin
1½ cups mushrooms, sliced thin
3 teaspoons cornstarch
⅓ cup water

Preheat oven to 350°F.

Rinse chicken, pat dry with paper towel, and set aside on a dish.

In a medium bowl, combine yogurt, garlic, tarragon, salt and pepper (to taste).

Place chicken in a large, shallow pan and spoon contents of bowl over the chicken. Let stand 7–8 minutes and then turn over and let stand again (7–8 minutes).

While chicken marinates, place oil in a large skillet and heat. Add onion and mushrooms and sauté (2 minutes).

In a small dish, combine cornstarch and water. Mix well. Pour into skillet with onion and mushrooms and stir until thickened.

Remove chicken from shallow pan and place into casserole or baking dish.

Add skillet contents to marinade and mix thoroughly. Pour over chicken, cover, and bake 25 minutes. Uncover, and bake until chicken is tender to the tines of a fork (10–15 minutes).

Serve with rice or noodles.

BLACK PEPPERCORN TUNA $\quad$ *Serves 4*

This wonderful peppery dish will wake up and delight any palate.

1 tablespoon crushed black pepper
2 tablespoons Teriyaki sauce
2 tablespoons lemon or lime juice

4 teaspoons olive oil
4 medium tuna steaks
¼ cup chicken broth
¼ cup dry white wine
4 thin lemon slices

Preheat broiler.

In a small bowl, combine pepper, Teriyaki sauce, and juice. Mix and set aside.

Coat thinly both sides of each steak with olive oil, place steaks on a broiling tray, and broil each side for 5–6 minutes. Turn off heat but leave tuna in oven.

In a large skillet over medium-high heat, combine pepper mixture, broth, and wine. Stirring continually, cook over high heat until sauce is light brown. Reduce heat to low, remove tuna from oven, and lay steaks in skillet and sauté 1 minute for each side.

Place steaks on plates, pour remaining sauce over steaks, and garnish with lemon slices.

SHRIMP IN WINE SAUCE $\quad$ *Serves 4*

One of the all-time favorites, shrimp can be used in so many creative ways to delight the taste.

2 teaspoons olive oil
1 medium onion, chopped
3 cloves garlic, cut in quarters
1 cup dry white wine
½ cup chicken broth

1 pound medium shrimp, shelled and deveined
Salt (or low-salt substitute)
Coarse black pepper
¼ cup lemon juice

In a large skillet over low heat, add oil, onion, and garlic, stir well, and cook over medium heat until onion begins to turn golden.

Mix in wine and broth, turn heat up full, and cook until liquid starts to boil. Reduce heat and simmer for 2 minutes.

Add shrimp and quickly mix, coating all shrimp. Cover and cook until shrimp all turn pink (4–5 minutes).

With slotted spoon, transfer shrimp to serving dish, add salt and pepper (to taste), and lemon juice, and pour contents of skillet over shrimp. Serve plain or with rice.

BAKED FISH WITH WINE   *Serves 4*

A perfect finish to a successful fishing venture in which you eat the one that "didn't get away."

1½ pounds fillets of fish	1 teaspoon Teriyaki sauce
4 tablespoons butter	(or low-salt substitute)
(or low-fat substitute)	12 medium mushroom caps
1 cup dry white wine	Sprigs of fresh parsley
1 clove garlic, minced	4 lemon wedges
Ground black pepper	

Preheat oven to 350°F.

Rinse off fillets and set aside.

Grease a large baking dish using 1 tablespoon butter.

Pour wine over all fillets, sprinkle with garlic and pepper (to taste), and dot each fillet with butter (2 tablespoons in total). Place tip of meat thermometer into the deepest part of thickest fillet and place dish into oven. Bake until done (thermometer reaches 140°F).

Add remaining butter to a medium skillet and melt over medium heat.

Cut mushroom caps in half and add, along with Teriyaki sauce, to the hot skillet. Sauté until mushrooms are soft (3–4 minutes).

Remove dish from oven, transfer fillets to serving plates, and pour dish liquid over fillets.

Garnish with mushrooms and parsley, and serve with lemon wedges.

BROILED LOBSTER TAILS   *Serves 4*

No matter how it is prepared, the best part of the lobster is the tail, and here is one simple way to enjoy this delicacy.

4 medium-large lobster tails
¼ cup lime juice
¼ cup olive oil
1 teaspoon mild paprika
1 teaspoon salt
    (or salt substitute)

1 clove garlic, minced
1 teaspoon dried tarragon
1 teaspoon dried sweet basil
1 tablespoon butter
    (or low-fat substitute)

Preheat broiler.

Using a strong scissors, carefully cut along both sides of the undercover of tail and remove.

In a large shallow dish, combine lime juice, olive oil, paprika, salt, garlic, tarragon, and basil. Mix well and marinate lobster tails for 3 hours.

Remove tails from marinade, slightly crack upper shell with a cleaver, and bend sides up so that tails will lie flat. Lightly coat the exposed meat with butter. Broil 5 minutes a side.

Place on plates and serve with melted butter and any desired side dishes.

BATTER FRIED SHRIMP   *Serves 6*

A restaurant favorite that can be prepared and served at home with little muss or fuss.

2 teaspoons salt
    (or salt substitute)
½ teaspoon coarse black
    pepper
1 clove garlic, minced
4 eggs, separated

2 tablespoons butter
    (or low-fat substitute),
    melted
1½ cups flat beer
2 pounds medium shrimp,
    shelled and deveined

In a medium bowl, combine salt, pepper, garlic, egg yolks, and melted butter. Mix thoroughly, cover, and refrigerate (4 hours or more). Just prior to use, beat egg whites and fold into batter. Preheat deep-fryer to 370°F.

Coat shrimp with batter and deep-fry until golden brown. Drain on paper towel, set on platter, and serve. You may wish to serve with lemon wedges, tartar sauce, or any relish that you find pleasing.

FILLETS OF SOLE WITH HERBS   *Serves 6*

From the Pacific Northwest to your table in a matter of 25–30 minutes of cooking time.

2 fillets of sole	½ teaspoon minced garlic
½ cup butter	2 tablespoons chopped chives
(or low-fat substitute)	Salt
2 tablespoons lime juice	Paprika
1 tablespoon dried tarragon	Parsley sprigs

Preheat oven to 350°F.

In a small skillet, melt butter and use half to brush on fillets. Sprinkle with lime juice.

Grease a large baking dish and arrange fillets in dish. Cover dish, place in oven, and cook until fish flakes at touch of fork tines (18–20 minutes).

To melted butter remaining in skillet, add tarragon, garlic, chives, and salt and paprika (to taste).

Serve fish, heat skillet contents slightly, and pour over fish. Garnish with parsley sprigs if desired.

BREADED FISH FILLETS

Serves 6

A quick and easy main course that is healthful and satisfying.

2 pounds fish fillets	6 tablespoons butter
1 egg	(or low-fat substitute)
½ cup seasoned dry bread	Parsley sprigs
crumbs, packaged	6 lemon wedges

Rinse fillets, pat dry on paper towel, and cut into serving-size pieces.

Spread bread crumbs on large dish or platter.

In a small dish, beat egg with fork. Dip fish in egg, moistening both sides, and then into crumbs, coating both sides well.

In large skillet heat butter until quite hot. Add enough fish pieces to cover the bottom of the skillet. Reduce heat to medium and sauté until golden brown (4–5 minutes). Turn pieces over and sauté other side (4–5 minutes).

Remove to serving platter, garnish with parsley and lemon wedges, and serve. You may add your favorite relish or sauce.

FRIED CLAMS

Serves 5–6

One of nature's greatest ocean bounties is the clam, and one of the best ways to serve clams is what we describe here.

2 cups sour cream	1 quart clams, shucked
(or low-fat substitute)	1 egg
4 tablespoons sweet pickle	¼ teaspoon paprika
relish	1 cup flavored dry bread
1 teaspoon salt	crumbs, packaged
(or salt substitute)	½ cup butter
½ teaspoon Tabasco sauce	(or low-fat substitute)
2 teaspoons garlic, minced	

In a small bowl, combine sour cream, sweet pickle relish, salt, Tabasco sauce, and minced garlic. Mix thoroughly.

Refrigerate sauce for 2 hours or more.

Drain clams and set aside. Reserve 2 tablespoons of clam liquid.

In a small bowl, combine clam liquid, egg, and paprika. Mix thoroughly.

In another small bowl, place the bread crumbs. Dip clams in egg mixture, then roll in bread crumbs.

In a large skillet, add butter and melt over medium heat. When butter is hot, sauté clams until done (3–4 minutes each side).

Drain on paper towel and serve with sour cream sauce.

Essential Balance Meals: Desserts

CREAM CHEESE CAKE   *Serves 12–14*

A creamy delight for either the family, a buffet, or a dessert party. It can be eaten plain or topped with your favorite glaze.

Crust:
2½ cups graham crackers, packed
¼ cup sugar
½ cup butter
(or low-fat substitute)

Filling:
3 large packages (8 ounces each) cream cheese (regular or low-fat)

3 tablespoons grated lemon peel
1 cup sugar
½ cup brown sugar, firmly packed
Butter for greasing pan (or low-fat substitute)
3 tablespoons flour
4 eggs
1 teaspoon vanilla
½ cup lemon juice

In medium bowl, combine cracker crumbs, sugar, and butter until thoroughly mixed.

Grease a baking dish (12 × 8 × 2 inches) and, with the back of a large spoon, press crumb mixture to the bottom and sides of the dish.

Preheat oven to 350°F.

In a large electric mixer bowl, gently beat softened cream cheese, lemon peel, sugar, and flour until well mixed.

Add eggs, vanilla, and lemon juice and mix until smooth.

Pour mixture into crust and bake until center of filling appears firm (35–40 minutes) when dish is shaken.

Cool completely, refrigerate for at least 4 hours, and serve.

BANANA FRITTERS
Serves 6

This wonderful dessert is worth the effort.

1 cup flour
1 tablespoon sugar
1 teaspoon baking powder
1 teaspoon salt
(or salt substitute)
2 eggs
½ cup milk
(regular or low-fat)
1 teaspoon corn oil
½ teaspoon vanilla

1 teaspoon grated lemon peel
3 large, semiripe bananas, peeled
1 tablespoon lemon juice
3 cups salad oil or vegetable shortening
Flour
Confectioners' sugar

In a small mixing bowl combine flour, sugar, baking powder, and salt, mixing thoroughly.

In medium mixing bowl, combine eggs, milk and corn oil, vanilla, and lemon peel, and mix thoroughly.

Mixing continually, slowly add the contents of the small bowl and mix until the mixture is smooth.

Slice bananas diagonally into ½-inch sections and sprinkle each chunk with lemon juice

Heat oil or shortening in a deep skillet (heated contents should be at least 2 inches deep) until a temperature of 375°F is reached (use deep-fry thermometer).

Coat banana chunks with flour; shake off excess. Use a fork to dip coated chunks into mixture in the bowl and then hold ½ inch above hot oil and, using a knife, gently dislodge the chunk so that it falls gently into the oil. Continue with all pieces.

Deep-fry until golden brown, remove with a slotted spoon, and drain on paper towels.

Sprinkle with confectioners' sugar and serve hot.

You may wish to add any topping of your choice.

RICE CUSTARD   *Serves 8*

This is a fine ending for any meal. Not too sweet but rich enough to make anyone feel satisfied.

4 cups water	3 eggs
⅓ cup uncooked regular white rice	½ cup sugar
	¼ cup brown sugar, firmly packed
5 cups milk (regular or low-fat)	2 teaspoons vanilla
1 teaspoon salt (or salt substitute)	¼ teaspoon ground cinnamon
	2 tablespoons sugar

Place water into the bottom of a double boiler. In the top of the double boiler combine rice, 4 cups milk, and salt; mix well.

Heat water to boiling and cook mixture until rice is tender (1 hour), stirring occasionally.

Preheat oven to 350°F. Grease a 2-quart casserole and place into a large baking pan.

In a large bowl, combine eggs, sugar, brown sugar, vanilla, and 1 cup milk. Mix well and then stir in hot rice mixture.

Pour mixture into prepared casserole and pour hot water into baking pan to form a 2-inch-deep layer around the casserole.

Mix cinnamon and sugar together, sprinkle over top of mixture in casserole, and bake uncovered about 1 hour, until the blade of a kitchen knife inserted 1 inch from any edge of the casserole comes out clean.

Remove casserole from water and cool. Then refrigerate at least 3 hours.

Serve plain or topped with whipped cream (or low-fat substitute).

APPLE COBBLER   *Serves 8–10*

Wonderful as a finish to a dinner on a cold winter evening, but also appropriate any time of year.

Filling:

5 cups peeled and sliced Granny Smith apples
1 tablespoon lemon juice
½ cup sugar
¼ brown sugar, firmly packed
2 tablespoons flour
1 teaspoon vanilla
½ teaspoon ground cinnamon
¼ teaspoon salt (or salt substitute)
¼ cup water

2 tablespoons butter (or low-fat substitute)

Crust:

½ cup flour
½ cup sugar
½ teaspoon baking powder
¼ teaspoon salt (or salt substitute)
2 tablespoons butter (or low-fat substitute)
1 egg, beaten lightly

Combine apples, lemon juice, sugar, brown sugar, flour, vanilla, cinnamon, salt, and water in medium bowl. Mix thoroughly.

Empty mixture into baking dish (8 × 8 × 2 inches), smooth out, and dot with butter. Set aside.

Preheat oven to 375°F.

Combine all crust ingredients in medium bowl and beat until smooth.

Drop 9 equally spaced portions of crust mixture onto the mixture in the baking dish. Do not worry about the results. The crust mix will spread during baking.

Bake until apples are tender and the crust is a golden brown (35–45 minutes).

Serve with cream or whipped cream (or low-fat substitutes).

FRESH PEARS IN WINE   *Serves 6*

A light and rewarding finish for the simplest to the most elegant meal.

½ cup water
6 large pears, peeled and
  cored
1 cup sugar

1 cup your favorite dry red
  wine
½ cup orange juice
Grated peel of 1 orange

Add water, pears, and sugar to a large saucepan and place over heat. Cover and simmer until pears are soft (about 30 minutes).

Remove from heat, add wine, juice, and orange peel, and serve hot, if desired, or chill and serve. A dash of whipped cream (or low-fat substitute) is optional.

ICED LEMON SOUFFLÉ   *Serves 6*

A chilled dessert that will warm the hearts of family and guests alike. It leaves a wonderful taste after the dinner is through.

1 tablespoon powdered gelatin
½ cup lemon juice
1 cup egg whites

1 cup sugar
1 cup heavy cream
  (or low-fat substitute)

In a mixing bowl, dissolve gelatin as directed on package.

Add lemon juice to gelatin mixture. Set aside.

In a medium bowl, beat egg whites until foamy only. Add sugar to whites and continue to beat until sugar is dissolved and whites are glossy. Set aside.

In a clean bowl, whip cream until stiff. Gently fold whites and whipped cream into gelatin mixture.

Divide mixture into 6 soufflé dishes and freeze until solid.

Serve plain or with your favorite topping.

APPLE CREAM PIE

Serves 8–10

This is an apple pie with a wonderful hint of cream that will have everyone asking for the recipe.

1 teaspoon sugar	4 Granny Smith apples, peeled
1¼ cups flour	and cored
6 tablespoons butter	½ cup sugar
(or low-fat substitute)	½ cup heavy cream
2 tablespoons vegetable	(or low-fat substitute)
shortening	1 egg
3 tablespoons cold water	1 teaspoon fruit liqueur

Preheat oven to 375°F.

In a medium bowl combine sugar, flour, butter, and shortening. Mix until crumbly. Add water and mix until the ingredients appear to hold together.

Using the back of a spoon, press ingredients into the sides and bottom of a 9-inch pie pan. Place pan into oven and bake until crust is light brown (15–20 minutes). Remove from the oven.

Slice apples into thin pieces, arrange neatly in the pan, and put back in the oven for 15 minutes. Remove from oven and set aside.

In a medium bowl, combine sugar, cream, egg, and fruit liqueur. Mix thoroughly and pour over the apples.

Return pan to oven and cook until custard sets (20 minutes). Cool on rack and sprinkle with cinnamon. Serve either at room temperature or chilled. Top with ice cream or sherbet if you wish.

CHOCOLATE RUGELACH (CHOCOLATE ROLLED COOKIES)

Serves 15–18

A favorite dessert that is always right and seems to disappear almost as fast as you set it out.

8 ounces cream cheese (or low-fat substitute)	⅔ cup ground walnuts
8 ounces butter (or low-fat substitute)	⅓ cup raisins
	2 teaspoons ground cinnamon
¼ cup confectioners' sugar	½ cup dark brown sugar, firmly packed
½ teaspoon vanilla	¼ cup semisweet chocolate chips
2½ cups flour	
Butter (or low-fat substitute)	¼ cup milk chocolate chips
2 tablespoons butter, melted	

Preheat oven to 375°F.

In a small bowl, combine cream cheese and butter. Add sugar and vanilla and mix thoroughly.

Add and mix in flour until mixture is no longer sticky.

Butter and flour the top of a large cookie sheet. Divide dough into three equal parts and roll each part into a circle about ⅛-inch thick.

Brush the top of each circle of dough with melted butter.

Sprinkle each circle with nuts, then raisins, then cinnamon, then sugar, then the semisweet chocolate chips, and finally the milk chocolate chips.

Cut each circle into 12 equal wedges and roll up each wedge (wide edge to narrowed point).

Place on cookie sheet and bake until golden brown (20 minutes).

CRÈME BRÛLÉE

Serves 6

This wonderful longtime French favorite will always be the height of elegance at any dinner.

2 cups heavy cream
(or low-fat substitute)
1 tablespoon vanilla

5 tablespoons sugar
4 egg yolks
Light brown sugar

In a medium saucepan combine cream and vanilla and heat until warm.

In a medium bowl, combine sugar and egg yolks and mix well.

Pour mixture into the saucepan and mix contents thoroughly. Divide mixture into 6 individual oven dishes. Place dishes into a shallow pan filled with 1 inch of water. Place pan into the oven and cook until set (40–50 minutes).

Remove from oven, sprinkle top with brown sugar, place in broiler, and broil until sugar is melted. Serve plain or with any topping that you may find an interesting twist.

LEMON-LIME MERINGUE PIE

Serves 8–10

A delectable classic old-fashioned pie with a little extra zip that will satisfy the sweet tooth and the tummy.

1 cup sugar
⅓ cup cornstarch
¼ teaspoon salt
(or salt substitute)
1 cup water
¾ cup lemon juice

¼ cup lime juice
4 egg yolks
1 tablespoon butter
(or low-fat substitute)
4 egg whites
¼ cup sugar

Prepare any standard pie crust and bake until golden brown. Set aside.

In a saucepan, combine sugar, cornstarch, salt, water, lemon juice, and lime juice. Place over medium heat and stir constantly until thick. Remove from heat.

Add the egg yolks while stirring constantly. Return pan to medium heat until mixture becomes thicker (2–4 minutes).

Remove from heat, add butter, and mix thoroughly, and then pour into crust. Set aside.

Preheat oven to 400°F.

Add egg whites to a clean bowl and beat until foamy. Add sugar and beat until the meringue peaks.

With a spoon, spread meringue over entire surface of pie and make peaks.

Place pie in oven and bake until meringue peaks are golden brown (5–6 minutes).

QUICK AND EASY MOCHA PIE   *Serves 6*

A breeze to prepare for the busy person who wants a quick and easy dessert with which to make friends and influence people.

1 chocolate crust, commercially prepared

1 quart coffee ice cream (or low-fat substitute), softened

4 small Heath English Toffee bars

2 cups whipped cream (or low-fat substitute)

1 tablespoon coffee liqueur

Place ice cream into crust and spread out evenly.

Place Heath bars into sturdy plastic bag and close securely.

With a hammer or some hard instrument, break the Heath bars into small pieces.

In a small bowl, mix the whipped cream and liqueur and then spoon into the crust.

Sprinkle broken Heath bar pieces over whipped cream, freeze (2 or more hours), and serve when ready.

RUM CAKE DELIGHT   *Serves 10–12*

This wonderful variation on a basic recipe is sure to make family and guests sit up and take notice.

Vegetable shortening
Flour
1 box yellow cake mix with pudding
3 eggs
½ cup cold water
⅓ cup vegetable oil

¾ cup rum (light or dark)
1 cup chopped pecans
¼ pound butter (or low-fat substitute)
¼ cup water
1 cup sugar

Preheat oven to 325°F.

Grease and flour a bundt pan.

In a large bowl, combine cake mix, eggs, water, oil, ½ cup rum, and nuts, and mix thoroughly.

Pour the mixture into the bundt pan and place in the oven until golden (1 hour). Set aside to cool.

In a medium saucepan, combine butter, water, sugar, and ¼ cup rum. Heat over medium heat, stirring continually, until butter is melted and sugar is dissolved.

Using fork tines, poke holes on all sides of the cake and spoon hot topping over the cake. Wait briefly between spoonings so as to allow topping to be absorbed into cake.

Serve with your favorite dessert beverage.

CHILLED CRANBERRY CAKE   *Serves 10–12*

An unusual combination of berries and cake that blends well and makes a fine finish to a meal.

2 cups fresh cranberries,
  chopped (or canned
  whole cranberries)
1 large slightly green banana,
  diced
⅔ cup sugar
2 cups crushed vanilla
  wafers

½ cup butter
  (or low-fat substitute)
1 cup confectioners' sugar
2 eggs
½ cup chopped pecans
  (or other nuts)
1 cup heavy cream
  (or low-fat substitute)

In a medium bowl, combine cranberries, diced banana, and sugar. Set aside.

In an 8-×-8-inch pan, add one half wafer crumbs and spread uniformly on the bottom.

In another medium bowl, combine butter and sugar, then add eggs. Mix thoroughly and spread over wafer crumbs.

Add cranberry-banana mixture and spread uniformly over wafer crumbs. Sprinkle chopped nuts over the top.

Whip cream until it forms peaks. Spread whipped cream over the top of the ingredients in the pan and sprinkle remaining wafer crumbs on top of the cream.

Refrigerate before serving (minimally, 4 hours).

CHOCOLATE FUDGE PIE
Serves 8

This one is for all of the chocolate lovers among your family and friends.

¼ cup flour	1 tablespoon vanilla extract
1 cup sugar	1 tablespoon almond
6 tablespoons cocoa	extract
2 eggs	Butter (or low-fat substitute)
½ cup mayonnaise	
(regular or low-fat)	

In a medium bowl, combine flour, sugar, and cocoa. Mix well.

In another medium bowl, beat eggs, then add mayonnaise and mix thoroughly. Add this mixture and the two extracts to the contents of the first bowl and mix everything thoroughly.

Heat oven to 375°F.

Butter an 8-inch pie pan and pour contents into the pan. Bake for 20 minutes.

Serve warm and plain or with your favorite topping for chocolate dishes.

PECAN PIE
Serves 8

A specialty that is easy to prepare.

1 uncooked standard 9-inch	¼ teaspoon salt
pie shell	(or salt substitute)
8 ounces cream cheese	1½ teaspoons vanilla
(regular or low-fat)	1 cup pecan halves
½ cup sugar	1 cup corn syrup
4 eggs	

Preheat oven to 375°F.

In a medium bowl, combine cream cheese, ¼ cup sugar, 1 egg, salt, and ½ teaspoon vanilla. Mix thoroughly until thick and smooth. Pour mixture into pie shell and cover with pecan halves.

In a small bowl, combine 3 eggs, remaining sugar, corn syrup, and remaining vanilla. Mix thoroughly and pour over mixture in pie shell.

Place in oven and bake until set (35–40 minutes).

CHOCOLATE CHIP COFFEE CAKE   *Serves 15–18*

A nice and light dessert that can be served plain or with your favorite topping.

½ cup butter (or low-fat substitute)	1 cup sour cream (or low-fat substitute)
1 cup sugar	2 cups flour
½ cup brown sugar, firmly packed	16 ounces semisweet chocolate chips
2 eggs	1 cup chopped pecans (or any other nuts)
1 teaspoon vanilla	1 teaspoon ground cinnamon
1 teaspoon baking powder	
1 teaspoon salt (or salt substitute)	

Preheat oven to 350°F.

In a medium bowl, combine butter and 1 cup sugar. Mix thoroughly, then add ¼ cup of the brown sugar, eggs, vanilla, baking powder, salt, and sour cream. Blend well.

Slowly add flour and mix until all lumps are gone.

In another medium bowl, combine ¼ cup of the brown sugar, chocolate chips, pecans, and cinnamon to form topping. Mix thoroughly.

Grease and flour a tube pan and sprinkle one fourth of topping on the bottom of the pan.

Alternate the following three times: Pour one third batter into pan and sprinkle surface with topping mixture.

Place in oven and bake (30–40 minutes) until a dry knife edge inserted into the cake comes out dry.

POUND CAKE
Serves 8–10

By itself, a wonderful dessert, but with a little imagination and daring, it can become the base for some of the fanciest endings to a meal.

¾ cup butter
(or low-fat substitute)
2 cups confectioners' sugar
3 large eggs

2 tablespoons brown sugar
1 teaspoon vanilla
1 teaspoon lemon juice
2 cups flour

Preheat oven to 325°F.

In a medium bowl, combine butter and confectioners' sugar and beat until fluffy. One at a time, add eggs and beat thoroughly.

Add vanilla and lemon juice and mix again.

Finally, slowly add flour and brown sugar and mix thoroughly.

Grease 9-×-5-×3-inch loaf pan and pour in the mixture.

Place into oven and bake until golden (1 hour).

Cool and serve plain or with your favorite topping, or glaze with your favorite glaze and serve. Play with ideas.

SCOTTISH PECAN SHORTBREAD
Serves 10–15

You don't need to have a burr or wear kilts to make this simple but wonderful dessert.

2 cups butter
(or low-fat substitute)
1 cup sugar

1 cup pecans, chopped
2 cups flour

Preheat oven to 300°F.

In a medium bowl, combine butter and sugar, mixing thoroughly. Add pecans and flour and mix again.

In your hands, knead dough until it appears blended.

Divide the dough into four equal parts.

Take one quarter of the dough and, on a floured board, roll into a 9-inch circle about ¼-inch thick. Cut the circle into 8 wedges immediately and transfer to a large greased cookie sheet. Using fork tines, prick each wedge several times.

Repeat the process for each remaining quarter. Use a second greased cookie sheet if necessary.

Place sheets in oven and bake until the wedge edges barely turn brown.

Essential Balance Meals:
Vegetarian Choices

VEGETARIAN "BEEF" CASSEROLE   *Serves 6*

This elegant casserole dish is guaranteed to satisfy dietary standards and the taste buds.

2 teaspoons olive oil	1 clove garlic, minced
3 large potatoes, peeled and quartered	1 cup fresh green peas
	½ cup chopped parsley
3 large turnips, peeled and quartered	Salt (or salt substitute)
	Ground black pepper
1 pound vegetarian "beefsteaks"	1 tablespoon butter (or low-fat substitute)
1 large onion, sliced thin	2 tablespoons flour
2 cups mushrooms, sliced	1 cup water
½ teaspoon dried rosemary	1 tablespoon Teriyaki sauce
½ teaspoon dried sweet basil	(or low-salt substitute)

Coat a large casserole with 1 teaspoon oil. Set aside. In a large pot of water, boil potatoes and turnips until tender to touch of fork tines. Remove, cool, and cut into semithin slices. Set aside.

Coat a large skillet with remainder of oil, heat over medium heat, and cook "beefsteaks" until light brown. Remove from skillet, place in small bowl, and set aside.

Preheat oven to 350°F. Place skillet back over medium-low heat, add all but 6 slices of onion to skillet, and heat until onions are soft.

Add mushrooms, rosemary, basil, and garlic. Continue cooking until mushrooms are tender. Stir in peas and parsley, "beefsteaks," and salt and pepper (to taste). Set aside.

Cover bottom of prepared casserole with a layer of one third potatoes and turnips, and top with half of onion-beef mixture. Repeat process once and end with last third of potatoes and turnips on top.

In a small saucepan over low heat, melt butter and mix in flour. When thoroughly mixed, add in water and Teriyaki and heat until thickened. Pour contents of saucepan over contents of casserole; top with remainder of onion slices, cover, and bake for 30 minutes.

Remove cover and bake until light brown (10 minutes). Serve piping hot.

FRIED LEMON VEGETARIAN "CHICKEN"

Serves 6

A tender and juicy dish inside and crisp and golden on the outside. Sure to delight family and guests alike.

3 eggs (or egg substitute)	½ cup oat bran
6 teaspoons lemon juice	Salt (or salt substitute)
½ teaspoon hot paprika	Ground black pepper
6 pieces vegetarian "chicken steaks" (3 ounces each)	1 teaspoon butter (or low-fat substitute)
1 teaspoon dried basil	6 lemon slices
1 teaspoon dried parsley	6 sprigs parsley
2 cups flavored bread crumbs	

In medium bowl, combine eggs, 3 teaspoons lemon juice, and paprika. Mix thoroughly.

Add "chicken steaks" and coat both sides, leaving "steaks" in bowl.

In a large shallow dish combine basil, parsley, bread crumbs, oat bran, and salt and pepper (to taste). Mix well.

Take "chicken" pieces from the egg mixture and dip into bread crumb mixture, coating both sides well. Place coated pieces on a platter and set aside. Preheat oven to 400°F.

Grease a large baking pan with butter and form a single layer of coated "chicken" in the pan. Place pan in oven and bake until golden brown (15 minutes). Remove pan, turn "chicken," and bake until golden brown (10 minutes).

Place "chicken" on serving platter; sprinkle with remaining lemon juice. Garnish with lemon slices and parsley and serve.

FLOUNDER WITH WILD RICE AND WATER CHESTNUTS
Serves 6–8

This tasty dish is worth the effort and goes well with any steamed vegetables such as asparagus, broccoli, or brussels sprouts.

2 cups wild rice	2 cups water chestnuts
6 cups water	½ cup slivered almonds
½ cup Teriyaki sauce (or low-salt substitute)	Salt (or salt substitute) Ground black pepper
3 tablespoons butter (or low-fat substitute)	2½ pounds flounder fillets (or sole fillets)
2 small onions, diced	2 teaspoons lemon juice
2 stalks celery, diced	¼ cup chopped parsley
2 cups mushrooms, sliced	

In a medium pot combine rice, 4 cups water, and Teriyaki sauce. Cook mixture until wild rice is tender (40–50 minutes).

Preheat oven to 350°F. Coat a large baking dish with 1 tablespoon butter and set aside.

Transfer rice and excess liquid to a large mixing bowl.

In a large skillet, over medium heat, melt remaining butter and add onion, celery, and mushrooms. Heat and stir until onions are light brown (3–4 minutes).

Add contents of skillet to bowl with rice. Add water chestnuts, almonds, and salt and pepper (to taste). Toss lightly.

Spoon mixture into greased baking dish, top with fish fillets, and sprinkle with lemon juice. Place in oven and bake until fish flakes with the touch of fork tines (12–15 minutes). Remove from oven, garnish with parsley, and serve immediately.

SEAFOOD-VEGETABLE DELIGHT *Serves 4*

A truly delicious combination dish of tomato stew containing shellfish and fish. Watch for the sighs of delight as your family or guests take their first taste.

1 tablespoon olive oil	1 bay leaf
1 large carrot, chopped	1 teaspoon hot sauce
1 large stalk celery, diced	1 teaspoon dried oregano
1 large green pepper, chopped	¾ pound shrimp, peeled and
1 large red pepper, chopped	deveined
4 large cloves garlic, chopped	3 dozen littleneck clams,
1 large onion, chopped	scrubbed
4 cups canned whole tomatoes,	10 green olives
chopped	10 black olives
1 cup dry red wine	¼ cup chopped parsley
2 small zucchini, sliced	Ground black pepper

In a large, deep skillet over medium-low heat, add oil and coat. Add carrot, celery, green pepper, red pepper, garlic and onion. Sauté until onion is soft (4–5 minutes).

Add tomatoes, wine, zucchini, bay leaf, hot sauce, and oregano. Mix well, raise heat, and cook until small bubbles appear. Reduce heat and simmer 15 minutes.

Add shrimp, clams, green olives, and black olives. Cover and simmer, gently shaking pan from time to time, until clams have been steamed open (5–8 minutes). Discard unopened clams.

Stir in parsley and pepper to taste.

Serve immediately.

VEGETABLE JOY   *Serves 6*

This elegant casserole is truly a vegetarian's joy to see, smell, and feast upon.

1 teaspoon sesame oil
1 tablespoon olive oil
1 cup French-cut green beans
1 small–medium zucchini
1 medium yellow squash
1 green pepper, cubed
1 large can (28 ounces) whole tomatoes
¼ teaspoon dried sweet basil

¼ teaspoon ground black pepper
¼ teaspoon dried marjoram
¼ teaspoon dried sage
¼ teaspoon dried savory
¼ cup dried thyme
½ teaspoon salt (or salt substitute)
6 slices Swiss cheese (regular or low-fat)

Preheat oven to 375°F.

To a large, deep skillet, over medium heat, add sesame oil and olive oil. Add beans, zucchini, squash, and pepper. Fry until tender. Do not overcook.

Add tomatoes with juice and cut tomatoes into pieces in the pan.

Add basil, black pepper, marjoram, sage, savory, thyme, and salt. Mix well, cover, and cook for 5 minutes.

Pour contents of skillet into large casserole, cover with cheese slices, and place into the oven to bake until brown (10–15 minutes).

Serve immediately.

FETTUCCINE WITH AVOCADOS AND VEGETARIAN "SAUSAGE"

Serves 6

A quick recipe that will spark the palate and perk up any family dinner or dinner party for friends.

1 teaspoon butter
(or low-fat substitute)
6 ounces vegetarian "sausage links," chopped
½ teaspoon salt
(or salt substitute)
4 cups water
8 ounces fettuccine, packaged or fresh
½ cup butter
(or low-fat substitute)

1 teaspoon flour
1 cup heavy cream
(or low-fat substitute)
2 avocados, peeled and chopped
1 avocado, peeled and sliced
Parmesan cheese
(or low-fat substitute), grated
Ground black pepper

In a medium skillet over medium heat, melt butter, add chopped "sausage," and cook until golden (4–5 minutes). Set aside.

In a medium pot, combine salt and water, heat to a boil, add fettuccine, and cook until al dente. Drain water and cover pot to keep fettuccine hot.

To a small saucepan over medium heat, add butter, and melt. Add flour, and stir. Add cream, and stir constantly while cooking for 5 minutes.

Briefly heat chopped "sausage" in skillet.

Remove fettuccine and place on serving platter. Pour cream sauce over fettuccine, add chopped avocado, three fourths of "sausage," three fourths of Parmesan cheese, and pepper (to taste).

Garnish with sliced avocado and remaining "sausage," and serve with remaining Parmesan cheese.

VEGETARIAN "BEEF" AND MACARONI CASSEROLE
Serves 4–5

A tantalizing and delightful vegetarian casserole that can be used for any festive occasion.

½ pound macaroni
¾ cup butter
   (or low-fat substitute)
½ cup grated Parmesan cheese
   (regular or low-fat)
4 eggs
½ large onion, chopped
¾ pound vegetarian "beef,"
   ground
¼ medium can tomato sauce

1½ teaspoons ground nutmeg
1 tablespoon dried sweet
   basil
4 tablespoons Teriyaki sauce
   (or low-salt substitute)
⅛ teaspoon ground black
   pepper
1½ tablespoons flour
2 cups milk
   (regular or low-fat)

Preheat oven to 350°F.

Following directions on the package, cook macaroni. Rinse in cold water and drain thoroughly.

In a small pan over medium heat, melt ¼ cup butter, turn off heat and cool. Add two well-beaten eggs. Mix well and stir mixture into macaroni. Set aside.

In a skillet over medium heat, melt ¼ cup butter, and add onion and "beef" and sauté. Add tomato sauce, 1 teaspoon nutmeg, basil, 2 tablespoons Teriyaki sauce, pepper, and ¼ cup Parmesan cheese. Stir constantly while simmering for 10 minutes.

Spoon half of macaroni over bottom of a large baking pan (18 × 12 × 3 inches). Then spoon in entire meat mixture and spread evenly. Cover with the remaining macaroni.

In a medium saucepan, melt ¼ cup butter, gradually stir in flour, and stir constantly and sauté until flour dissolves. Slowly add milk and bring to a low boil while stirring constantly. Cook until sauce thickens (3–5 minutes). Stir in remaining Teriyaki sauce and cool.

Add remaining eggs, one at a time, beating well after each addition.

Pour sauce uniformly over the macaroni and shake the baking pan to allow sauce to distribute below the surface.

Sprinkle surface with remaining Parmesan cheese and nutmeg. Place in oven and bake until custard forms and becomes puffed, firm, and brown (1–1½ hours).

PACIFIC ISLAND VEGETARIAN "CHICKEN"
Serves 6–8

A tropical delight that turns a plain vegetarian dish into a gourmet entrée, bringing on thoughts of tropical palms and warm waves lapping on the beach.

3 pounds vegetarian "chicken"	1½ tablespoons cornstarch
1 cup flour	¾ cup brown sugar, firmly packed
1½ teaspoons salt (or salt substitute)	1½ tablespoons Teriyaki sauce
¼ pound butter (or low-fat substitute)	2 cups cubed papaya
2 cups orange juice	2 cups diced pineapple
3 tablespoons lemon juice	2 cups sliced banana
	1 cup water chestnuts

Preheat oven to 350°F.

In a large plastic bag, combine serving-size pieces of "chicken," flour, and salt. Shake until "chicken" is thoroughly coated.

Grease shallow baking pan with 1 tablespoon butter, and at the bottom of the pan, form a single layer of coated "chicken" pieces.

Melt remaining butter and sprinkle over top of "chicken."

Place pan in oven and bake for 45–50 minutes.

In the meantime, in a large saucepan combine orange juice, lemon juice, cornstarch, sugar, and Teriyaki sauce. Heat over medium flame, continually stirring, until sauce becomes thick and clear.

Add papaya, pineapple, banana, and water chestnuts and mix thoroughly. When baking is finished, remove pan from oven, pour fruit sauce over "chicken" in pan, and return to oven for 10 more minutes.

Serve plain or over a bed of white or brown rice.

BRANDIED VEGETARIAN "BEEF"   *Serves 4*

A wonderful pan-broiled dish that is not only a contrast in flavors but quick and easy to prepare.

4 serving-size pieces of
   vegetarian "beef"
1 tablespoon coarse ground
   black pepper
1½ tablespoons butter
   (or low-fat substitute)
1½ tablespoons olive oil
2 cups sliced mushrooms
½ cup chopped scallion

½ teaspoon hot sauce
½ teaspoon Teriyaki sauce
   (or low-salt substitute)
¼ teaspoon lemon juice
1 teaspoon flour
½ cup dry red wine
2 tablespoons brandy
4 sprigs parsley

Sprinkle both sides of each piece of "beef" with pepper and gently pat in with fingers.

In a large skillet over high heat, add butter and olive oil. When butter foams but does not smoke, lower to moderate heat and sauté "beef" on one side, then turn and do the same on the other side (3–4 minutes per side).

Set "beef" on platter and reduce heat to medium-low. Add to skillet the mushrooms, scallion, hot sauce, Teriyaki sauce, and lemon juice. Stir constantly while cooking for 1 minute.

Add flour and mix well. Add wine and brandy and stir while rapidly bringing to a boil until sauce is slightly thickened (2 minutes).

Place "beef" on serving plates and pour sauce over the "beef."

Garnish with parsley and serve.

VEGETARIAN "BEEF-SAUSAGE" LOAF

Serves 4

Not an ordinary meat loaf, this marvelously satisfying vegetarian dish is rich in fiber and low in calories and fat.

1½ teaspoons olive oil
2 cloves garlic, chopped
2 large scallions, chopped
1 medium tomato, chopped, with juice
⅓ cup chopped fresh basil
½ teaspoon dried oregano
4 tablespoons dry red wine
1 small zucchini, chopped
1 medium green pepper, chopped

½ teaspoon hot sauce
½ pound vegetarian "beef," broken up
½ pound vegetarian "sausage," broken up
¼ cup rolled oats
3 tablespoons oat bran
2 large egg whites, beaten
Salt (or salt substitute)
Coarse black pepper

Preheat oven to 350°F.

Coat loaf pan with ½ teaspoon olive oil. Set aside.

In a saucepan over medium-low heat, combine remaining olive oil, garlic, and scallions, and cook for 3 minutes. Stir several times during cooking.

Add tomato with juice, 2 tablespoons basil, oregano, and wine. Simmer for 10 minutes, stirring occasionally.

In a large bowl, combine contents of saucepan with zucchini, green pepper, hot sauce, "beef," "sausage," rolled oats, oat bran, egg whites, and salt and pepper (to taste). Mix thoroughly.

Transfer to loaf pan and spread uniformly.

Place in oven and cook until golden brown on top (1 hour).

Serve hot or cold. Garnish with remaining basil.

SWEET AND PUNGENT FISH   *Serves 6*

A sweet, spicy, aromatic treat that makes fine use of a fresh catch or purchase.

1 large onion, sliced	1 clove garlic, diced
1 teaspoon minced ginger root	2 large carrots, sliced
3 tablespoons Teriyaki sauce	1 medium onion, diced
¼ teaspoon salt	1 green pepper, diced
(or salt substitute)	¾ cup brown sugar, firmly
¼ teaspoon ground black	packed
pepper	½ cup vinegar
1 teaspoon cooking sherry	1 cup water
6 medium fish fillets	1 tablespoon ketchup
3 tablespoons cornstarch	3 cups vegetable oil
2 teaspoons olive oil	

In a medium bowl, combine onion, ginger root, 1 tablespoon Teriyaki sauce, salt, pepper, and sherry. Mix thoroughly.

Rub mixture on both sides of fillets and let stand 30 minutes.

Sprinkle 2 tablespoons cornstarch on a plate and coat both sides of each fillet. Let stand an additional 5 minutes. Reserve remaining cornstarch.

In a large skillet over medium heat, combine 1 teaspoon olive oil and garlic. Cook until light brown. Add carrots, onion, and green pepper. Fry until just tender to touch of fork tines.

In a small bowl, combine sugar, vinegar, and ½ cup water. Pour mixture into skillet with vegetables and heat to boiling.

In a small bowl, combine remaining cornstarch and water, mix well, and add to skillet. Cook with continual stirring until sauce is thick and clear. Stir in ketchup. Remove from heat.

In another large skillet, heat vegetable oil to 375°F, checking temperature with deep-fry thermometer.

Place fish fillets into oil and fry until golden brown, then turn fillets over and continue until second sides are golden brown.

Drain and serve with sauce over fillets.

VEGETARIAN "CHICKEN" AND BEANS

Serves 6–8

A wonderful variation that is fine for parties or small gatherings.

3 quarts water
1½ cups small white beans
1 large onion, sliced
4 cloves garlic, minced
12 vegetarian "chicken" slices

1½ teaspoons salt (or salt substitute)
½ teaspoon ground black pepper
½ teaspoon paprika

In a large saucepan, combine water and beans. Soak overnight.
Drain water and add fresh water to just cover beans. Add onion and garlic, and cook over medium heat (1½ hours).
Add "chicken" slices, salt, pepper, and paprika. Cook 1 hour more.

VEGETARIAN "SCALLOP" NEWBURG

Serves 4

A delectable dish that can be enjoyed over and over again.

4 tablespoons butter (or low-fat substitute)
2 cups vegetarian "scallops"
⅓ teaspoon ground nutmeg
½ teaspoon paprika
3 egg yolks, beaten

1 cup heavy cream (or low-fat substitute)
¼ cup cooking sherry
Salt (or salt substitute)
Ground black pepper

In a double boiler, melt butter, mix in "scallops," and cook 3–4 minutes.
Add nutmeg and paprika, and cook for 1–2 minutes longer.
Add egg yolks and heavy cream. Stir and cook (do not boil) until liquid is thick.
Add sherry, salt and pepper (to taste), and serve over buttered and toasted bread of your choice.

VEGETARIAN SPAGHETTI WITH "SAUSAGE" AND TOMATO SAUCE

Serves 4–6

A wonderfully tasty dish with a hearty flavor.

2 large cans (28 ounces) whole tomatoes
1 can (12 ounces) tomato sauce
1 large onion, sliced
1 medium clove garlic, minced
½ teaspoon ground allspice
6 whole cloves
2 teaspoons dried sweet basil
1 tablespoon sugar

2 bay leaves
1 teaspoon celery seeds
8 vegetarian "sausage" patties
4 tablespoons olive oil
Salt (or salt substitute)
Coarse ground black pepper
1 pound spaghetti (or other pasta)

In a large saucepan over medium heat, combine tomatoes, tomato sauce, onion, garlic, allspice, cloves, basil, sugar, bay leaves, and celery seeds. Reduce heat and simmer for 1 hour.

In a medium bowl, combine "sausage," 2 tablespoons olive oil, and salt and pepper (to taste).

In a large skillet, heat 1 tablespoon of remaining olive oil. Form "sausage" mixture into balls about 1½ inches in diameter and fry in the oil.

Add "sausage" balls to large saucepan with simmering sauce. Cover and simmer for 1 hour, stirring occasionally. Uncover and simmer for an additional hour, stirring occasionally. If sauce is too thick, add a little water.

In a medium pot of boiling water, add remaining olive oil and spaghetti and cook until your favorite texture is reached.

Serve spaghetti and "sausage" balls on large plates or in large bowls. Add your favorite grated cheese (regular or low-fat).

BAKED MACARONI AND TOMATO DELIGHT

Serves 6

A specialty that is fun to prepare and a delight to eat.

1 large can (28 ounces) whole tomatoes
1 small can tomato paste
½ tablespoon sugar
   Salt (or salt substitute)
   Ground black pepper
1 clove garlic, minced
⅛ teaspoon dried sweet basil
⅛ teaspoon dried chervil

⅛ teaspoon dried marjoram
⅛ teaspoon dried oregano
3 teaspoons olive oil
1 large onion, sliced thin
1 large green pepper, sliced thin
1 pound elbow macaroni
   Thin slices of Swiss cheese (regular or low-fat)

In large frying pan over low heat, combine tomatoes, tomato paste, sugar, salt and pepper (to taste), garlic, basil, chervil, marjoram, and oregano. Cook uncovered for 1 hour.

Preheat oven to 350°F.

In a small frying pan over medium heat, combine 1 tablespoon olive oil, onion, and green pepper. Sauté for 3 minutes.

Cook elbow macaroni according to directions on package. Rinse in cold water.

Use remaining olive oil to coat inside of large casserole. Add in layers the macaroni, sauce, and cheese slices until casserole is full. End with sauce and cheese on top.

Place in oven and bake uncovered until cheese melts (20–30 minutes).

Serve piping hot and sprinkle on your favorite grated cheese.

RISK-REDUCING PERCENTAGE CHART*

Total of Option Points for the Week

Total Profactor-H Self-Evaluation Score

	1–10	11–20	21–30	31–40	41–50	51–60	61–70	71–80	81–90	91-100
96–100	6%	16%	26%	36%	46%	57%	67%	77%	87%	97%
91–95	6%	17%	27%	38%	49%	60%	70%	81%	92%	Optimal Status
86–90	6%	18%	29%	40%	51%	63%	74%	86%	97%	Optimal Status
81–85	7%	19%	31%	43%	53%	67%	79%	91%	Optimal Status	Optimal Status
76–80	7%	20%	33%	46%	58%	71%	84%	97%	Optimal Status	Optimal Status
71–75	8%	21%	35%	49%	62%	76%	90%	Optimal Status	Optimal Status	Optimal Status
66–70	8%	23%	38%	52%	67%	82%	96%	Optimal Status	Optimal Status	Optimal Status
61–65	9%	25%	40%	56%	72%	88%	Optimal Status	Optimal Status	Optimal Status	Optimal Status
56–60	9%	27%	44%	61%	78%	96%	Optimal Status	Optimal Status	Optimal Status	Optimal Status
51–55	10%	29%	48%	67%	86%	Optimal Status	Optimal Status	Optimal Status	Optimal Status	Optimal Status
46–50	11%	32%	53%	74%	95%	Optimal Status	Optimal Status	Optimal Status	Optimal Status	Optimal Status
41–45	13%	36%	59%	83%	Optimal Status	Optimal Status	Optimal Status	Optimal Status	Optimal Status	Optimal Status
36–40	14%	41%	67%	93%	Optimal Status	Optimal Status	Optimal Status	Optimal Status	Optimal Status	Optimal Status
31–35	17%	47%	77%	Optimal Status	Optimal Status	Optimal Status	Optimal Status	Optimal Status	Optimal Status	Optimal Status
26–30	20%	55%	91%	Optimal Status	Optimal Status	Optimal Status	Optimal Status	Optimal Status	Optimal Status	Optimal Status

*Risk-Reduction Percentages are relative and are based on the continuation and combination of Risk-Reducing Options. Calculations have been based on the scientific data we have found available.

REFERENCES

Abraham, A. S.; Sonnenblick, M.; Eini, M.; Shemesh, O.; and Batt, A. P. "The effect of chromium on established atherosclerotic plaques in rabbits." *Am J Clin Nutr* 33:2294–2298, 1980.

Alemany, M. "The etiological basis for the classification of obesity." *Prog Food Nutr Sci* 13(1):46–66, 1989.

Altomare, E.; Vendemiale, G.; Chicco, D.; Procacci, V.; and Cirelli, F. "Increased lipid peroxidation in type 2 poorly controlled diabetic patients." *Diabetes Metab* 18(4):264–271, 1992.

Anderson, J. W. "Nutrition Management of Diabetes Mellitus." In *Modern Nutrition in Health and Disease.* 7th ed., edited by M. E. Shils and V. R. Young, pp. 1204–1229. Philadelphia: Lea and Febiger, 1988.

Anderson, R. A. "Nutritional role of chromium." *The Sci of the Tot Environ* 17:13–29, 1981.

Anderson, R. A.; Polansky, M. M.; Bryden, N. A.; Roginsk, E. E.; Patterson, K. Y.; and Reamer, D. C. "Effect of exercise (running) on serum glucose, insulin, glucagon, and chromium excretion." *Diabetes* 31:212–216, 1982.

Anderson, R. A. "Chromium metabolism and its role in disease processes in man." *Clin Physiol Biochem* 4:31–41, 1986.

Anderson, R. A.; Polansky, M. M.; Bryden, N. A.; and Guttman, H. N.

"Strenuous exercise may increase dietary needs for chromium and zinc." *Sports, Health and Nutrition*. Edited by F. I. Katch, vol. 2:83–88, 1986.

Anderson, R. A.; Polansky, M. M.; Bryden, N. A.; Bhathena, S. J.; and Canary, J. J. "Effects of supplemental chromium on patients with symptoms of reactive hypoglycemia." *Metab* 36(4):351–355, 1987.

Anderson, R. A. "Selenium, chromium, and manganese: (b) chromium." In *Modern Nutrition in Health and Disease*. 7th ed., edited by M. E. Shils and V. R. Young, pp. 268–273. Philadelphia: Lea and Febiger, 1988.

Anderson, R. A. "Essentiality of chromium in humans." *The Sci of the Tot Environ* 86(1–2):75–81, 1989.

Anderson, R. A.; Bryden, N. A.; Polansky, M. M.; and Reisner, S. "Urinary chromium excretion and insulinogenic properties of carbohydrates." *Am J Clin Nutr* 51(5):864–868, 1990.

Anke, M. "Role of trace elements in the dynamics of atherosclerosis." *Z Gesamte Inn Med* 41(4):105–111, 1986.

Anselmo, J.; Vaz, F.; Correia, L. G.; Pereira, E.; Lima de Silva, F.; Pires, M. T.; and Nunes-Correa, J. C. "Influence of body fat topography on glucose homeostasis and serum lipid levels." *Acta Med Port* 3(6):341–346, 1990.

Aparicio, M.; Gin, H.; Potaux, L.; Bouchet, J. L.; Morel, D.; and Aubertin, J. "Effect of a ketoacid diet on glucose tolerance and tissue insulin sensitivity." *Kidney Int* (suppl 27):S231–S235, 1989.

Aronow, W. S.; Ahn, C.; Kronzon, I.; and Koenigsberg, M. "Congestive heart failure, coronary events and atherothromic brain infarction in elderly blacks and whites with systemic hypertension and with and without echocardiographic and electrocardiographic evidence of left ventricular hypertrophy." *FASEB J* 67:295–299, 1991.

Assimacopoulos, F., and Jeanrenaud, J. B. "The hormonal and metabolic basis of experimental obesity." *Clin Endocrinol Metab* 5(2):337–365, 1976.

Bagdade, J. D., and Dunn, F. L. "Effects of insulin treatment on lipoprotein composition and function in patients with IDDM." *Diabetes* 41 (suppl 2):107–110, 1992.

Bantam Medical Dictionary, The. New York and London: Bantam Books, 1982.

Barrett-Connor, L. "Obesity, atherosclerosis, and coronary heart disease." *Annals Intern Med* 103 (6 pt 2):1010–1019, 1985.

Beck-Nielsen, H.; Nielsen, O. H.; Damsbo, P.; Vaag, A.; Handberg, A.; and Henriksen, J. E. "Impairment of glucose tolerance: mechanism of action and impact on the cardiovascular system." *Am J Obstel Gynecol* 163(1 pt 2):292–295, 1990.

Berne, C. "Insulin in hypertension—a relationship with consequences?" *J Intern Med Suppl* 735:65–73, 1991.

Beverly, C. "Sugary foods may be hazardous for those who have breast cancer." *Natural Healing Newsletter* 3(1G):5, 1991.

Bhathena, S. J.; Aparicio, P.; Revett, K.; Voyles, N.; and Recant, L. "Effect of dietary carbohydrates on glucagon and insulin receptors in genetically obese female Zucker rats." *J Nutr* 117(7):1291–1297, 1987.

Bhathena, S. J.; Berlin, E.; Judd, J. T.; Jones, J.; Kennedy, B. W.; Smith, P. M.; Jones, D. Y.; Taylor, P. R.; and Campbell, W. S. "Dietary fat and menstrual-cycle effects on the erythrocyte ghost insulin receptor in premenopausal women." *Am J Clin Nutr* 50:460–464, 1989.

Bierman, E. L., and Chait, A. "Nutrition and diet in relation to hyperlipidemia and atherosclerosis." In *Modern Nutrition in Health and Disease*. 7th ed., edited by M. E. Shils and V. R. Young, pp. 1283–1297. Philadelphia: Lea and Febiger, 1988.

Bjorntorp, P. "Obesity and adipose tissue distribution as a risk factor for the development of disease. A review." *Infusionstherapie* 17(1):24–27, 1990.

Black, H. R. "The coronary artery disease paradox: the role of hyperinsulinemia and insulin resistance and its implications for therapy." *J Cardiovasc Pharmacol* 15(suppl 5):S26–S38, 1990.

Blackburn, G. L. "Medical treatment of obesity." In *Treatment of Obesity: A Multidisciplinary Approach*. Edited by G. L. Blackburn; P. N. Benotti; and E. A. Mascioli. Presented through the Department of Education at Harvard Medical School, November 7–9, 1991.

Bland, Jeffrey. *Nutraerobics*. San Francisco: Harper and Row, 1983.

Blendis, L. M., and Jenkins, D. J. A. "Nutrition and diet in management of diseases of the gastrointestinal tract." In *Modern Nutrition in Health and Disease*. 7th ed., edited by M. E. Shils and V. R. Young, pp. 1182–1200. Philadelphia: Lea and Febiger, 1988.

Block, G.; Dresser, C.; Hartman, H.; and Carol, M. D. "Nutrient sources in the American diet: Quantitative data from the HANES II survey. I Vitamins and minerals." *Am J Epidemiol* 122:13–40, 1985.

Boden, G.; Jadali, F.; White, J.; Liang, Y.; Mozzoli, M.; Chen, X.; and Coleman, E.; and Smith, C. "Effects of fat on insulin-stimulated carbohydrate metabolism in normal men." *J Clin Invest* 88(3):960–966, 1991.

Bogardus, C.; Lillioja, S.; Foley, J.; Christin, L.; Freymond, D.; Nyomba, B.; Bennett, P. H.; Reaven, G. M.; and Salans, L. "Insulin resistance predicts the development of non-insulin dependent diabetes mellitus in Pima Indians." *Diabetes* 36 (suppl #1):47A (abstract), 1987.

Bottermann, P., and Classen, M. "Diabetes mellitus and arterial hypertension. In search of the connecting link." *Z Gesamte Inn Med* 46(15):558–562, 1991.

Brands, M. W., and Hall, J. E. "Insulin resistance, hyperinsulinemia, and obesity-associated hypertension." *J Am Soc Nephrol* 3(5):1064–1077, 1992.

Bray, G. A. "Obesity: historical development of scientific and cultural ideas." *Int J Obes* 14(11):909–926, 1990.

Bray, G. A. "Obesity, a disorder of nutrient partitioning: The MONA LISA hypothesis." *J Nutr* 121:1146–1162, 1991.

Brindley, D. N., and Rolland, Y. "Possible connections between stress, diabetes, obesity, hypertension and altered lipoprotein metabolism that may result in atherosclerosis." *Clin Sci* 77(5):453–461, 1989.

Brindley, D. N. "Mode of action of benfluorex. Recent data." *Presse Med* 21(28):1330–1335, 1992.

Broughton, D. L., and Taylor, R. "Review: deterioration of glucose tolerance with age: the role of insulin resistance." *Aging* 20(3):221–225, 1991.

Bruning, P. F.; Bonfrer, J. M.; van Noord, P. A.; Hart, A. A.; de Jong-Bakker, M.; and Nooijen, W. J. "Insulin resistance and breast cancer risk." *Int J Cancer* 52(4):511–516, 1992.

Buchanan, T. A. "Glucose metabolism during pregnancy: normal physiology and implications for diabetes mellitus." *Isr J Med Sci* 27(8–9):432–441, 1991.

Buhler, F. R. "Cardiovascular risk factors—an integrated sympathetic viewpoint." *Schweiz Med Wochenschr* 121(49):1793–1802, 1991.

Bunker, V. W.; Lawson, M. S.; Delves, H. T.; and Clayton, B. E. "The uptake and excretion of chromium by the elderly." *Am J Clin Nutr* 39:797–802, 1984.

Butler, P.; Kryshak, E.; and Rizza, R. "Mechanism of growth hormone–induced postprandial carbohydrate intolerance in humans."

Am J Physiol 260 (4 pt 1):E513–E520, 1991. [pub erratum appears in *Am J Physiol* 261 (6 pt 1):E677.]

Cabrijan, T.; Levanat, S.; Pekic, P.; Pavelic, J.; Spaventi, R.; Frahm, H.; Zjacic-Rotkvic, V.; Goldoni, V.; Vrbanec, D.; Misjak, M.; et al. "The role of insulin-related substance in Hodgkin's disease." *J Cancer Res Clin Oncol* 117(6):615–619, 1991.

Campbell, W. W., and Anderson, R. A. "Effects of aerobic exercise and training on the trace minerals chromium, zinc and copper." *Sports Med* 4(1):9–18, 1987.

Ceriello, A.; Quatraro, A.; Caretta, F.; Varano, R.; and Giugliano, D. "Evidence for the possible role of oxygen free radicals in the abnormal function of arterial vasomotor in insulin dependent diabetes." *Diabetes Metab* 16(4):318–322, 1990.

Chandrasekhar, Y.; Heiner, J.; Osuamkpe, C.; and Nagamani, M. "Insulin-like growth factor I and II binding in human myometrium and leiomyomas." *Am J Obstet Gynecol* 166 (1 pt 1):64–69, 1992.

Chaouloff, F.; Laude, D.; Merino, D.; Serrurier, B.; and Elghozi, J. L. "Peripheral and central consequences of immobilization stress in genetically obese Zucker rats." *Am J Physiol* 256 (2 pt 2):R435–R442, 1989.

Clark, M. G.; Rattigan, S.; and Clark, D. G. "Obesity with insulin resistance: experiential insights." *Lancet* 1236–1240, Nov. 26, 1983.

Contreras, R. J., and Williams, V. L. "Dietary obesity and weight cycling: effects on blood pressure and heart rate in rats." *Am J Physiol* 256 (6 pt 2):R1209–R1219, 1989.

Conway, G. S.; Agrawal, R.; Betteridge, D. J.; and Jacobs, H. S. "Risk factors for coronary artery disease in lean and obese women with the polycystic ovary syndrome." *Clin Endocrinol* (Oxf) 37(2): 119–125, 1992.

Conway, G. S.; Clark, P. M.; and Wong, D. "Hyperinsulinemia in the polycystic ovary syndrome confirmed with a specific immunoradiometric assay for insulin." *Clin Endocrinol* (Oxf) 38(2):219–222, 1993.

Coulston, A. M.; Liu, G. C.; and Reaven, G. M. "Plasma glucose, insulin and lipid responses to high-carbohydrate low-fat diets in normal humans." *Metab* 32(1):52–56, 1983.

Coulston, A. M.; Hollenbeck, C. B.; Swislocki, A. L. M.; Chen, Y-D. I.; and Reaven, G. M. "Deleterious metabolic effects of high-carbohydrate, sucrose-containing diets in patients with non-insulin-dependent diabetes mellitus." *Am J Med* 82 (Feb):213–220, 1987.

Creutzfeldt, W.; Ebert, R.; Willms, B.; Frefichs, H.; and Brown, J. C. "Gastric inhibitory polypeptide (GIP) and insulin in obesity: Increased response to stimulation and defective feedback control of serum levels." *Diabetologia* 14:15–24, 1978.

Daly, P. A., and Landsberg, L. "Hypertension in obesity and NIDDM. Role of insulin and sympathetic nervous system." *Diabetes Care* 14(3):240–248, 1991.

DeFronzo, R. A., and Ferrannini, E. "Insulin resistance. A multifaceted syndrome responsible for NIDDM, óbesity, hypertension, dyslipidemia, and atherosclerotic cardiovascular disease." *Diabetes Care* 14(3):173–194, 1991.

Del Prato, S. "Hyperinsulinemia. Causes and mechanisms." *Presse Med* 21(28):1312–1317, 1992.

Devlin, J. T., and Horton, E. S. "Hormone and nutrient interactions." In *Modern Nutrition in Health and Disease.* 7th ed., edited by M. E. Shils and V. R. Young, pp. 570–584. Philadelphia: Lea and Febiger, 1988.

Dietz, W. H. "Obesity." *J Am Coll Nutr* 8(suppl):13S–21S, 1989.

Di Pietro, S., and Suraci, C. "Metabolic abnormalities in first-degree relatives of type 2 diabetics." *Boll Soc Ital Biol Sper* 66(7):631–638, 1990.

Doeden, B., and Rizza, R. "Use of a variable insulin infusion to assess insulin action in obesity: defects in both kinetics and amplitude of response." *J Clin Endocrinol Metab* 64(5):902–908, 1987.

Dorner, G.; Plagemann, A.; Ruckert, J.; Gotz, F.; Rohde, W.; Stahl, F.; Kurschner, U.; Gottschalk, J.; Mohnike, A.; and Steindel, E. "Teratogenic maternofoetal transmission and prevention of diabetes susceptibility." *Exp Clin Endocrinol* 91(3):247–258, 1988.

Drash, A. "Relationship between diabetes mellitus and obesity in the child." *Metab* 22(2):337–34, 1973.

Du Cailar, G.; Ribstein, J.; Pasquie, J. L.; Simandoux, V.; and Mimran, A. "Left systolic ventricular function and metabolic disorders in untreated hypertensive patients." *Arch Mal Coeur Vaiss* 85(8):1071–1073, 1992.

Dustan, H. "Obesity and hypertension." *Ann Int Med* 103 (6 pt 2):1047–1049, 1985.

Dyer, K. R., and Messing, A. "Peripheral neuropathy associated with functional islet cell adenoma in SV40 transgenic mice." *J Neuropathol Exp Neurol* 48(4):399–412, 1989.

Dzurik, R.; Malkova, J.; and Spustova, V. "Essential hypertension and insulin resistance." *Cor Vasa* 33(4):294–300, 1991.

Eaton, S. B., and Konner, M. J. "Stone age nutrition: implications for today." *ASDC J Dent Child* 53(4):300–303, 1986.

Eaton, S. B.; Konner, M.; and Shostak, M. "Stone agers in the fast lane: chronic degenerative diseases in evolutionary perspective." *New Eng J Med* 84(4):739–749, 1988.

Einhorn, D., and Landsberg, L. "Nutrition and diet in hypertension." In *Modern Nutrition in Health and Disease.* 7th ed., edited by M. E. Shils and V. R. Young, pp. 1269–1282. Philadelphia: Lea and Febiger, 1988.

Ellis, E. N.; Kemp, S. K.; Frindik, J. P.; and Elders, M. J. "Glomerulopathy in patients with Donohue syndrome (leprechaunism)." *Diabetes Care* 14(5):413–414, 1991.

Ellison, R. C.; Newburger, J. W.; and Gross, D. M. "Pediatric aspects of essential hypertension." *J Am Diet Assoc* 80:21–25, 1982.

Epstein, M., and Sowers, J. R. "Diabetes mellitus and hypertension." *Hypertension* 19(5):403–418, 1992.

Eriksson, L. S.; Thorne, A.; and Wahren, J. "Diet-induced thermogenesis in patients with liver cirrhosis." *Clin Physiol* 9(2):131–141, 1989.

Facchini, F.; Chen, Y. D.; Hollenbeck, C. B.; and Reaven, G. M. "Relationship between resistance to insulin-mediated glucose uptake, urinary uric acid clearance, and plasma uric acid concentration." *JAMA* 266(21):3008–3011, 1991.

Farquhar, J. W.; Frank, A.; Gross, R. C.; and Reaven, G. M. "Glucose, insulin, and triglyceride responses to high and low carbohydrate diets in man." *J Clin Invest* 45(10):1648–1656, 1966.

Feraille, E.; Krempf, M.; Chabonnel, B.; Bouhour, J. B.; and Nicolas, G. "Arterial hypertension in patients with obesity. Role of hyperinsulinism and insulin resistance." *Rev Med Interne* 11(4):293–296, 1990.

Ferrari, P.; Weidmann, P.; Shaw, S.; Giachino, D.; Riesen, W.; Allemann, Y.; and Heynen, G. "Altered insulin sensitivity, hyperinsulinemia, and dyslipidemia in individuals with a hypertensive parent." *Am J Med* 91(6):589–596, 1991.

Fisher, J. A. *The Chromium Program.* New York: Harper and Row, 1990.

Flack, J. M., and Sowers, J. R. "Epidemiologic and clinical aspects of insulin resistance and hyperinsulinemia." *Am J Med* 91(1A): 11S–21S.

Flodin, N. W. "Atherosclerosis: An insulin-dependent disease?" *J Amer Coll Nutr* 5:417–427, 1986.

Fontbonne, A., and Eschwege, E. "Diabetes, hyperglycemia, hyperinsulinemia and atherosclerosis: epidemiological data." *Diabetes Metab* 13 (3 pt 2):350–353, 1987.

Fontbonne, A.; Charles, M.A.; Thibult, N.; Richard, J. L.; Claude, J. R.; Warnet, J. M.; Rosselin, G. E.; and Eschwege, E. "Hyperinsulinemia as a predictor of coronary heart disease mortality in a healthy population: the Paris Prospective Study, 15-year follow-up." *Diabetologia* 34(5):356–361, 1991.

Fontbonne, A., and Eschwege, E. "Insulin and cardiovascular disease. Paris Prospective Study." *Diabetes Care* 14(6):461–469, 1991.

Foster, D. W. "Insulin resistance—a secret killer?" *New Eng J Med* 320(11):733–734, 1989.

Friedman, J. M., and Leibel, R. L. "Tackling a weighty problem." *Cell* 69:217–220, 1992.

Fuh, M. M-T.; Shieh, S-M.; Wu, D-A.; Chen, Y-D. I.; Reaven, G. M. "Abnormalities of carbohydrate and lipid metabolism in patients with hypertension." *Arch Intern Med* 147(Jun):1035–1038, 1987.

Fujimoto, S. "Studies on the relationships between blood trace metal concentrations and the clinical status of patients with cerebrovascular disease, gastric cancer, and diabetes mellitus." *Hokkaido Igaku Zasshi* 62(6):913–932, 1987.

Garg, A.; Helderman, J. H.; Koffler, M.; Ayuso, R.; Rosenstock, J.; and Raskin, P. "Relationship between lipoprotein levels in vivo insulin action in normal young white men." *Metabolism* 37(10):982–987, 1988a.

Garg, A.; Bonanome, A.; Grundy, S. M.; Zhang, Z.; and Unger, R. H. "Comparison of a high-carbohydrate diet with a high-monounsaturated-fat diet in patients with non-insulin-dependent diabetes." *New Eng J Med* 319:829–834, 1988b.

Garg, A.; Grundy, S. M.; and Unger, R. H. "Comparison of effects of high and low carbohydrate diets on plasma lipoproteins and insulin sensitivity in patients with mild NIDDM." *Diabetes* 41(10):1278–1285, 1992.

Geiselman, P. J. "Sugar-induced hyperphagia: Is hyperinsulinemia, hypoglycemia, or any other factor a 'necessary' condition?" *Appetite* 11 (suppl 1):26–34, 1988.

Geiselman, P. J., and Novin, D. "The role of carbohydrates in appetite, hunger and obesity." *Appetite: J Intake Res* 3:203–223, 1982.

Ginsberg, H.; Olefsky, J. M.; Kimmerling, G.; Crapo, P.; and Reaven, G. M. "Induction of hypertriglyceridemia by a low-fat diet." *J Clin Endocrinol Metab* 42:729–735, 1976.

Gong, E. J., and Heald, F. P. "Diet, nutrition, and adolescence." In *Modern Nutrition in Health and Disease.* 7th ed., edited by M. E. Shils and V. R. Young, pp. 969–981. Philadelphia: Lea and Febiger, 1988.

Grimaldi, A.; Sachon, C.; Bosquet, F.; and Doumith, R. "Intolerance to carbohydrates: the seven questions." *Rev Med Interne* 11(4): 297–307, 1990.

Groop, L. C., and Eriksson, J. G. "The etiology and pathogenesis of non-insulin-dependent diabetes." *Ann Med* 24(6):483–489, 1992.

Grugni, G.; Moreni, G.; Guzzaloni, G.; Ardizzi, A.; De Medici, C.; Sartorio, A.; and Morabito, F. "No correlation between insulinemic levels and arterial hypertension in obese females." *Minerva Endocrinol* 15(2):141–143, 1990.

Gwinup, G., and Elias, A. N. "Hypothesis: Insulin is responsible for the vascular complications of diabetes." *Med-Hypotheses* 34(1):1–6, 1991.

Haenel, H. "Phylogenesis and nutrition." *Nahrung* 33(9):867–887, 1989.

Haffner, S. M.; Stern, M. P.; Hazuda, H. P.; Mitchel, B. D.; and Patterson, J. K. "Incidence of type II diabetes in Mexican Americans predicted by fasting insulin and glucose levels, obesity, and body-fat distribution." *Diabetes* 39:283–288, 1990.

Haffner, S. M.; Stern, M. P.; Hazuda, H. P.; Mitchel, B. D.; and Patterson, J. K. "Cardiovascular risk factors in confirmed prediabetic individuals. Does the clock for coronary heart disease start ticking before the onset of clinical diabetes?" *JAMA* 263(21):2893–2898, 1990.

Haffner, S. M.; Ferrannini, E.; Hazuda, H. P.; and Stern, M. P. "Clustering of cardiovascular risk factors in confirmed prehypertensive individuals." *Hypertension* 20(1):38–45, 1992.

Hallfrisch, J. "Metabolic effects of dietary fructose." *FASEB J* 4(9):2652–2660, 1990.

Heaton, K. W.; Marcus, S. N.; Emmett, P. M.; and Bolton, C. H. "Particle size of wheat, maize, and oat test meals: effects on plasma glucose and insulin responses and on the rate of starch digestion in the liver." *Am J Clin Nutr* 47(4):675–682, 1988.

Heber, D. "The endocrinology of obesity." In *Treatment of Obesity: A Multidisciplinary Approach.* Edited by G. L. Blackburn; P. N. Benotti; and E. A. Mascioli. Presented through the Department of Education at Harvard Medical School, November 7–9, 1991.

Himsworth, H. P. "Diabetes mellitus: its differentiation into insulin-sensitive and insulin-insensitive types." *Lancet* 127–130, 1936.

Himsworth, H. P., and Kerr, R. B. "Insulin-sensitive and insulin-insensitive types of diabetes mellitus." In *Clinical Science Incorporating Heart.* Edited by Thomas Lewis. Vol. 4, pp. 119–152. London: Shaw and Sons Ltd, 1939.

Hollenbeck, C., and Reaven, G. M. "Variations in insulin-stimulated glucose uptake in healthy individuals with normal glucose tolerance." *J Clin Endocrinol Metab* 64:1169–1173, 1987.

Hollenbeck, C.; Coulston, A. M.; and Reaven, G. M. "Effects of sucrose on carbohydrate and lipid metabolism in NIDDM patients." *Diabetes Care* 12(1):62–66, 1989.

Hrnciar, J.; Jakubikova, K.; and Okapcova, J. "How should we implement the basic principles of treatment of type 2 diabetes mellitus from the aspect of the hormone-metabolic syndrome X (5H)?" *Vnitr Lek* 38(8):729–737, 1992.

Hubner, G.; von Dorsche, H. H.; and Zuhlke, H. "Morphological studies of the effect of chromium-III-chloride on the islet cell organ in rats under the conditions of high and low fat diets." *Anat Anz* 167(5):389–391, 1988.

Hud, J. A., Jr.; Cohen, J. B.; Wagner, J. M.; and Cruz, P. D., Jr. "Prevalence and significance of acanthosis nigricans in an adult obese population." *Arch Dermatol* 128(7):941–944, 1992.

Ishiguro, T.; Sato, Y.; Oshida, Y.; Yamanouchi, K.; Okuyama, M.; and Sakamoto, N. "The relationship between insulin sensitivity and weight reduction in simple obese and obese diabetic patients." *Nagoya J Med Sci* 49:61–69, 1987.

Janka, H. U.; Ziegler, A. G.; Standl, E.; and Mehnert, H. "Daily insulin dose as a predictor of macrovascular disease in insulin treated non-insulin-dependent diabetics." *Diabetes Metab* 13 (3 pt 2):359–364, 1987.

Jeejeebhoy, K. N.; Chu, R. C.; Marliss, E. B.; Greenburg, G. R.; and Bruce-Robertson, A. "Chromium deficiency, glucose intolerance and neuropathy reversed by chromium supplementation in a patient receiving long term total parenteral nutrition." *Am J Clin Nutr* 30:531–538, 1977.

Jenkins, D. J. A. "Nutrition and diet in management of diseases of the gastrointestinal tract: (D) colon." In *Modern Nutrition in Health and Disease.* 7th ed., edited by M. E. Shils and V. R. Young, pp. 1023–1066. Philadelphia: Lea and Febiger, 1988.

Jenkins, D. J. A.; Shapira, N.; Greenberg, G.; Jenkins, A. L.; Collier, G. R.; Poduch, C.; Wolever, T. M.; Anderson, R. A.; and Blendis, L. M. "Low glycemic index foods and reduced glucose, amino acid, and endocrine responses in cirrhosis." *Am J Gastroenterol* 84(7):732–739, 1989.

Jern, S. "Effects of acute carbohydrate administration on central and peripheral hemodynamic responses to mental stress." *Hypertension* 18(6):790–797, 1991.

Kakar, F.; Hursting, S. D.; Henderson, M. M.; and Thronquist, M. D. "Dietary sugar and breast cancer: Epidemiologic evidence." *Clin Nutr* 9:68–71, 1990.

Kakar, F.; Thornquist, M. D.; Henderson, M. M.; Klein, R. D.; Kozawa, S. M.; Santisteben, G. A.; Hursting, S. D.; and Urban, N. D. "The effect of dietary sugar and dietary antioxidants on mammary tumor growth and lethality in BALB/c mice." *Clin Nutr* 9:62–67, 1990.

Kannel, W. B.; Wilson, P. W.; and Zhang, T. J. "The epidemiology of impaired glucose tolerance and hypertension." *Am Heart J* 121 (4 pt 2):1268–1273, 1991.

Kaplan, N. M. "The deadly quartet: Upper-body obesity, glucose intolerance, hypertriglyceridemia, and hypertension." *Arch Intern Med* 149:1514–1520, 1989.

Kazumi, T.; Yoshino, G.; Matsuba, K.; Iwai, M.; Iwatani, I.; Matsushita, M.; Kasama, T.; Hosokawa, T.; Numano, F.; and Baba, S. "Effects of dietary glucose or fructose on the secretion rate and particle size of triglyceride-rich lipoproteins in Zucker fatty rats." *Metab* 40(9):962–966, 1991.

Klurfeld, D. M.; Lloyd, L. M.; Welch, C. B.; Davis, M. J.; Tulp, O. L.; and Kritchevsky, D. "Reduction of enhanced mammary carcinogenesis in LA/N-cp (corpulent) rats by energy restriction." *Proc Soc Exp Biol Med* 196(4):381–384, 1991.

Koop, C. E. *The Surgeon General's Report on Nutrition and Health*. U. S. Department Health and Human Services, Publication No. 88-50210, 1988.

Koppel, J. D. "Nutrition, diet, and the kidney." In *Modern Nutrition in Health and Disease*. 7th ed., edited by M. E. Shils and V. R. Young, pp. 1230–1268. Philadelphia: Lea and Febiger, 1988.

Kornhuber, H. H.; Kornhuber, J.; Wanner, W.; Kornhuber, A.; and Kaiserauer, C. H. "Alcohol, smoking and body build: obesity as a result of the toxic effect of 'social' alcohol consumption." *Clin Physiol Biochem* 7(3–4):203–216, 1989.

Kozlovsky, A. S.; Moser, P. B.; Reisner, S.; and Anderson, R. A. "Effects of diets high in simple sugars on urinary chromium losses." *Metab* 35(6):515–518, 1986.

Kumpulainen, J. T.; Wolf, W. R.; Veillon, C.; and Mertz, W. "Determination of chromium in selected United States diets." *J Agric Food Chem* 27(3):490–494, 1979.

Laakso, M.; Sarlund, H.; Salonen, R.; Suhonen, M.; Pyörälä, K.; Salonen, J. T.; and Karhapää, P. "Asymptomatic atherosclerosis and insulin resistance." *Atheroscler and Thromb* 11:1068–1076, 1991.

Landin, K.; Tengborn, L.; and Smith, V. "Treating insulin resistance in hypertension with metformin reduces both blood pressure and metabolic risk factors." *J Intern Med* 229(2):181–187, 1991.

Landsberg, L. "Obesity, metabolism, and hypertension." *Yale J Biol Med* 62(5):511–519, 1989.

Landsberg, L. "Insulin resistance, energy balance and sympathetic nervous system activity." *Clin Exp Hypertens* 12(5):817–830, 1990.

Lange, J.; Arends, J.; and Willms, B. "Alcohol-induced hypoglycemia in type 1 diabetes." *Medizinische Klinik* 86(11):551–554, 1991.

Lefebvre, P. J., and Scheen, A. J. "Hypoglycemia." In *Diabetes Mellitus, Theory and Practice*, edited by H. Rifkin and D. Porte, Jr., pp. 896–910. New York: Elsevier Sci. Pub. Co., Inc., 1990.

Leibel, R. *Obesity and Nutrient Metabolism*. Presented at the American Association for the Advancement of Science, May 26, 1984.

Leiter, E. H. "Control of spontaneous glucose intolerance, hyperinsulinemia, and islet hyperplasia in nonobese C3H.SW male mice by Y-linked locus and adrenal gland." *Metab* 37(7):689–696, 1988.

Leutenegger, M. "Theoretical aspects of the relationship between diabetic macroangiopathy and hyperinsulinism." *Presse Med* 21(28): 1324–1329, 1992.

Lillioja, S.; Mott, D. M.; Howard, B. V.; Bennett, P. H.; Yki-Jarvinen, H.; Freymond, D.; Nyomba, B. L.; Zurlo, F.; Swinburn, B.; and Bogardus, C. "Impaired glucose tolerance as a disorder of insulin action: Longitudinal and cross-sectional studies in Pima Indians." *New Eng J Med* 318:1217–1225, 1988.

Linscheer, W. G., and Vergroesen, A. J. "Lipids." In *Modern Nutrition in Health and Disease*. 7th ed., edited by M. E. Shils and V. R. Young, pp. 72–107. Philadelphia: Lea and Febiger, 1988.

Lithell, H. "Insulin resistance and cardiovascular drugs." *Clin Exp Hypertens* 14(1–2):151–162, 1992.

Liu, G.; Coulston, A.; Hollenbeck, C.; and Reaven, G. "The effect of sucrose content in high and low carbohydrate diets on plasma glucose, insulin, and lipid responses in hypertriglyceridemic humans." *J Clin Endocrinol Metab* 59(4):636–642, 1984.

Lutz, W. "Life expectancy—the Japanese experience." *Wein Med Wochenschr* 141(7):148–150, 1991.

Mahler, R. J. "Diabetes and hypertension." *Horm Metab Res* 22(12): 599–607, 1990.

Marshall, S.; Garvey, W. T.; and Traxinger, R. R. "New insights into the metabolic regulation of insulin action and insulin resistance: role of glucose and amino acids." *FASEB J* 5:3031–3036, 1991.

Marston, R. W., and Peterkin, B. B. "Nutrient content of the national food supply." *Natl Food Rev* 9:21–25, 1980.

MacDonald, I. "Carbohydrates." In *Modern Nutrition in Health and Disease*. 7th ed., edited by M. E. Shils and V. R. Young, pp. 38–51. Philadelphia: Lea and Febiger, 1988.

Melchoir, J. C.; Rigaud, D.; Colas-Linhart, N.; Petiet, A.; Girard, A.; and Apfelbaum, M. "Immunoreactive beta-endorphin increases after an aspartame chocolate drink in healthy human subjects." *Physiol Behav* 50(5):941–944, 1991.

Modan, M.; Halkin, H.; Almog, S.; Lusky, A.; Eshkol, A.; Sheft, M.; Shitrit, A.; and Fuchs, Z. "Hyperinsulinemia. A link between hypertension obesity and glucose intolerance." *J Clin Invest* 75:809–817, 1985.

Modan, M.; Halkin, H.; Lusky, A.; Segal, P.; Fuchs, Z. and Chetrit, A. "Hyperinsulinemia is characterized by jointly distributed plasma VLDL, LDL, and HDL levels. A population study." *Atheroscler and Thromb* 8(3):227–236, 1988.

Modan, M., and Halkin, H. "Hyperinsulinemia or increased sympathetic drive as links for obesity and hypertension." *Diabetes Care* 14(6):470–487, 1991.

Molnar, D. "Insulin secretion and carbohydrate tolerance in childhood obesity." *Klin Padiatr* 202(3):131–135, 1990.

Morgan, J. B.; York, D. A.; Wasilewska, A.; and Portman, J. "A study of the thermic responses to a meal and to a sympathomimetic drug (ephedrine) in relation to energy balance in man." *Brit J Nutr* 47:21–32, 1982.

Mountjoy, K. G., and Holdaway, I. M. "Effect of insulin receptor down regulation on insulin-stimulated thymidine incorporation in cultured human fibroblasts and tumor cell lines." *Cancer Biochem Biophys* 12(2):117–126, 1991.

Nader, S. "Polycystic ovary syndrome and the androgen-insulin connection." *Am J Obstet Gynecol* 165(2):346–348, 1991.

Niijima, A.; Togiyama, T.; and Adachi, A. "Cephalic-phase insulin release induced by taste stimulus of monosodium glutamate (umami taste)." *Physiol Behav* 48(6):905–908, 1990.

Nobels, F., and Dewailly, D. "Puberty and polycystic ovarian syndrome: the insulin/insulin-like growth factor I hypothesis." *Fertil Steril* 58(4):655–666, 1992.

Noberasco, G.; Odetti, P.; Boeri, D.; Maiello, M.; and Adezati, L. "Malondialdehyde (MDA) level in diabetic subjects. Relationship with blood glucose and glycosylated hemoglobin." *Biomed Pharmacother* 45(4–5):193–196, 1991.

O'Dea, K. "Westernization and non-insulin-dependent diabetes in Australian aborigines." *Ethn Dis* 1(2):171–187, 1991.

O'Dea, K. "Westernization, insulin resistance and diabetes in Australian Aborigines." *Med J Aust* 155(4):258–264, 1991.

O'Donnell, M. J., and Dodson, P. M. "The non-drug treatment of hypertension in the diabetic patient." *J Hum Hypertens* 5(4):287–294, 1991.

Oh, W.; Gelardi, N. L.; and Cha, C. J. "Maternal hyperglycemia in pregnant rats: its effects on growth and carbohydrate metabolism in the offspring." *Metab* 37(12):1146–1151, 1988.

Ohlson, L. O.; Larsson, B.; Bjorntorp, P.; Eriksson, H.; Szardsudd, K.; Welin, L.; Tibblin, G.; and Wilhelmsen, L. "Risk factors for type 2 (non-insulin-dependent) diabetes mellitus. Thirteen and one-half years of follow-up of the participants in a study of Swedish men born in 1913." *Diabetologia* 31(11):798–805, 1988.

Olefsky, J. M. "Obesity." In *Harrison's Principles of Internal Medicine.* 12th ed., edited by J. D. Wilson; D. Braunwald; K. J. Isselbacher; R. G. Petersdorf; J. B. Martin; A. S. Fauci; and R. K. Root. Vol. 1, pp. 411–417. New York: McGraw-Hill, Inc., Health Professions Division, 1991.

Oral Contraceptives. Mead Johnson Laboratories. OVCON®50 OVCON®35 (Norethindrone and ethinyl estradiol tablets, UPS). A Bristol-Meyers Squibb Co. Evansville, Ind. 47721, 1990.

Pedersen, O. "Insulin resistance—a pathophysiological condition with numerous sequelae: non-insulin-dependent diabetes mellitus (NIDDM), android obesity, essential hypertension, dyspipidemia and atherosclerosis." *Ugeskr Laeger* 154(20):1411–1418, 1992.

Petrides, A. S., and DeFronzo, R. A. "Glucose metabolism in cirrhosis." *H Hepatol* 8(1):107–114, 1989.

Pi-Sunyer, F. X. "Obesity." In *Modern Nutrition in Health and Disease.* 7th ed., edited by M. E. Shils and V. R. Young, pp. 795–816. Philadelphia: Lea and Febiger, 1988.

Pollare, T.; Vessby, B.; and Lithell, H. "Lipoprotein lipase activity in skeletal muscle is related to insulin sensitivity." *Atheroscler and Thromb* 11(5):1192–1203, 1991.

Pontremoli, R.; Zavaroni, I.; Mazza, S.; Battezzati, M.; Massarino, F.; Tixianello, A.; and Reaven, G. M. "Changes in blood pressure, plasma triglyceride and aldosterone concentration, and red cell cation concentration in patients with hyperinsulinemia." *Am J Hypertens* 4 (2 pt 1):159–163, 1991.

Poulter, N. R. "Treatment of hypertension: a clinical epidemiologist's view." *J Cardiovasc Pharmacol* 18(suppl 2):S35–S38, 1991.

Prelevic, G. M.; Wurzburger, M. I.; Balint-Peric, L.; and Ginsberg, J. "Twenty-four-hour serum growth hormone, insulin, c-peptide and blood glucose profiles and serum insulin-like growth factor-I concentrations in women with polycystic ovaries." *Horm Res* 37(4–5): 125–131, 1992.

Proctor, C. A.; Proctor, T. B.; and Proctor, B. "Etiology and treatment of fluid retention (hydrops) in Menière's syndrome." *Ear Nose Throat J* 71(12):631–635, 1992.

Randolph, J. F.; Kipersztok, S.; Ayers, J. W.; Ansbacher, R.; Peegel, H.; and Menon, K. M. "The effect of insulin on aromatase activity in isolated human endometrial glands and stroma." *Am J Obstet Gynecol* 157(6):1534–1539, 1990.

Ravussin, E., and Bogardus, C. "Energy expenditure in the obese: Is there a Thrifty Gene?" *Infusionstherapie* 17:108–112, 1990.

Ravussin, E. "Energy metabolism in obesity. Studies in the Pima Indians." *Diabetes Care* 16(1):232–238, 1993.

Reaven, G. M. "Role of insulin resistance in human disease." *Diabetes* 37:1595–1607, 1988.

Reaven, G. M., and Hoffman, B. B. "Hypertension as a disease of carbohydrate and lipoprotein metabolism." *Am J Med* 87(6A): 2S–6S, 1989.

Reaven, G. M. "Insulin resistance and compensatory hyperinsulinemia: role in hypertension, dyslipidemia, and coronary heart disease." *Am Heart J* 121 (4 pt 2):1283–1288, 1991.

Reaven, G. M. "Insulin resistance, hyperinsulinemia, and hypertriglyceridemia in the etiology and clinical course of hypertension." *Am J Med* 90(2A):7S–11S, 1991.

Reaven, G. M. "Role of insulin resistance in human disease." *Diabetes* 37:1595–1607, 1991.

Reaven, G. M. "Relationship between insulin resistance and hypertension." *Diabetes Care* 14 (suppl 4):33–38, 1991.

Reiser, S.; Bickard, M. C.; Hallfrisch, J.; Michaelis, O. E., IV; and Prather, E. S. "Blood lipids and their distribution in lipoproteins in hyperinsulinemic subjects fed three different levels of sucrose." *J Nutr* 111:1045–1057, 1981.

Reiser, S.; Powell, A. S.; Scholfield, D. J.; Panda, P.; Ellwood, K. C.; and Canary, J. J. "Blood lipids, lipoproteins, apoproteins, and uric acid in men fed diets containing fructose or high-amylose cornstarch." *Am J Clin Nutr* 49(5):832–839, 1989.

Ri, K. "Study on insulin resistance in rats treated with estrogen and progesterone—assessment with euglycemic clamp technique." *Nippon Naibunpi Gakkai Zasshi* 63(6):798–808, 1987.

Rimm, I. J., and Rimm, A. A. "Association between juvenile onset obesity and severe obesity in 73,532 women." *Am J Public Health* 66:479–481, 1976.

Rodin, J. "Insulin levels, hunger, and food intake: An example of feedback loops in body weight regulation." *Health Psychol* 4:1–18, 1985.

Rönnemaa, T.; Laakso, M.; Pyörälä, K.; Kallio, V.; and Puukka, P. "High fasting plasma insulin is an indicator of coronary heart disease in non-insulin-dependent diabetic patients and nondiabetic subjects." *Atheroscler and Thromb* 11(1):80–90, 1991.

Rossi-Fanelli, F.; Cascino, A.; and Muscaritoli, M. "Abnormal substrate metabolism and nutritional strategies in cancer management." *J Parenter Enteral Nutr* 15(6):680–683, 1991.

Ruderman, N. "Exercise in therapy and prevention of type II diabetes. Implications for blacks." *Diabetes Care* 13(11):1163–1168, 1990.

Rupp, H. "Insulin resistance, hyperinsulinemia, and cardiovascular disease. The need for novel dietary prevention strategies [editorial]." *Basic Res Cardiol* 87(2):99–105, 1992.

Saad, M. F.; Knowler, W. C.; Pettitt, D. J.; Nelson, R. G.; Mott, D. M.; and Bennett, P. H. "The natural history of impaired glucose tolerance in the Pima Indians." *New Eng J Med* 319:1500–1506, 1988.

Salomaa, V. V.; Tuomilehto, J.; Jaucianien, M.; Korhonsen, H. J.; Stengard, J.; Uusitupa, M.; Pitkanen, M.; and Penttilla, I. "Hypertriglyceridemia in different degrees of glucose intolerance in a Finnish population-based study." *Diabetes Care* 15(5):657–665, 1992.

Sato, Y.; Shiraishi, S.; Oshida, Y.; Ishiguro, T.; and Sakamoto, N. "Experimental atherosclerosis-like lesions induced by hyperinsulinism in Wistar rats." *Diabetes* 38:91–96, 1989.

Scallet, A. C.; Faris, P. L.; Beinfeld, M. C.; and Olney, J. W. "Hypothalamic neurotoxins alter the contents of immunoreactive cholecystokinin in pituitary." *Brain Res* 407(2):390–393, 1987.

Schneider, D. J., and Sobel, B. E. "Augmentation of synthesis of plasminogen activator inhibitor type 1 by insulin and insulin-like growth factor type I: implications for vascular disease in hyperinsulinemic states." *Proc Natl Acad Sci USA* 88(22):9959–9963, 1991.

Schroeder, H. A. "The role of chromium in mammalian nutrition." *Am J Clin Nutr* 21(6):230–244, 1968.

Schumann, D. "Post-operative hyperglycemia: clinical benefits of insulin therapy." *Heart-Lung* 19(2):165–173, 1990.

Schwarz, K., and Mertz, W. "A glucose tolerance factor and its differentiation from factor 3." *Arch Biochem Biophys* 72:515–518, 1957.

Sechi, L. A.; Melis, A.; Pala, A.; Marigliano, A.; Sechi, G.; and Tedde, R. "Serum insulin, insulin sensitivity, and erythrocyte sodium metabolism in normotensive and essential hypertensive subjects with and without overweight." *Clin Exp Hypertens* [A] 13(2):261–272, 1991.

Sharma, A. M.; Ruland, K.; Spies, K. P.; and Distler, A. "Salt sensitivity in young normotensive subjects is associated with a hyperinsulinemic response to oral glucose." *J Hypertens* 9(4):329–335, 1991.

Shelepov, V. P.; Chekulaev, V. A.; and Pasha-Zade, G. R. "Effect of putrescine on carbohydrate and lipid metabolism in rats." *Biomed Sci* 1(6):591–596, 1990.

Shelmet, J. J.; Reichard, G. A.; Skutches, C. L.; Hoeldtke, R. D.; Owen, O. E.; and Boden, G. "Ethanol causes acute inhibition of carbohydrate, fat, and protein oxidation and insulin resistance." *J Clin Invest* 81(4):1137–1145, 1988.

Shils, M. E. "Enteral (tube) and parenteral nutrition support." In *Modern Nutrition in Health and Disease.* 7th ed., edited by M. E. Shils and V. R. Young, pp. 1023–1066. Philadelphia: Lea and Febiger, 1988.

Sicree, R. A; Zimmet, P. Z.; King, H. O. M.; and Coventry, J. S. "Plasma insulin response among Nauruans: Prediction of deterioration in glucose tolerance over 6 yr." *Diabetes* 36:179–186, 1987.

Sidey, F. M. "Role of the adrenal medulla in stress-induced hyperinsulinemia in normal mice and in mice infected with Bordetella pertussis or treated with pertussis toxin." *J Endocrinol* 118(1): 135–140, 1988.

Simonson, D. C. "Hyperinsulinemia and its sequelae." *Horm Metab Res Suppl* 22:17–25, 1990.

Singer, P., and Baumann, R. "Glucose-induced or postprandial hyperinsulinemia in mild essential hypertension—an underestimated biochemical risk factor." *Med Hypotheses* 34(2):57–64, 1991.

Skouby, S. O.; Andersen, O.; Saurbrey, N.; and Kuhl, C. "Oral contraception and insulin sensitivity: in vivo assessment in normal women and in women with previous gestational diabetes." *J Clin Endocrinol Metab* 64:519–526, 1987.

Skouby, S. O.; Andersen, O.; Petersen, K. R.; Molsted-Pedersen, L.; and Kuhl, C. "Mechanism of action of oral contraceptives on carbohydrate metabolism at the cellular level." *Am J Obstet Gynecol* 163 (1 pt 2):343–348, 1990.

Smith, U.; Gudbjornsdottir, S.; and Landin, K. "Hypertension as a metabolic disorder—an overview." *J Intern Med Suppl* 735:1–7, 1991.

Sowers, J. R. "Is hypertension an insulin-resistant state? Metabolic changes associated with hypertension and antihypertensive therapy." *Am Heart J* 122 (3 pt 2):932–935, 1991.

Sowers, J. R.; Standley, P. R.; Ram, J. L.; Zemel, M. B.; and Resnick, L. M. "Insulin resistance, carbohydrate metabolism, and hypertension." *Am J Hypertens* 4(7 pt 2):46S–472S, 1991.

Spring, B.; Chiodo, J.; Harden, M.; Bourgeois, M. J.; Mason, J. D.; and Lutherer, L. "Psychobiological effects of carbohydrates." *J Clin Psychiatry* 50 (5 suppl):27–33, 1989.

Spustova, V. "Insulin resistance as a risk factor in atherosclerosis." *Vnitr Lek* 38(11):1105–1110, 1992.

"Statistical Bulletin. Hypertension in the United States: 1960 to 1980 and 1987 estimates." Statistical Bulletin, 13–17, 1989.

"Statistical Bulletin. Life expectancy remains at record level." Statistical Bulletin, 26–30, 1989.

"Statistical Bulletin. Diabetes mortality update." Statistical Bulletin, 24–35 (Oct.–Dec.), 1989.

Staub, H. W.; Reussner, G.; and Thiessen, R., Jr. "Serum cholesterol reduction by chromium in hypercholesterolemic rats." *Sci* 165:746–747, 1969.

Stern, M. P., and Haffner, S. M. "Body fat distribution and hyperinsulinemia as risk factors for diabetes and cardiovascular disease." *Atheroscler and Thromb* 6:123–130, 1986.

Stern, M. P.; Knapp, J. A. A.; Hazuda, H. P.; Haffner, S. M.; Patterson, J. K.; and Mitchell, B. D. "Genetic and environmental determinants of type II diabetes in Mexican Americans. Is there a 'descending limb' to the modernization/diabetes relationship?" *Diabetes Care* 14(7):649–654, 1991.

Stock, S.; Granstrom, L.; Backman, L.; Matthiesen, A. S.; and Uvnas-Moberg, K. "Elevated plasma levels of oxytocin in obese subjects before and after gastric banding." *Int J Obes* 13(2):213–222, 1989.

Stolar, M. W. "Atherosclerosis in diabetes: the role of hyperinsulinemia." *Metab* 37 (2 suppl 1):1–9, 1988.

Stoll, B. A., and Secreto, G. "New hormone-related markers of high risk to breast cancer." *Ann Oncol* 3(6):435–438, 1992.

Storlien, L. H.; Kraegen, E. W.; Jenkins, A. B; and Chisholm, D. J. "Effects of sucrose vs. starch diets on in vivo insulin action, thermogenesis, and obesity in rats." *Am J Clin Nutr* 47(3):420–427, 1988.

Storlien, L. H.; Oakes, N. D.; Pan, D. A.; Kusunoki, M.; and Jenkins, A. B. "Syndromes of insulin resistance in the rat. Inducement by diet and amelioration with benfluorex." *Diabetes* 42(3):457–462, 1993.

Stout, R. W. "Overview of the association between insulin and atherosclerosis." *Metab* 34(12):7–12, 1985.

Stout, R. W. "Insulin and atheroma. 20-year perspective." *Diabetes Care* 13(6):631–654, 1990.

Stout, R. W. "Insulin and atherogenesis." *Eur J Epidemiol* 8 (suppl 1): 134–135, 1992.

Striffler, J. S.; Polansky, M. M.; and Anderson, R. A. "Dietary chromium improves IVGTT insulin and glucose responses in sucrose-fed Cr-deficient rats." Abs 6285 in *FASEB J* 4/5–4/9): A2022, 1992.

Sugiyama, Y. "The role of insulin in reproductive endocrinology and perinatal medicine." *Nippon Sanka Fujinka Gakkai Zasshi* 42(8): 791–799, 1990.

Telander, R. L.; Wolf, S. A.; Simmons, P. S.; Zimmerman, D.; and Haymond, M. W. "Endocrine disorders of the pancreas and adrenal cortex in pediatric patients." *Mayo Clin Proc* 61(6):459–466, 1986.

Thomas, D. E.; Brotherhood, J. R.; and Brand, J. C. "Carbohydrate feeding before exercise: effect of glycemic index." *Int J Sports Med* 12(2):180–186, 1991.

Thomassen, A.; Neilsen, T. T.; Bagger, J. P.; and Henningsen, P. "Effects of intravenous glutamate on substrate availability and utilization across the human heart and leg." *Metab* 40(4):378–384, 1991.

Toepfer, E. W; Mertz, W.; Roginski, E. E.; and Polansky, M. M. "Chromium in foods in relation to biological activity." *J Agr Food Chem* 21(1):69–73, 1973.

Troisi, R. J.; Weiss, S. T.; Parker, D. R.; Sparrow, D.; Young, J. B.; and Landsberg, L. "Relation of obesity and diet to sympathetic nervous system activity." *Hypertens* 17(5):669–677, 1991.

Tufts University Diet and Nutrition, vol. 11, no. 5, July 1993.

Tweng, C. H., and Tai, T. Y. "Risk factors for hyperinsulinemia in chloropropamide-treated diabetic patients: a three-year follow-up." *J Formos Med Assoc* 91(8):770–774, 1992.

Unterberger, P.; Sinop, A.; Noder, W.; Berger, M. R.; Fink, M.; Edler, L.;

Schmahl, D.; and Ehrhart, H. "Diabetes mellitus and breast cancer. A retrospective follow-up study." *Onkologie* 13(1):17–20, 1990.

Urdl, W.; Desoye, G.; Schmon, B.; Hofmann, H. M.; and Ralph, G. "Interaction between insulin and insulin-like growth factor I in the pathogenesis of polycystic ovarian disease." *Ann NY Acad Sci* 626:177–183, 1991.

Vaaler, S. "Carbohydrate metabolism, insulin resistance, and metabolic cardiovascular syndrome." *J Cardiovasc Pharmacol* 20 (suppl 8): S11–S14, 1992.

Vaisman, N.; Sklan, D.; and Dayan, Y. "Effect of semi-starvation on plasma lipids." *Int J Obes* 14(12):989–996, 1990.

Valensi, P. "Pathogenic role of hyperinsulinism in macroangiopathy. Epidemiological data." *Presse Med* 21(28):1307–1311, 1992.

Van der Walt, J. G., and Linington, M. J. "A review of energy metabolism in producing ruminants. 2. Control of nutrient partitioning." *J S Afr Vet Assoc* 61(2):78–80, 1990.

Van Itallie, T. B. "Health implications of overweight and obesity in the United States." *Ann Intern Med* 103 (6 pt 2):983–988, 1985.

Velek, J.; Karasova, L.; Pelikanova, T.; Sosna, T.; and Skibova, J. "Blood pressure and insulin resistance in type 2 diabetics." *Vnitr Lek* 37(9–10):752–760, 1991.

Weaver, J. U.; Kopelman, P. G.; and Hitman, G. A. "Central obesity and hyperinsulinemia in women are associated with polymorphism in the 5' flanking region of the human insulin gene." *Eur J Clin Invest* 22(4):265-270, 1992.

Wendorf, M. "Diabetes, the ice free corridor, and the Paleoindian settlement on North America." *Am J Phys Anthropol* 79(4):503–520, 1989.

Wendorf, M., and Goldfine, I. D. "Archeology of NIDDM. Excavation of the 'thrifty' genotype." *Diabetes* 40(2):161–165, 1991.

Wendorf, M. "Archeology and the "thrifty" non insulin dependent diabetes mellitus (NIDDM) genotype." *Adv Perit Dial* 8:201–207, 1992.

White, P. J.; Cybulski, K. A.; Primus, R.; Johnson, D. F.; Collier, G. H.; and Wagner, G. C. "Changes in macronutrient selection as a function of dietary tryptophan." *Physiol and Behav* 43:73–77, 1988.

Wicklmayr, M.; Rett, K.; Baldermann, H.; and Dietze, G. "The kallikrein/kinin system in the pathogenesis of hypertension in diabetes mellitus." *Diabetes Metab* 15 (5 pt 2):306–310, 1989.

Woods, S. C.; Porte, D., Jr.; Bobbioni, E.; Ionescu, E.; Sauter, J. F.; Rohner-Jeanrenaud, F.; and Jeanrenaud, B. "Insulin: its relationship to the central nervous system and to the control of food intake and body weight." *Am J Clin Nutr* 42:1063–1071, 1985.

Woteki, C. E.; Walsh, S. O.; Raper, N.; et al. "Recent trends and levels of dietary sugars and other caloric sweeteners." In *Metabolic Effects of Utilizable Dietary Carbohydrates*. Edited by S. Reiser. New York: Marcel Dekker, 1982.

Yam, D.; Fink, A.; Nir, I.; and Budowski, P. "Insulin-tumor interrelationships in thymoma bearing mice. Effects of dietary glucose and fructose." *Br J Cancer* 64(6):1043–1046, 1991.

Young, I. S.; Torney, J. J.; and Trimble, E. R. "The effect of ascorbate supplementation on oxidative stress in the streptozotocin diabetic rats." *Free Radic Biol Med* 13(1):41–46, 1992.

Zavaroni, I.; Bonora, E.; Pagliara, M.; Dall'Aglio, E.; Luchetti, L.; Buonanno, G.; Bonati, P. A.; Bergonzani, M.; Gnudi, L.; Passeri, M.; and Reaven, G. "Risk factors for coronary artery disease in healthy persons with hyperinsulinemia and normal glucose tolerance." *New Eng J Med* 320(11):702–706, 1989.

INDEX

A NOTE ON THE TYPE

The typeface used in this book is one of many versions of Garamond, a modern homage to—rather than, strictly speaking, a revival of—the celebrated fonts of Claude Garamond (c.1480–1561), the first founder to produce type on a large scale. Garamond's type was inspired by Francesco Griffo's *De Ætna* type (cut in the 1490s for Venetian printer Aldus Manutius and revived in the 1920s as Bembo), but its letter forms were cleaner and the fit between pieces of type improved. It therefore gave text a more harmonious overall appearance than its predecessors had, becoming the basis of all romans created on the Continent for the next two hundred years; it was itself still in use through the eighteenth century. Besides the many "Garamonds" in use today, other typefaces derived from his fonts are Granjon and Sabon (despite their being named after other printers).